Fostering Social Work Gerontology Competence: A Collection of Papers from the First National Gerontological Social Work Conference

Fostering Social Work Gerontology Competence: A Collection of Papers from the First National Gerontological Social Work Conference has been co-published simultaneously as *Journal of Gerontological Social Work*, Volume 48, Numbers 1/2 2006, and 3/4 2007.

Monographs from the *Journal of Gerontological Social Work*™

For additional information on these and other Haworth Press titles, including descriptions, tables of contents, reviews, and prices, use the QuickSearch catalog at http://www.HaworthPress.com.

1. *Gerontological Social Work Practice in Long-Term Care,* edited by George S. Getzel, DSW, and M. Joanna Mellor, DSW (Vol. 5, No. 1/2, 1983). *"Veteran practitioners and graduate social work students will find the book insightful and a valuable prescriptive guide to the dos and don'ts of practice in their daily work." (The Gerontologist)*

2. *A Healthy Old Age: A Sourcebook for Health Promotion with Older Adults,* edited by Stephanie FallCreek, MSW, and Molly K. Mettler, MSW (Vol. 6, No. 2/3, 1984). *"An outstanding text on the 'how-tos' of health promotion for elderly persons." (Physical Therapy)*

3. *The Uses of Reminiscence: New Ways of Working with Older Adults,* edited by Marc Kaminsky (Vol. 7, No. 1/2, 1984). *"Rich in ideas for anyone working with life review groups." (Guidepost)*

4. *Gerontological Social Work in Home Health Care,* edited by Rose Dobrof, DSW (Vol. 7, No. 4, 1984). *"A useful window onto the home health care scene in terms of current forms of service provided to the elderly and the direction of social work practice in this field today." (PRIDE Institute Journal)*

5. *Gerontological Social Work Practice in the Community,* edited by George S. Getzel, DSW, and M. Joanna Mellor, DSW (Vol. 8, No. 3/4, 1985). *"A wealth of information for all practitioners who deal with the elderly. An excellent reference for faculty, administrators, clinicians, and graduate students in nursing and other service professions who work with the elderly." (American Journal of Care for the Aging)*

6. *Social Work and Alzheimer's Disease,* edited by Rose Dobrof, DSW (Vol. 9, No. 2, 1986). *"New and innovative social work roles with Alzheimer's victims and their families in both hospital and non-hospital settings." (Continuing Education Update)*

7. *Gerontological Social Work Practice with Families: A Guide to Practice Issues and Service Delivery,* edited by Rose Dobrof, DSW (Vol. 10, No. 1/2, 1987). *An in-depth examination of the importance of family relationships within the context of social work practice with the elderly.*

8. *Gerontological Social Work: International Perspectives,* edited by Merl C. Hokenstad, Jr., PhD, and Katherine A. Kendall, PhD (Vol. 12, No. 1/2, 1988). *"Makes a very useful contribution in examining the changing role of the social work profession in serving the elderly." (Journal of the International Federation on Ageing)*

9. *Twenty-Five Years of the Life Review: Theoretical and Practical Considerations,* edited by Robert Disch, MA (Vol. 12, No. 3/4, 1989). *This practical and thought-provoking book examines the history and concept of the life review.*

10. *Health Care of the Aged: Needs, Policies, and Services,* edited by Abraham Monk, PhD (Vol. 15, No. 3/4, 1990). *"The chapters reflect firsthand experience and are competent and informative. Readers . . . will find the book rewarding and useful. The text is timely, appropriate, and well-presented." (Health & Social Work)*

11. *Vision and Aging: Issues in Social Work Practice,* edited by Nancy D. Weber, MSW (Vol. 17, No. 3/4, 1992). *"For those involved in vision rehabilitation programs, the book provides practical information and should stimulate readers to revise their present programs of care." (Journal of Vision Rehabilitation)*

12. *Geriatric Social Work Education,* edited by M. Joanna Mellor, DSW, and Renee Solomon, DSW (Vol. 18, No. 3/4, 1992). *"Serves as a foundation upon which educators and fieldwork instructors can build courses that incorporate more aging content." (SciTech Book News)*

13. *New Developments in Home Care Services for the Elderly: Innovations in Policy, Program, and Practice*, edited by Lenard W. Kaye, DSW (Vol. 24, No. 3/4, 1995). *"An excellent compilation. . . . Especially pertinent to the functions of administrators, supervisors, and case managers in home care. . . . Highly recommended for every home care agency and a must for administrators and middle managers." (Geriatric Nursing Book Review)*

14. *Special Aging Populations and Systems Linkages*, edited by M. Joanna Mellor, DSW (Vol. 25, No. 1/2, 1996). *"An invaluable tool for anyone working with older persons with special needs." (Irene Gutheil, DSW, Associate Professor, Graduate School of Social Service, Fordham University)*

15. *Social Work Response to the White House Conference on Aging: From Issues to Actions*, edited by Constance Corley Saltz, PhD, LCSW (Vol. 27, No. 3, 1997). *"Provides a framework for the discussion of issues relevant to social work values and practice, including productive aging, quality of life, the psychological needs of older persons, and family issues." (Jordan I. Kosberg, PhD, Professor and PhD Program Coordinator, School of Social Work, Florida International University, North Miami, FL)*

16. *Intergenerational Approaches in Aging: Implications for Education, Policy and Practice*, edited by Kevin Brabazon, MPA, and Robert Disch, MA (Vol. 28, No. 1/2/3, 1997). *"Provides a wealth of concrete examples of areas in which intergenerational perspectives and knowledge are needed." (Robert C. Atchley, PhD, Director, Scribbs Gerontology Center, Miami University)*

17. *Dignity and Old Age*, edited by Harry R. Moody, PhD, Rose Dobrof, DSW, and Robert Disch, MA (Vol. 29, No. 2/3, 1998). *"Challenges us to uphold the right to age with dignity, which is embedded in the heart and soul of every man and woman." (H. James Towey, President, Commission on Aging with Dignity, Tallahassee, FL)*

18. *Latino Elders and the Twenty-First Century: Issues and Challenges for Culturally Competent Research and Practice*, edited by Melvin Delgado, PhD (Vol. 30, No. 1/2, 1998). *Explores the challenges that gerontological social work will encounter as it attempts to meet the needs of the growing number of Latino elders utilizing culturally competent principles.*

19. *Grandparents as Carers of Children with Disabilities: Facing the Challenges,* edited by Philip McCallion, PhD, ACSW, and Matthew Janicki, PhD (Vol. 33, No. 3, 2000). *Here is the first comprehensive consideration of the unique needs and experiences of grandparents caring for children with developmental disabilities. The vital information found here will assist practitioners, administrators, and policymakers to include the needs of this special population in the planning and delivery of services, and it will help grandparents in this situation to better care for themselves as well as for the children in their charge.*

20. *Social Work Practice with the Asian American Elderly,* edited by Namkee G. Choi, PhD (Vol. 36, No. 1/2, 2001). *"Encompasses the richness of diversity among Asian Americans by including articles on Vietnamese, Japanese, Chinese, Taiwanese, Asian Indian, and Korean Americans." (Nancy R. Hooyman, PhD, MSW, Professor and Dean Emeritus, University of Washington School of Social Work, Seattle)*

21. *Gerontological Social Work Practice: Issues, Challenges, and Potential,* edited by Enid Opal Cox, DSW, Elizabeth S. Kelchner, MSW, ACSW, and Rosemary Chapin, PhD (Vol. 36, No. 3/4, 2001). *This book gives you an essential overview of the role, status, and potential of gerontological social work in aging societies around the world. Drawing on the expertise of leaders in the field, it identifies key policy and practice issues and suggests directions for the future. Here you'll find important perspectives on home health care, mental health, elder abuse, older workers' issues, and death and dying, as well as an examination of the policy and practice issues of utmost concern to social workers dealing with the elderly.*

22. *Advancing Gerontological Social Work Education*, edited by M. Joanna Mellor, DSW, and Joann Ivry, PhD (Vol. 39, No. 1/2, 2002). *Examines the current status of geriatric/gerontological education; offers models for curriculum development within the classroom and the practice arena.*

23. *Older People and Their Caregivers Across the Spectrum of Care,* edited by Judith L. Howe, PhD (Vol. 40, No. 1/2, 2002). *Focuses on numerous issues relating to caregiving and social work assessment for improving quality of life for the elderly.*

24. ***Gerontological Social Work in Small Towns and Rural Communities,*** edited by Sandra S. Butler, PhD, and Lenard W. Kaye, DSW (Vol. 41, No. 1/2 and 3/4, 2003). *Provides a range of intervention and community skills aimed precisely at the needs of rural elders.*

25. ***Group Work and Aging: Issues in Practice, Research, and Education,*** edited by Robert Salmon, DSW, and Robert Graziano, DSW (Vol. 44, No. 1/2, 2004). *Although there is a considerable amount of writing on both group work and social work with the elderly, there is surprisingly little about applying this practice method to this specific age group.* Group Work and Aging: Issues in Practice, Research, and Education *fills this gap by presenting penetrating articles about a mutual aid approach to working with diverse groups of older adults with varied needs. Respected experts and gifted researchers provide case studies, practice examples, and explanations of theory to illustrate this practice method with aging adults, their families, and their caregivers. Each well-referenced chapter delivers high quality, up-to-date social group work practice strategies to prepare practitioners for the needs of the growing population of elderly in the near future.*

26. ***Religion, Spirituality, and Aging: A Social Work Perspective,*** edited by Harry R. Moody, PhD (Vol. 45, No. 1/2 and 3, 2005). *"From the definitive opening chapter by the eminent social gerontologist David Moberg to the erudite final chapter by Eugene Bianchi, the breadth and depth of this collection of essays provide a major contribution to the understanding of religion, spirituality, aging, and social work. These essays will both inform and challenge the reader." (Dr. Melvin A. Kimble, PhD, Professor Emeritus of Pastoral Theology and Director, Center for Aging, Religion, and Spirituality, Luther Seminary, St. Paul, Minnesota; Editor of* Viktor Frankl's Contribution to Spirituality and Aging)

27. ***Elder Abuse and Mistreatment: Policy, Practice, and Research,*** edited by M. Joanna Mellor, DSW, and Patricia Brownell, PhD (Vol 46, No. 3/4, 2006). *"Important. . . . Rarely does a single book offer the reader the wealth of information and the multidimensional perspective of this collection. The contributors are academicians and practitioners in the variety of fields whose involvement is now understood to be vital to an effective response to a growing problem. Their contributions provide practical tools to professionals in several disciplines, and put forward concrete methodologies for screening, assessment, and intervention." (Betty F. Malks, MSW, CSW, Director, Santa Clara County Department of Aging and Adult Services, San Jose, California; North American Regional Representative, International Network for the Prevention of Elder Abuse)*

Fostering Social Work Gerontology Competence: A Collection of Papers from the First National Gerontological Social Work Conference

Catherine J. Tompkins, MSW, PhD
Anita L. Rosen, MSW, PhD
Editors

Fostering Social Work Gerontology Competence: A Collection of Papers from the First National Gerontological Social Work Conference has been co-published simultaneously as *Journal of Gerontological Social Work*, Volume 48, Numbers 1/2 2006, and 3/4 2007.

The Haworth Press, Inc.

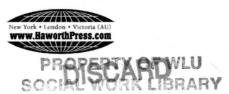

New York • London • Victoria (AU)
www.HaworthPress.com

Fostering Social Work Gerontology Competence: A Collection of Papers from the First National Gerontological Social Work Conference has been co-published simultaneously as *Journal of Gerontological Social Work,*™ Volume 48, Numbers 1/2 2006, and 3/4 2007.

Library of Congress Catalog-in-Publication Data

National Gerontological Social Work Conference (1st : 2003 : Atlanta, Ga.) Fostering social work gerontology competence : a collection of papers from the First National Gerontological Social Work Conference / Catherine J. Tompkins, Anita L. Rosen, editors.
    p. cm.
    "Co-published simultaneously as Journal of gerontological social work, Volume 48, numbers 1/2 2006, and 3/4 2007."
    Includes bibliographical references and index.
    ISBN 13: 978-0-7890-3413-7 (hard cover : alk. paper)
    ISBN 10: 0-7890-3413-1 (hard cover : alk. paper)
    ISBN 13: 978-0-7890-3414-4 (soft cover : alk. paper)
    ISBN 10: 0-7890-3414-X (soft cover : alk. paper)
    1. Social work with older people–United States–Congresses. 2. Social work education–Congresses. 3. Older people–United States–Congresses. 4. Gerontology–Congresses. I. Tompkins, Catherine J. II. Rosen, Anita L. III. Journal of gerontological social work. IV. Title.
HV1461.N3644 2003
362.6–dc22
                                                                            2006038352

Indexing, Abstracting & Website/Internet Coverage

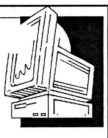

This section provides you with a list of major indexing & abstracting services and other tools for bibliographic access. That is to say, each service began covering this periodical during the year noted in the right column. Most Websites which are listed below have indicated that they will either post, disseminate, compile, archive, cite or alert their own Website users with research-based content from this work. (This list is as current as the copyright date of this publication.)

Abstracting, Website/Indexing Coverage . . . . Year When Coverage Began

- *Abstracts in Social Gerontology: Current Literature on Aging (Sage)* . . **1989**
- *Academic Search Premier (EBSCO) <http://www.epnet.com/ academic/acasearchprem.asp>* **1993**
- *AgeInfo CD-Rom (Centre for Policy on Ageing) <http://www.cpa.org.uk>* **1995**
- *AgeLine Database (AARP) <http://research.aarp.org/ageline>* **1978**
- *Alzheimer's Disease Education & Referral Center (ADEAR) (Combined Health Information Database)* **1994**
- *Applied Social Sciences Index & Abstracts (Cambridge Scientific Abstracts) (ASSIA) (Online: ASSI via Data-Star) (CDRom: ASSIA Plus) <http://www.csa.com>* **1987**
- *Behavioral Medicine Abstracts* **1992**
- *British Library Inside (The British Library) <http://www.bl.uk/services/current/inside.html>* **2006**
- *Cabell's Directory of Publishing Opportunities in Psychology > (Bibliographic Access) <http://www.cabells.com>* **2006**
- *Cambridge Scientific Abstracts (A leading publisher of scientific information in print journals, online databases, CD-ROM, and via the Internet) <http://www.csa.com>* **2006**

(continued)

(continued)

(continued)

*Special Bibliographic Notes related to special journal issues
(separates) and indexing/abstracting:*

- indexing/abstracting services in this list will also cover material in any "separate" that is co-published simultaneously with Haworth's special thematic journal issue or DocuSerial. Indexing/abstracting usually covers material at the article/chapter level.
- monographic co-editions are intended for either non-subscribers or libraries which intend to purchase a second copy for their circulating collections.
- monographic co-editions are reported to all jobbers/wholesalers/approval plans. The source journal is listed as the "series" to assist the prevention of duplicate purchasing in the same manner utilized for books-in-series.
- to facilitate user/access services all indexing/abstracting services are encouraged to utilize the co-indexing entry note indicated at the bottom of the first page of each article/chapter/contribution.
- this is intended to assist a library user of any reference tool (whether print, electronic, online, or CD-ROM) to locate the monographic version if the library has purchased this version but not a subscription to the source journal.
- individual articles/chapters in any Haworth publication are also available through the Haworth Document Delivery Service (HDDS).

Fostering Social Work Gerontology Competence: A Collection of Papers from the First National Gerontological Social Work Conference

CONTENTS

ABOUT THE EDITORS

Catherine J. Tompkins, MSW, PhD, is Assistant Professor and BSW Program Director, George Mason University. She has been the undergraduate social work program director at George Mason University since August, 2003. Dr. Tompkins has many administrative responsibilities and teaches three courses over the academic year. Her teaching interests include social work and aging, research, social welfare and human behavior. She was also a consultant for the Council on Social Work Education's Gero Ed Center. Her responsibilities included curriculum development, reviewing manuscripts and organizing a textbook review project. Prior to coming to George Mason, Dr. Tompkins was the project director for the CSWE SAGE-SW project. She was instrumental in organizing and running faculty development institutes to teach social work faculty from across the country how to infuse aging content throughout the social work curriculum. For three years, she was Director of the Association for Gerontology in Higher Education, where she gained skills in grant writing, fund raising, strategic planning, board development, volunteer coordination and budget management. Prior to moving to the DC area, Dr. Tompkins was Assistant Professor at James Madison University, Harrisonburg, VA. She taught four classes each semester and was involved with various community activities and organizations. Dr. Tompkins has served on the board of the Virginia Mennonite Retirement Community in Harrisonburg, VA and two national boards: Secretary, Association for Gerontology in Higher Education and member-at-large for the Association for Gerontology Education in Social Work. Her current research interests include exploring the long-term relationship between grandmothers and granddaughters where the grandmother is the primary careprovider for the granddaughter and examining the importance of faith communities in ethical decision making for Alzheimer's patients and their care providers.

Anita L. Rosen, MSW, PhD, is the Special Projects Advisor at the Council on Social Work Education (CSWE). She also served as the CSWE Project Manager for the John A. Hartford Foundation of New York City's SAGE-SW gerontology initiative at CSWE. Dr. Rosen represents CSWE to other associations, government agencies and professional organizations, and takes responsibility to strengthen social workers' capacity to serve a growing aging population through resource and curriculum development. Dr. Rosen serves on the Board of Directors of the American Society on Aging (ASA) and is Chair of the Mental Health and Aging Network (MHAN) of the American Society on Aging. She also serves on the Executive Committee of the National Coalition on Mental Health and Aging, and is a Reviewer for the *Journal of Gerontological Social Work* and *Families in Society*. She also serves as an expert consultant in mental health and social work curriculum.

Prior to her work at CSWE, she was the Senior Staff Associate for Aging at the National Association of Social Workers, where she was responsible for policy and practice issues for aging and long-term care, and was a delegate to the 1995 White House Conference on Aging. She has served on expert panels and committees for government agencies such as HFCA, SAMSHA, AHRQ, and the Centers for Mental Health Services. Other work experience includes 14 years of full-time teaching and 5 years of adjunct status in social work and health care administration. She also has experience in public health and international health care financing and management.

Dr. Rosen is the author of over 40 journal articles, book chapters or textbooks and has presented over 60 symposia, papers or workshops at major national meetings, including the Council on Social Work Education, the American Public Health Association, National Council on the Aging, Gerontological Society of America, Association of Gerontology in Higher Education, and the American Society on Aging. Her primary areas of expertise are long-term care services and financing, community-based services, interdisciplinary training, social work education, and mental health and aging policy.

Acknowledgements

The editors would like to express their gratitude to the John A. Hartford Foundation for their support of the first National Gerontological Social Work Conference (NGSWC) and their continued work in supporting Gerontological/Geriatric Social Work since the first NGSWC.

A special thanks goes out to Angela Curl, a doctoral student at Case Western Reserve University's Mandel School of Applied Social Science. Angela provided a tremendous amount of work and editorial support to the editors for which we are immensely grateful.

Lastly, we would like to thank all of the authors for their fantastic contributions and their patience throughout this process. Both of the editors experienced life events that caused delays to the publication of this volume and we are eternally grateful to all of the authors for their patience and support.

Foreword

It is no secret that the demographic imperative of increasing numbers of persons over the age of 65 in the United States will demand an ever-increasing number of social workers to work with older persons in the future. It has been clear for some time that the number of existing geriatric/gerontological social workers is insufficient to meet the needs of the current older population and the provider-client gap will only widen unless action is taken.

Several leading gerontologists, notably Dr. Rose Dobrof, editor of *JGSW*, have worked tirelessly to bring aging into the mainstream consciousness of social work. As a result, NASW now has a vibrant section on aging and AGE-SW has grown enormously in the last few years. The John A. Hartford Foundation, Inc. is a key player in this push to prepare social workers to work with older persons and its funding of CSWE's Strengthening Aging and Gerontology Education for Social Work (CSWE/SAGE) project led directly to the first National Gerontological Social Work Conference (NGSWC), now a regular section of the CSWE annual program meeting. All the articles in this special volume were presented as papers at this first NGSWC. The introductory chapter by editors Catherine Tompkins and Anita Rosen provides a clear picture of the genesis of the conference. It is a mark of the impact made by the Hartford Foundation's promotion of gerontological social work education that roughly half of the articles in this issue report on programs funded by the Foundation. At least 8 articles speak to the infusion of aging content into social work education with each approaching the subject within different settings and from different perspectives.

In spite of the headways that are being made in promoting gerontological social work, there is much to be accomplished. Recent surveys show that there has actually been a decline in the number of aging specialties and courses offered by

[Haworth co-indexing entry note]: "Foreword." Mellor, M. Joanna. Co-published simultaneously in *Journal of Gerontological Social Work* (The Haworth Press, Inc.) Vol. 48, No. 1/2, 2006, pp. xxvii-xxviii; and: *Fostering Social Work Gerontology Competence: A Collection of Papers from the First National Gerontological Social Work Conference* (ed: Catherine J. Tompkins, and Anita L. Rosen) The Haworth Press, Inc., 2007, pp. xxi-xxii. Single or multiple copies of this article are available for a fee from The Haworth Document Delivery Service [1-800-HAWORTH, 9:00 a.m. - 5:00 p.m. (EST). E-mail address: docdelivery@haworthpress.com].

xxi

the schools of social work over the past decade. It is more than time for a renewed focus on aging content in social work learning.

There is something for everyone in this special collection. There are articles dealing with teaching research, community collaboration, and social work competencies while several focus on special populations and issues in aging, e.g., elder abuse, end-of-life, spirituality, and mental health. Education is the overarching theme and clearly this volume is valuable to all those who educate future social workers or lead staff training sessions, and/or teach continuing education courses in aging. But there is something for everyone–practitioner, researcher, administrator or educator in the field. Rose Dobrof and I know that you will find much to both inspire and affirm you in your own endeavors in educating, supervising and acting as role models for the social workers of tomorrow.

M. Joanna Mellor, DSW

Developing Visibility for Aging in Social Work: The First NGSWC

Catherine J. Tompkins, MSW, PhD
Anita L. Rosen, PhD

SUMMARY. In March 2001, the Council on Social Work Education's (CSWE) Strengthening Aging and Gerontology Education for Social Work (SAGE-SW) project published an action agenda for social work and aging (CSWE/SAGE-SW, 2001). CSWE SAGE-SW, funded by the John A. Hartford Foundation from 1998 to 2004, had several charges in the first phase of funding, including the gathering of data through a thorough review of literature, focus groups, surveys and a variety of activities to garner expert input. This agenda, often referred to as the *Blueprint*, identified a number of serious issues regarding the lack of attention, preparation, leadership and interest in aging within the social work profession. It also provided some recommended actions to address these issues and help set the stage for the creation of the National Gerontological Social Work Conference. What were the issues at hand and why might a National Gerontological Social Work Conference (NGSWC) address some of these issues? doi: 10.1300/J083v48n01_01 *[Article copies available for a fee from The Haworth Document Delivery Service: 1-800-HAWORTH. E-mail address: <docdelivery@haworthpress.com> Website: <http://www.HaworthPress.com> © 2006 by The Haworth Press, Inc. All rights reserved.]*

[Haworth co-indexing entry note]: "Developing Visibility for Aging in Social Work: The First NGSWC." Tompkins, Catherine J., and Anita L. Rosen. Co-published simultaneously in *Journal of Gerontological Social Work* (The Haworth Press, Inc.) Vol. 48, No. 1/2, 2006, pp. 1-8; and: *Fostering Social Work Gerontology Competence: A Collection of Papers from the First National Gerontological Social Work Conference* (ed: Catherine J. Tompkins, and Anita L. Rosen) The Haworth Press, Inc., 2007, pp. 1-8. Single or multiple copies of this article are available for a fee from The Haworth Document Delivery Service [1-800-HAWORTH, 9:00 a.m. - 5:00 p.m. (EST). E-mail address: docdelivery@haworthpress.com].

KEYWORDS. Social work, education, gerontology, conference, aging

BACKGROUND

A variety of authors and studies have indicated that social work appeared ill-prepared to meet the needs of a growing aging population (Berkman, Dobrof, Damron-Rodriguez & Harry, 1997; Scharlach, Damron-Rodriguez, Robinson & Feldman, 2000; Rosen & Zlotnik, 2001). Faculty were largely disinterested in aging and few social work students were provided aging skills and knowledge in textbooks, in the classroom, or the field. In fact, it was suggested in both the *Blueprint* (2001) and by other authors (Scharlach, Damron-Rodriguez, Robinson & Feldman, 2000) that there was a lack of visibility for aging in social work. This lack of interest was evident in social work foundation textbooks for both BSW and MSW students, foundation curricula, social work publications and equity in acceptance of paper presentations at non-aging social work conferences (Austin & Moan, 1999). Few social work educators, deans or directors had interest or knowledge in aging and academe provided few opportunities, resources, incentives or forums to increase the visibility and respect for aging in social work. In addition, neither faculty nor national organizations had been able to take leadership to change this social work culture that "generally failed to mount a significant effort to better prepare its future practitioners for a growing aging population" (Rosen, Zlotnik & Singer, 2002, p. 26).

Of the many ways that the CSWE SAGE-SW program sought to increase the basic competence of all social work students in aging and increase the visibility of aging in social work, the NGSWC was seen as a genuine opportunity to attempt to create an ongoing, nationally visibile forum on "gerontological social work policy, practice and education" (CSWE/SAGE-SW 2001, p. 3).

WHY A NATIONAL GERONTOLOGICAL SOCIAL WORK CONFERENCE?

A national social work and aging conference, held in conjunction with another national conference (the Annual Program Meeting of the Council on Social Work Education) and self-sustaining, was seen as a way to create visibility and interest for aging among social work educators, administrators and field practica supervisors and to help in the development of an aging and social work community. Theoretical constructs of community change and development (Homan, 2004; Brueggemann, 2002) suggested that CSWE could build on certain assets within the social work education community, connect people and groups, foster more positive attitudes toward aging, create collaborations among individuals and groups, build a self-sustaining conference and ultimately enhance the quality of life of older adults through increasing interest, competence and activity in gerontological social work.

CSWE SAGE-SW could attempt to use its power and resources to create a new entity, the NGSWC to not only increase the visibility and respect for aging in social work, but to increase or enhance the positive interaction, social engagement and feelings of belonging of social work educators in relation to aging. This last concept is quite similar to conceptions of social capital as described by Putnam (1993, 1995, 2000) and Homan (2004).

Community change and development models informed the entire process of the development of the NGSWC that is described in this paper. Rothman and Tropman (1987) and Dolgoff, Feldstein and Skolnick (1997) provide structure and models that suggest important notions of linking people with shared interest, changing conditions and environment, enhancing resources and redistributing "power." In effect, the NGSWC was a successful community development process with an objective to develop a visible, inclusive gerontological social work education community of interest that was self sustaining in order to strengthen the capacity of social work education to prepare all BSW and MSW practitioners for a growing aging population.

DEVELOPING THE NATIONAL GERONTOLOGICAL SOCIAL WORK CONFERENCE

The NGSWC was one of several tasks in the second phase of the CSWE SAGE-SW project. Though the actual format and logistics of such a conference were not pre-defined, there were several clear overall objectives for having such a conference. Among the most important, based on the *Blueprint* (2001) and other works were:

- Transforming the perceptions and interest in gerontological social;
- Providing a visible and respected forum for presenting resources for infusing aging content into the social work curricula;
- Presenting an inclusive and creative venue for communication, networking, and mentoring in social work and aging; and
- Creating an environment conducive to linking and promoting a variety of groups and organizations with interest in or supportive of the overall goals of the CSWE SAGE-SW program.

Though the original John A. Hartford grant conceived of the NGSWC as a free-standing, and independent national conference, the staff of the CSWE

SAGE-SW program along with its Executive Committee quickly determined that it would be more advantageous to link the NGSWC with another national social work education conference. The rationale for this decision was based on several important points. First, holding the conference in conjunction with another national conference would greatly conserve resources, both for potential attendees and for CSWE SAGE-SW. Social work faculty often have funds only to attend one conference per year so that they could benefit if the NGSWC were to "piggy back" on a conference that faculty already attend. The NGSWC would benefit by eliminating duplication for conference planning time, marketing and promotion, communication, and a variety of expenses.

A second but even more compelling benefit to holding the NGSWC in conjunction with another national social work education conference was that a joint conference would give exposure to aging and the presenters, to deans, directors and the vast majority of social work faculty with little knowledge or interest in aging.

The decision was made to hold the NGSWC jointly with the Annual Program Meeting (APM) of CSWE which averages about 2,300 attendees per conference and is known throughout social work education. It should be noted that though there was agreement to hold the two conferences jointly and to share staff and resources, the NGSWC requested and received permission to organize its own planning committee, conduct its own call for presentations, select its own proposal review committees, and to have a variety of presentation and meeting venues that may be quite different than that of the APM. This later request was made in order to clearly demonstrate that the NGSWC was seeking to be very inclusive and was an alternative to what was perceived as "ageist" presentation selection processes of social work education conferences. In addition, it was intended to provide venues that could more readily encourage first time presenters, allow a focus on curriculum change and resources, and encourage BSW, MSW and PhD student participation.

INNOVATIONS

The new conference created several features that differed from the APM. One such innovation was the poster presentation. It was felt that in order to encourage first time presenters, such as doctoral students or new faculty, the poster session would be an ideal format. In addition, the poster sessions were planned to be held in the Exhibit Hall at times when there would be a coffee break or when there would be heavier traffic. The poster session was a positive way to address several of the NGSWC's purposes–visibility for aging, mentoring, creating a less stressful presentation format to first time presenters, and creating interest in aging. It should be noted that the success of this first poster session offering was noted by CSWE APM and the concept was subsequently adopted by APM.

The NGSWC printed and distributed to all joint conference participants an abstract book of all NGSWC presentations. APM had not offered such a publication. CSWE SAGE-SW incurred the expense of creating and printing the Abstract Book in keeping with its efforts to create visibility for aging in social work with the wider social work education community and to feature an encourage those who did present at the conference. Presenters were pleased to have this book to use for tenure and promotion dossiers.

The NGSWC staff also sought to gain outside funding from a grant or foundation. Though the first efforts presented some difficulties, the staff was able to obtain a grant from the Health Care Georgia Foundation. Both Health Care Georgia and the John A. Hartford Foundation were publicly noted at the conference for their contributions.

THE FIRST NGSWC

February 27 – March 2, 2003 marked the first NGSWC held in conjunction with the CSWE's 49th APM in Atlanta, Georgia, and was attended by 2,600 participants. Planning and preparation for the conference involved social work faculty from across the country, CSWE and SAGE-SW staff and the CSWE president. A unique Faculty Development Institute (FDI) was a pre-conference feature. Over 55 participants attended the NGSWC FDI entitled, "Making Infusing Less Confusing: A Lifespan Approach to Practice and Field Curriculum," were a blend of Field Instructors and Practice Faculty. The opening plenary session of CSWE's Annual Program Meeting included recognition and support for the NGSWC as well as an excellent presentation by 91-year-old Katherine Kendall, one of the first leaders of the Council on Social Work Education.

Some data and information on the NGSWC include the following:

- The overall conference evaluations supported the qualitative feedback marking the success of the NGSWC. For example, out of 635 participants providing an evaluation, 544 respondents stated that attending special presentations, such as those offered by the NGSWC was an important feature in their choice to attend the joint conference.
- The NGSWC had 82 paper, symposia, roundtable and workshop presentations, 36 poster presentations and 4 special sessions for a total of 122 presentations.
- A total of 272 first, second, third and fourth listed author names were assigned to these papers.

- The first-time Poster Session format was rated at High or Excellent quality by 71.4% of respondents evaluating the conference.
- NGSWC Roundtable Sessions were rated at High or Excellent quality by 72.9% of respondents evaluating the conference.
- Special Sessions were well received by respondents. Special sessions included: "How to Find External Support for Your Social Work Program: Working with Funders 101"; rated High or Excellent by 72.9% of respondents; "Ask the Experts: A Dialogue on Social Work Education in Aging"; rated High or Excellent by 74.5% of respondents; "Creating Aging-Enriched Social Work Education"; rated High or Excellent by 87.2% of respondents; and "Models for Using CSWE SAGE-SW Aging Competencies in Education" rated High or Excellent by 73.2% of respondents.
- The NGSWC Abstract book was rated as High Quality or Excellent by 81% of respondents.

In addition to formal presentations, there were extensive opportunities for networking including interacting with staff and participants in all five of the John A. Hartford Foundation's Geriatric Social Work Initiative projects: The Faculty Scholars, Doctoral Fellows Practicum Partnership, Geriatric Enrichment and the Faculty Development projects. More than 120 people attended a jointly sponsored SAGE-SW and Association for Gerontology Education in Social Work (AGE-SW) event that included roundtable discussions lead by national experts, award presentations, and a reception, partially supported by CSWE SAGE-SW. The newly formed Aging Committee of the Association for Baccalaureate Social Work Program Directors (BPD) held a meeting at the conference which was well attended and cosponsored by SAGE-SW. The National Association of Deans and Directors of Schools of Social Work also held a very large and well attended meeting at the NGSWC. These three sessions created many networking and mentoring opportunities including very positive exposure for the BPD and NADD Aging Committees and AGE-SW.

The joint conference created high visibility for aging. Every participant of the CSWE APM and the NGSWC received a tote bag that had bold purple letters announcing the conference and an NGSWC presentation abstract book. This meant that faculty, practitioners and students who were among the 2600 + participants who were not focused on gerontological social work, had a tremendous opportunity to be positively exposed to aging and to obtain knowledge relative to the issues and concerns social workers face when working with older adults. The second NGSWC was already planned for the following year with a call for presentations in the conference program book.

SELECTED ARTICLES FROM THE FIRST NGSWC

Each of the twenty-eight articles that follow the foreword in this special collection resulted from a presentation done at the first National Gerontological Social Work Conference. These manuscripts were selected as being well representative of issues presented at the first NGSWC. There are many articles that focus on the infusion of aging content throughout the social work curriculum with some focusing on undergraduate education and others focusing on graduate education, a particular content area (such as human behavior, research and field education) or the infusion of intergenerational content specifically. There are two articles that focus on the development of gerontological social work competencies (one article that focuses on competencies that help guide curriculum infusion and resource development throughout the curriculum and another one that focuses on building gerontological social work competencies specifically for social work field education). It is important to also explore the articles that discuss the transformation of social work education to include gerontology/geriatric content as well as how to sustain this transformation.

The first NGSWC went beyond gerontological social work education to include presentations on end-of-life care, elder abuse, the effects of spirituality and social support on the well-being of older adults, grief counseling, mental health, cultural diversity and cultural competence. There are manuscripts on each one of these topic areas in this volume (which includes two issues of the *Journal of Gerontological Social Work*).

The Council on Social Work Education's National Center for Gerontological Social Work Education is planning for the fourth NGSWC (under the new name of the Gero Ed Forum). In 2005, due to the visibility of aging and the NGSWC, there were more than 200 presenters from over 80 social work education programs taking part in 69 paper, symposia, and special presentations; 8 workshops; 10 roundtable discussions; and 34 poster presentations. The NGSWC (Gero-Ed Forum) continues to be held in conjunction with the Council on Social Work Education's Annual Program Meeting and brings together hundreds of educators, students and practitioners eager to learn more about gerontological social work. Conference highlights encompass well-known keynote speakers, evidence-based paper presentations, student poster sessions, and informal networking opportunities (http://depts.washington.edu/geroctr/Center2/sub2_3_1NGSWC.html).

It is with great pride that we were a part of the implementation of the first NGSWC and that a conference where social work educators and practitioners can come together to share ideas on how to ensure that all social workers who graduate from either an undergraduate or graduate program in aging have a certain level of competence and are being exposed to a diverse array of issues, still continues today! You will learn something new from each of the articles in this volume so please enjoy and share the information with your colleagues.

REFERENCES

Austin, C. & Moan, P. (1999). Coverage of aging issues in eight peer reviewed journals. Manuscript.

Berkman, B., Dobrof, R., Damron-Rodriguez, J. & Harry, L. (1997). Social work. In S. M. Klein (Ed.), *A national agenda for geriatric education: White papers* (pp. 53-85). New York: Springer.

Brueggemann, W.G. (2002). *The practice of macro social work (2nd ed.)*. Chicago: Nelson-Hall.

Council on Social Work Education's National Center for Gerontological Social Work Education (2005). http://depts.washington.edu/geroctr/Center2/sub2_3_1NGSWC.html. Retrieved on-line on September 5, 2005.

CSWE/SAGE-SW (2001). *Strengthening the impact of social work to improve the quality of life for older adults and their families: A blueprint for the new millennium*. Alexandria, VA: Council on Social Work Education.

Dolgoff, R., Feldstein, D., & Skolnik, L. (1997). *Understanding social welfare* (4th ed.). White Plains, NY: Longman.

Homan, M. (2004). *Promoting community change*: *Making it happen in the real world*. (3rd ed.). Belmont, CA: Thomson Brooks/Cole.

Putnam, R.D. (1993). The prosperous community: Social capital and economic growth. *The American Prospect*, 35-42.

Putnam, R.D. (1995). Bowling alone: America's declining social capital. *Journal of Democracy*, 6 (1), 65-78.

Putnam, R.D. (2000). *Bowling alone: The collapse and revival of American community*. New York: Simon & Shuster.

Rosen, A. & Zlotnik, J.L. (2001). Social work's response to a growing older population. *Generations*, 25 (1), 69-71.

Rosen, A., Zlotnik, J.L. & Singer, T. (2002). Basic gerontological competence for all social workers: The need to "gerontologize" social work education. *Journal of Gerontological Social Work*, 39 (1/2), 25-36.

Rothman, J. & Tropman, J. (1987) Models of community organization and macro practice perspectives. Their mixing and phasing. In F.M. Cox, J.L. Erlich, J. Rothman & J.E. Tropman (eds). *Strategies of community organization: Macro practice* (4th ed, pp. 3-26). Itasca, IL: Peacock.

Scharlach, A., Damron-Rodriguez, J., Robinson, B. & Feldman, R. (2000). Educating Social Workers for an Aging Society: A Vision for the 21st Century. *Journal of Social Work Education*, 36 (3), 521-538.

doi: 10.1300/J083v48n01_01

Creating Aging-Enriched Social Work Education: A Process of Curricular and Organizational Change

Nancy Hooyman, PhD
Suzanne St. Peter, MSW

SUMMARY. The CSWE Geriatric Enrichment in Social Work Education Project, funded by the John A. Hartford foundation, aimed to change curricula and organizational structure in 67 GeroRich projects so that all students would graduate with foundation knowledge and skills to work effectively with older adults and their families. The emphasis was on change processes to infuse and sustain gerontological competencies and curricular resources in foundation courses. This article presents lessons learned and strategies for engaging faculty, practitioners and students in the curriculum and organizational change process. doi: 10.1300/J083v48n01_02 *[Article copies available for a fee from The Haworth Document Delivery Service: 1-800-HAWORTH. E-mail address: <docdelivery @haworthpress.com> Website: <http://www.HaworthPress.com> © 2006 by The Haworth Press, Inc. All rights reserved.]*

KEYWORDS. Infusion, foundation, organizational and curricular change, sustainability

---

[Haworth co-indexing entry note]: "Creating Aging-Enriched Social Work Education: A Process of Curricular and Organizational Change." Hooyman, Nancy, and Suzanne St. Peter. Co-published simultaneously in *Journal of Gerontological Social Work* (The Haworth Press, Inc.) Vol. 48, No. 1/2, 2006, pp. 9-29; and: *Fostering Social Work Gerontology Competence: A Collection of Papers from the First National Gerontological Social Work Conference* (ed: Catherine J. Tompkins, and Anita L. Rosen) The Haworth Press, Inc., 2007, pp. 9-29. Single or multiple copies of this article are available for a fee from The Haworth Document Delivery Service [1-800-HAWORTH, 9:00 a.m. - 5:00 p.m. (EST). E-mail address: docdelivery@haworthpress.com].

OVERVIEW

The Geriatric Enrichment in Social Work Education (GeroRich[1]) Program, funded by the John A. Hartford Foundation and the Council on Social Work Education, provided resources and technical support to 67 GeroRich Projects in social work programs nationally. These projects aimed to implement curricular changes to increase aging-rich learning opportunities for all social work students. The long-term goal is to prepare all social workers with foundation gerontological knowledge, skills, and values to work effectively with older adults and their families in a wide range of practice contexts.

GeroRich projects engaged in processes of organizational development and curricular change oriented toward the dual goals of:

- Gerontological pervasiveness (e.g., all students will graduate with foundation knowledge, skills, and values needed to work with older adults and their families);
- Sustainability or the institutionalization of gerontological content, pedagogy, and experiential learning opportunities after funding ends; and
- Infusing gerontological content and transforming foundation learning experiences (e.g., classroom, field practica, service learning, modules) are the overall strategies toward achieving these goals.

A fundamental assumption is that an intensive planning process to engage the support of key stakeholders (e.g., deans, directors, faculty, students, practicum instructors, and older adults) increases the likelihood of sustainability and institutionalization of change. In other words, the process of change, rather than specific outcomes per se, is critical to long term sustainability. Within this overall framework of organizational change, this article (1) identifies the need; (2) presents different curricular models (specialization, integration, infusion, and transformation) and the rationale for the GeroRich emphasis on infusion and curriculum transformation; and (3) outlines strategies used by individual GeroRich projects to engage primary constituencies in organizational processes for creating and sustaining age-enriched changes. Although Hartford funding was the catalyst to organizational and curricular change, many of these strategies are nevertheless transferable, typically on an incremental basis, to unfunded settings.

THE NEED FOR CURRICULAR AND ORGANIZATIONAL CHANGE

The historical pattern of too few faculties prepared to teach gerontological social work content, too few students interested in gerontological careers, too few gerontological social work practitioners, and too little outcomes-based gerontological research is well documented. (CSWE SAGE-SW, 2001; Cummings & Galambos, 2003; Damron-Rodriguez & Lubben, 1997; Gibelman & Schervish, 1997; Kropf, 2002; Kropf, Schneider & Stahlman, 1993; Lubben, Damron-Rodriquez, & Beck, 1992; Rosen & Zlotnik, 2001; Scharlach, Damon-Rodriguez, Robinson, & Feldman, 2000). In fact, this pattern has characterized the social work profession for over three decades, even though the demand for gerontological social workers is growing (Scharlach, Simon, & Dal Santo, 2002; Takamura, 2001). For example, in the late 1970s, the Administration on Aging and the National Institutes on Mental Health funded demonstration and training grants in social work to recruit students to the field. In the early 1980s, the Council on Social Work Education sponsored the development of model gerontological social work course syllabi (Schneider, 1984; Schneider, Decker, Freeman, & Syran, 1984a, 1984b). These were not widely adopted for a variety of reasons, including limited funding and competing interests (Rosen, Zlotnik, & Singer, 2002). In 1981, a group of approximately 12 social work faculty members formed the Association for Gerontology Education in Social Work (AGE-SW) and agreed to do "whatever it takes to promote gerontology at our program" (Schneider, 2001). Fortunately, that small group of faculty has now grown to an AGE-SW membership of over 250 educators and researchers, and the support of deans, directors and faculty for gerontological social work has increased dramatically. This progress is largely due to the support and funding provided by the John A. Hartford Foundation through the Hartford Geriatric Social Work Initiative (GSWI).

This article describes one of these five initiatives–the Geriatric Enrichment in Social Work Education Program (e.g., GeroRich program). The GeroRich Program is distinguished from the second Hartford-supported curricular initiative, CSWE Strengthening Aging and Gerontology Education for Social Work (SAGE-SW), which focused on individual faculty development and the dissemination of state of the art teaching materials. With its emphasis on the process of curricular and organizational change, the GeroRich Program's priority has been the *infusion* of gerontological content into the foundation courses. This intensive change process of infusion is conceptualized as laying the foundation for *curricular transformation*.

MODELS OF CURRICULUM CHANGE

A brief review of four models of curricular change articulates the rationale for the GeroRich Program's priority on curriculum infusion and transformation. A common model of curricular change is specializations or concentrations in aging at the MSW level, and the inclusion of some content on aging in undergraduate courses, such as Human Behavior and the Social Environment (HBSE) or Introduction to Social Work. Because of the absence of gerontological content throughout the social work curriculum, few graduate social work students receive knowledge or skills to work with older adults unless they specialize in gerontology, through either an advanced practice concentration or a certificate program (Gleason Wynn, 1995; Kropf, Schneider, & Stahlman, 1993; Lubben, Damron-Rodriguez, & Beck, 1992). Nevertheless, most graduate programs do not offer a separate specialization in aging, partially because of limited resources, competing advanced practice domains, and low student interest; when an advanced gerontology specialization is available, slightly less than four percent of MSW students choose it (CSWE SAGE-SW, 2001; Damron-Rodriquez, Villa, Tseng, & Lubben, 1997; Lennon, 1999).

The barriers to students' specializing in aging include their primary interest in working with children and (young) families, which stems in part from ageism within our culture; their resistance to practice with older adults, partially because of stereotypes of fragility and illness; and the number of competing specializations in most MSW programs. When only a small percentage of students choose an aging specialization, cancellation or infrequent offering of courses is likely, further fueling faculty perceptions that "students are not interested in aging."

Although specialization can be a desirable direction for the depth inherent in graduate education for advanced practice, it can also segregate or isolate aging content from the rest of the curriculum, or create separate courses that compete with one another for students. When such fragmentation occurs, the majority of students graduate with little or no knowledge of aging content, ill-prepared to practice in our society characterized by rapid demographic changes and health disparities. Specialization is ill-suited for the reality that nearly all social workers encounter older adults in a wide range of settings, and therefore require foundation gerontological competence to meet their clients' needs (Damron-Rodriguez & Lubben, 1997; Peterson & Wendt, 1990). In sum, while specialization offers advanced content to those who choose to focus their studies on aging, it does not prepare bachelors and masters level social workers with foundation gerontological knowledge to work effectively with clients of all ages across the life span.

Integration is another curricular model in which aging content is strategically placed throughout the curriculum (Singer, 2000). Examples of an integrative approach are the addition of a single course on aging or social gerontology, guest lectures, or readings in the foundation HBSE course, some readings in a practice course, or the formation of student special interest groups or colloquia on aging. Delivering a brief curriculum module, for example, can increase knowledge, but typically has less impact on attitudes (Olson, 2002). Overall, an integrative approach may be limited by its compensatory "add on" nature. The addition of discussions, guest lectures, or readings onto existing courses may not fundamentally alter students' learning experiences in ways to change attitudes. With both specialization and integration, aging tends to be treated in separate units, rather than embedded in the curriculum and the organizational culture; not surprisingly, with such models, gerontology tends to remain somewhat invisible, secondary, and peripheral to the social work curriculum as a whole.

A number of structural factors underlie an "add on" curricular approach. A primary factor is accreditation expectations to include content on older people as one population among a long list of diverse groups. As a result, faculty often feels that too many content demands are placed on an already crowded curriculum. This can result in minimal attempts–if any–to meet accreditation expectations related to diversity in terms of age (e.g., invite an older person as a guest speaker in the foundation cultural diversity course or discuss illness, death and dying in the last HBSE class). At the undergraduate level, aging may be briefly discussed in generalist courses such as contemporary social problems or introduction to social work. In both instances, models of illness and frailty rather than strengths and resilience are typically portrayed. With specialization or integration, the pedagogy, structure and organization of courses are unlikely to be changed, and aging is generally not an organizing curriculum theme. Of even greater concern is that these approaches are unlikely to improve students' attitudes toward aging, excite them about the contributions they could make by working with older people, or recruit them to the field. As a result, the pattern of students' inadequate preparation for work with older clients across a wide range of settings continues.

THE RATIONALE UNDERLYING CURRICULUM INFUSION AND TRANSFORMATION

A basic premise of the GeroRich Program is that all social work graduates, regardless of field of practice, will interact in some way with older adults and their families. In fact, a national study of NASW members found that 62% of survey respondents worked in some capacity with older adults but had not been prepared to do so, and indicated their need for more aging knowledge. Similarly, less than 5 percent of NASW members indicate that they have expertise in gerontology (Damron-Rodriguez & Lubben, 1997; Gibelman & Schervish, 1997; Gleason Wynn, 1995; Peterson & Wendt, 1990).

The percent of social workers interacting with older adults has undoubtedly increased in the past decade, given the growth of both the older population and multigenerational families, such as grandparents caring for grandchildren. In fact, it can be argued that nearly every practice setting involves interaction with older adults and their families. For example, social workers in child welfare and school settings work with grandparents who are primary caregivers for grandchildren; those in hospitals or community-based health clinics encounter younger family members caring for aging relatives or older parents caring for adult children with developmental disabilities. Aging issues and older adults are linked with all fields of practice–substance abuse, mental health, health care, child welfare, domestic violence, or corrections. In other words, aging across the life course is inextricably intertwined with all that social workers do.

Given this pattern, the GeroRich Program concentrates on the foundation or generalist content areas within both MSW and BSW programs: practice, HBSE, social policy, research, and practicum/field. In fact, GeroRich projects were discouraged from investing resources in the development of specializations, minors, or certificate programs that would reach only a minority of students. Instead, projects were expected to utilize infusion and transformation models to allow for maximum sustained change.

Curriculum Infusion

Infusion suggests that content on aging be "poured into" the curriculum to permeate and alter every aspect of the curriculum, including program and course objectives, subject areas, reading assignments and outcomes assessment categories (Bogolub, 1998; Cummings & Kropf, 2000; Kropf, 1996; Rosen, Zlotnik, & Singer, 2002; Singer, 2000). For example, instead of adding one lecture or reading assignment to the last session of a practice or HBSE class, the course as a whole would be assessed to identify strategic locations for infusing aging content throughout the course and each class session. Through the CSWE SAGE-SW project as well as the work of other gerontologists (Richardson, 1999), a wide range of contemporary materials is now available for infusion.

In contrast to specialization or integration, one or only a few faculty members cannot accomplish curricular infusion. Instead, all key stakeholders–faculty, deans/directors, students, community practitioners, and elders–need to be involved in the process of planning, implementing, and sustaining the curricular changes. Organizational development and culture change, a labor and time intensive process, is essential to engage key stakeholders in the curricular change. In fact, the GeroRich program coordinating team assumed that model syllabi developed in the past (Schneider, 1984; Schneider et al., 1984a,

1984b; Greene, 1988; Richardson, 1999) may not have been widely utilized, because programs did not engage in an organizational change process to obtain constituencies' buy-in. In other words, providing faculty with syllabi and other course materials, while a necessary first step, fails to address attitudinal barriers, faculty's lack of expertise on how best to use gerontological resources, and limited incentives for changing teaching and research. Through some of the inevitable tensions, sources of resistance and other barriers inherent in organizational and curricular change, project directors were motivated by a visual image to avoid well-developed course syllabi or other teaching materials sitting untouched on office shelves!

Curricular Transformation

The term "curriculum transformation" is widely used in higher education, most frequently with regard to embedding multiculturalism and diversity with organizational environments. Specific to gerontological social work, curriculum transformation goes beyond merely creating a course or a module on geriatric social work, to developing ways to fundamentally alter curriculum structure, organization, and pedagogy to support gerontological learning competencies and outcomes. With such structural modifications, aging-based learning experiences can move from isolated examples to *a way of life* institutionalized and embedded in social work programs. A guiding question for curriculum transformation is: how can the face of social work education, research, and practice be transformed over time so that age is a central organizing principle, not secondary or relatively invisible? Alternatively, what would be the central themes and questions of foundation courses if age were a primary reference?

Through curriculum transformation, program-learning experiences are realigned with the desired (changed) outcome related to gerontological social work. It is recognized that there is no one right way to organize the curriculum; instead, the focus is on the fit between the learning experiences needed to achieve desired outcomes within the social work program's organizational culture, not only in discrete courses or in class sections. Potential transformative approaches to gerontological social work learning opportunities are illustrated as follows:

- Life span and multigenerational relationships become organizing principles for the whole curriculum, cross cutting a wide range of substantive areas (e.g., child welfare, mental health, health, and substance abuse). A multi- or intergenerational lens to learning highlights the reciprocity of social support, caregiving, well-being, and interdependence among generations across the life span. For instance, gerontology and early childhood education departments might create an intergenerational studies program (Rosebrook, Haley, & Larkin, 2001).

- Social justice, multiculturalism, feminism, and life span become organizing constructs, congruent with CSWE accreditation requirements related to diversity. A social work program's central themes and goals are transformed if older adults, women, people of color, persons with disabilities, and the poor are the primary reference, rather than viewed as specialized "interest" groups competing with curricular space and student interest. Under such a transformative approach, race, culture, class, gender, disability, sexual orientation, and age are discussed in the broader contexts of person-environment, the strengths perspective, and empowerment, rather than only in the context of oppression, poverty, and social problems. Accordingly, women, older adults, persons of color, persons with disabilities and the poor are conceptualized as active creative agents of social change and continuity, not as victims. Such a reconceptualization moves away from a more traditional focus on frailty, severe impairment and death in old age.
- The HBSE sequence would be turned "upside down" or conceptualized as a "spiral," beginning with aging and the end of life, rather than leaving any discussion of old age until the end of the course, and with continuous interactions across different age groups. The older person could be traced back through young-old age, middle adulthood, adolescence, youth, childhood, and infancy rather than beginning with the early years. This approach articulates the interconnections among early and later life experiences, and how inequities in early life and across the life span become exacerbated in old age.

Regardless of the particular transformative approach, interconnections are built across other curricular areas (e.g., mental health, health, substance abuse, child welfare, women's issues, multiculturalism and cultural diversity) and new partnerships formed within the social work program and the academic institution as a whole. Gerontological learning opportunities are not isolated, but pervade all relevant learning experiences for students: classroom, practica or fieldwork, service learning, and the classroom. Content on aging is no longer considered "unusual" or a "population at risk" but normative and inextricable to quality social work education and practice.

The line between curriculum infusion and transformation is blurred, since both fall along a continuum of curricular and organizational change. In the GeroRich program, infusion in the foundation courses is conceptualized as the first phase of a long-term change process and achievable within the two years of funding. As GeroRich projects succeed in infusing aging content, they build the framework for long range, more fundamental curricular transformation. Nevertheless, both infusion and transformation are grounded in the process of change, especially for obtaining key stakeholders' buy-in and support.

THE PROCESS OF CHANGE

The GeroRich Program assumes that curriculum change cannot be effected without a labor-intensive planning process that includes attention to the organizational context and that engages key stakeholders (Meredith & Watt, 1994; Watt, 1996; Watt & Meredith, 1995). To lay the groundwork for implementing curricular and organizational changes, the GeroRich projects engaged in an intensive eight-month planning process. Projects were expected to conduct a thorough organizational analysis and "environmental scan," which involved assessing the organization's readiness for change. Project directors were asked to conceptualize guiding principles for the change process and clarify the rationale or why underlying their activities. After completing this macro analysis, change strategies were formulated to address organizational barriers (e.g., time, resources, other curricular demands, accreditation self study, and diverse faculty teaching styles) and to be congruent with the program's organizational culture. Since infused content must fit and flow coherently with the social work program's mission, values, curricular goals and objectives, GeroRich projects conducted individual course analyses; this involved audits of course syllabi, agreed upon by faculty, and focus groups, surveys and/or individual interviews with all key stakeholders. After interpreting and discussing such data, some GeroRich projects involved faculty in articulating and agreeing upon competencies–knowledge, skills, and values essential to working with older adults and their families. Sets of foundation competencies developed by both CSWE SAGE-SW project and advanced competencies developed Practicum Partnership Project through the New York Academy of Medicine were modified by individual projects to be congruent with their own course structure, goals, and objectives. This clarification of competencies is a time consuming, difficult process, but helps to determine "how much infusion is enough," and enhances long-term faculty investment in the outcomes.

The essence of change, however, is mobilizing others and obtaining their commitment to act differently, e.g., to buy in to curricular change. Given this, the remainder of this article describes strategies effectively used by GeroRich projects for mobilizing primary constituencies and building partnerships or teams to bring about change. All GeroRich projects, regardless of their size or extent of constituencies' support, were faced with how to connect with stakeholders' different levels of motivation, and to utilize such differences as a source of strength within their organizational culture.

STRATEGIES FOR ENGAGING FACULTY

Since curriculum is the faculty's domain, they must share in the assumption that gerontological social work content needs to be infused throughout the foundation curricula. An earlier gerontological curricula infusion initiative in Canada, for example, emphasized that sustainable curricular change and the incentives for change must be rooted in the research and education interests of individual faculty responsible for courses (Meredith & Watt, 1994; Watt & Meredith, 1995). The planning process is thus conceptualized as a time to educate and then non-judgmentally and collectively surface multiple needs and interests. Even if faculty are unable to commit to making changes themselves, their buy-in regarding the need for aging-based infusion is essential.

Not surprisingly, faculty generally are resistant to including new content, given their own teaching loads, expertise, a full curriculum and perhaps prior negative experiences with curriculum change initiatives. In fact, a common response is that the curriculum "bucket" is way too full, and already crowded courses cannot absorb any more content (Lubben, Damron-Rodriguez, & Beck, 1992). Identifying and understanding the reasons for resistance, including the pressures on faculty, is a first and critical step to engaging them. Some faculties resist altering broadly written social work program goals and objectives that are perceived as accommodating accreditation guidelines for curriculum breadth. Others think that infusion of content on specific populations, groups, and/or fields of practice create inequities and competitiveness across curricular areas. Resistance, however, is not always active and conscious. As noted by one project director, the laws of physics regarding inertia have corollaries in systemic change processes.

Framing a curriculum change initiative as an open and inclusive faculty process, rather than one required by an outside project, enhances buy-in. Faculty support is more likely to be garnered when asked specifically about what they would like to see occur in the change process. For example, many GeroRich projects surveyed faculty regarding their research interests related to gerontology, their perceptions of potential barriers to curriculum change, and resources they needed to enrich their teaching with gerontological content, if they chose to do so. Others conducted one-on-one or small group interviews with faculty; although time-consuming, such personal contacts are effective in building trust and learning about faculty's gerontological knowledge, degree of comfort in teaching such content, and willingness to modify didactic and experiential class activities and assignments. These personal interactions with faculty also create opportunities to show them evidence of curricular needs based on course audits and student, practitioner and faculty surveys and focus groups. Some GeroRich projects in small social work programs sponsored weekly dialogues with faculty to address their ideas and concerns. Regardless of the specific strategy used, even relatively small amounts of time invested with faculty can lead to their broader engagement with the process.

In these interactions with faculty, project directors tried to connect the need for gerontological learning opportunities to the faculty stakeholders' existing areas of teaching and research interest. Listening openly to faculty's suggestions about possible curricular change, surfaced their own teaching expertise and passions. This process is conceptualized as finding a hook into a faculty's current interest and "hanging" new material onto that hook (Watt, 1996). Listening and responding, without judgment, to faculty's perspectives are more important in the long run than citing data about the need for gerontological social workers. Fostering reciprocity in such interactions–a willingness to learn more about the kinship care challenges facing the child welfare system, for example–and then finding common areas of interest can build bridges across faculty with diverse areas of expertise and engage faculty who heretofore may have been resistant. Although it appears self-evident, basic social work skills of eliciting feedback and then listening to and acting upon such input are essential to effective curriculum and organizational change.

Project directors were creative in developing supports and benefits to faculty willing to "gerontologize" both content and pedagogy. Some GeroRich projects provided resources organized by foundation course content and individualized to faculty members' specific interests and teaching needs. Materials for infusion (e.g., modules, class exercises, assignments) also took account of faculty's diverse teaching styles and needs. Creating curricular resources and then expecting faculty to use them on their own is generally unrealistic, however. Each project assessed whether the best approach was to prepare tailored course materials for faculty adoption or to provide incentives and recognition for faculty to develop their own materials for infusion into their own courses. Regardless, faculty members typically required additional training or development opportunities, often obtained through the CSWE SAGE-SW Faculty Development Institutes. A training the trainers or developmental approach with faculty avoids over-reliance on one or two gerontological "experts" to "take care of aging" by guest lecturing in foundation courses (Kropf, 2002).

Faculty members' developing their own resource typically leads to a greater sense of ownership and reduced reliance on the gerontological faculty as "experts"; however, this approach generally requires an honorarium or workload credit to provide the space and incentive for such course development. Some GeroRich projects provided a modest honorarium (typically $500) as tangible recognition of the extra work involved in this curriculum change. Other projects linked a national or regional gerontological consultant with each faculty member who indicated a willingness to develop content to infuse into his/her course. Regardless of the specific approach to course development, faculty need to be encouraged to talk across and within foundation areas to avoid duplication and repetition of gerontological content and to coordinate assignments, class exercises and use of media. As noted by one GeroRich project director, our infusion goals are not well served if students see the video "Big Mama" in every foundation course!

Regardless of specific strategies, being proactive, modeling how to use resources, consulting with faculty about what is useful to them and then providing feasible learning opportunities and resources that fit faculty's schedules and teaching strengths are basic. In general, personal contact with instructors and assistance with concentrated infusion of materials are more effective than minimal contact and extensive teaching materials without consultation on their potential use. Faculty often become engaged when personal connections are made, such as through sharing stories about caregiving for older relatives, posting photos of their parents or grandparents on the program's GeroRich website, or volunteering with programs that serve older adults. Such personal connections are likely to increase faculty's willingness to make changes in their course content, structure, and teaching methods.

These personal connections were generally coupled with opportunities for professional faculty development, such as travel to national or regional gerontological meetings, support to attend a CSWE SAGE-SW Faculty Development Institute, regional or statewide conferences on aging, or other gerontological training opportunities. Some GeroRich project directors asked faculty to co-present at conferences to connect them professionally with gerontological research and teaching; this approach especially benefited junior faculty faced with promotion and tenure pressures. In addition, expanding faculty research interests to include aging or intergenerational issues helps build sustainability (Watt, 1996).

Timelines need to be realistic. Expecting faculty to infuse content on aging immediately is not feasible, particularly given the pressures of an academic calendar year. Faculty need time: to process their own issues related to aging, learn new course content, and confront preconceived notions that students are not interested in gerontological social work. And few faculty are likely to devote their summer to plan geriatric infusion in their courses. Being realistic and then targeted about what can be accomplished within the nine-month academic calendar can itself generate faculty goodwill toward the effort entailed. In addition, strategically placed initiatives among selected courses may be more effective in the first year of curriculum implementation than attempts to modify all foundation courses too quickly. A targeted selective approach toward a small number of foundation courses appears to be more realistic for large programs with multiple sections and instructors, including adjunct or auxiliary faculty, for foundation courses. Last, thanking and publicly acknowledging faculty (e.g., at faculty meetings, through newsletters, postings on a website) who begin to infuse gerontological social work content also helps generate faculty investment and willingness to sustain implementation. Such appreciation publicly recognizes the bottom line that curricular and organizational change is time consuming and often unrewarded.

STRATEGIES FOR RECRUITING STUDENTS

Even programs with a critical mass of gerontological social work faculty still encounter challenges recruiting students. Only about 10 percent of MSW students select an aging course during their program of study, and less than 5 percent of BSW students express in interest in working with older adults (Damron-Rodriguez & Lubben, 1997; Damron-Rodriguez et al., 1997; Kosberg & Kaufman, 2002; Kropf, 2002; Kropf, Schneider, & Stahlman, 1993). After repeatedly citing the demographics of aging, gerontology faculty may feel that this forecast of the future is falling on deaf ears. Many of the GeroRich projects recognized the importance of first surveying students and then carefully interpreting what they learn to understand the sources of their disinterest in working with older adults. Although really listening to students' views may initially not seem "innovative," a process to ensure that students' suggestions and concerns are valued may be overlooked by busy faculty faced with multiple pressures and time constraints.

Understanding the nature and source of students' resistance to aging is the first step–just as it is with engaging other key stakeholders. Many students, especially those who are younger, often have little contact or life experience with older adults. Even if they have close interactions with grandparents, they may view their relatives as an exception and "not old." Aging is an unknown for most students, which understandably creates anxieties, discomfort, and negative attitudes (Damron-Rodriquez et al., 1997; Cummings, Kropf, & DeWeaver, 2000).

Many students with limited contact have negative stereotypes about older adults–as sick, non-communicative, unable to change, or dying. They also may not be exposed to aging as a field of practice, and may never have considered working with elders. On the other hand, students are unlikely to be interested in careers in aging, no matter how good the job market, if their negative attitudes are not addressed. Sometimes students do not really need more information about gerontological social work career and placement opportunities; rather, it may be more helpful to show them how their interests in other substantive areas, such as mental health, women's issues, or child welfare, intersect with aging. Providing specific examples of practice with older adults in diverse settings may serve to recruit students otherwise unaware of such interconnections.

By taking time to understand the sources of student resistance, strategies responding to both professional and personal concerns can be implemented. Student focus groups and surveys can help identify sources of student disinterest and check out their assumptions about older adults. The open-ended nature of small focus groups tends to yield richer data by probing and better understanding students' negative perceptions than is possible with surveys. Doing so can uncover causes of resistance, such as earlier negative experiences with older family members; feeling too "young" to work effectively with elders; fears of aging or the unknown; or lack of contact with older adults.

Conceptualizing gerontology as pedagogy, most GeroRich project directors recognize the need for innovative teaching approaches that connect with students personally and professionally. Experiential activities best address anxieties, negative attitudes, and lack of experience with older adults. In fact, in some instances, interaction with older adults, when carefully planned and guided by the faculty member, can foster positive attitudes toward older adults (Kane, 1999; Paton, Sar, Barber, & Holland, 2001; Tan, Hawkins, & Ryan, 2001). Foundation practice courses may require students to interview an elder and reflect on their learning in a paper or journal/log. This experience has greatest impact when instructors provide students with guidelines for the interview, suggests focused topics to explore, and address issues of confidentiality. This experience can be framed as a collaborative dialogue with the elder, not an "interview subject." In general, opportunities for students to work with diverse groups of elders, not only frail elders with chronic illness, increase their chances of preparing for practice with older adults.

Some GeroRich projects created simulations of age-related sensory and physical changes. As an example, students put cotton in their ears, Vaseline on eyeglasses, thick gloves on their hands, and then try to open or read the directions on a pill bottle. Dried beans in their shoes simulate the feeling of walking with arthritic feet. A chance to debrief and reflect on such simulations–and their implications for practice–is essential to the quality of students' learning experiences. When students start sharing such positive learning experiences, the "student grapevine percolates" and the organizational culture related to aging starts to change. Some projects, in collaboration with alumni, developed board games on elder care, which can be a fun way to obtain background information about aging and to interest students in the field.

Service learning provides a more focused level of personal interaction with older adults. Most academic institutions now have service learning options, although only recently in social work programs (Dorfman, Murty, Ingram, & Evans, 2002; Kropf & Tracey, 2000). Intergenerational service learning opportunities are growing, which allow students to volunteer with older adults, without the intensive requirements and supervision associated with their practicum. Service learning for credit in the sophomore or junior year is a good way to prepare students for the more intensive required practicum experience. Students who participate in service learning tend to show more positive attitudes toward the members of the group with whom they interact and in some instances, increased interest in a gerontological social work career (Hamon & Way, 2001; Hegeman, 1999; Jarrott, 2001; Weinreich, 2003).

Recruiting students to commit to a field practicum with older adults remains a challenge. Students who hold negative attitudes may mistakenly assume that clinical or therapeutic skills cannot be acquired in work with older adults. Or they may fear that clients will be sick and dying, unwilling to invest time and energy in a relationship with a social work student. Students need to be informed of the possibilities for successful change and the meaning and wisdom of elders' lives, no matter what stage of the life span. Time must be invested in educating students about the clinical and macro level competencies inherent in the diversity and richness of aging-relevant placements. Job-conscious students may be "hooked" by opportunities to acquire highly valued skills and quality supervision in aging-rich placements.

Another way to "hook" students is to involve them in leadership roles. Students included as members of the GeroRich curriculum change team in one social work program became more invested in learning about gerontology. Other GeroRich projects engaged students through their advisory boards, thus ensuring that students' perspectives on the curriculum are heard by board members and exposing students to the wide range of competencies and experiences possible in gerontological social work practice.

Due to limited exposure and interaction, students also may hold negative attitudes toward gerontological social work practitioners. As a way to create opportunities for students to learn more and interact with geriatric social workers, some GeroRich projects programs invited alumni to speak at student brown bags, in classes, and as mentors in order to open up new possibilities for students. Alternatively, photos and brief descriptors of gerontological social work alumni are posted on the GeroRich or program websites and encourage students to contact alumni. In general, gerontological-savvy alums are willing to speak to students in small groups, such as brownbag colloquia, or individually and thus become an accessible link to learning more about gerontological social work.

Although experiential learning hooks students emotionally, other options advance their professional goals. For example, some GeroRich projects fund students to present papers at national gerontological conferences, or provide research assistant or work-study opportunities on aging-relevant research projects. If resistance to aging content is high, requiring students to attend aging-related conferences as a basis for classroom or practicum credit may be helpful. Overall, providing students with a range of diverse learning options congruent with multiple learning styles is more effective than focusing on only one type of activity. As with any field of practice, stipends for field practica are a highly effective recruitment incentive, even for the most resistant students. Incentives do not necessarily need to be financial, however. For example, the status of a Gerontology Fellow who is committed to pursuing a career in aging can convey distinction and reward.

ENGAGING COMMUNITY PRACTITIONERS AND OLDER ADULTS

All social work programs face challenges of how best to involve community practitioners and clients in curriculum change initiatives and the program's organizational life. Faculty members vary in their degree of openness to practitioner's input into a curricular change process when they perceive the curriculum as the faculty's primary domain. Many of the GeroRich projects developed effective partnerships with both practitioners and elders that benefit all involved. Such partnerships are models for future curriculum change efforts in social work education generally.

A strong advisory board can help ensure accountability and continuity in the curriculum change process. In addition, a board's multiple and diverse perspectives tend to result in more effective program implementation than when only one constituency shapes its development. The composition and selection criteria of gerontological social work advisory boards require careful planning. Boards composed of relatively equal numbers of faculty, practitioners, students, and elders are viable, especially when members are able to listen carefully to ensure that that each is heard and respected. It is important, however, that members are involved due to their commitment to social work education, not to satisfy an external requirement of a funded project.

Reciprocity of benefits among advisory board members is essential. Community-based members can explicate what students need to know (HBSE, practice and policy) and identify practicum or service learning sites. Engagement with faculty, students, and the social work program through a well-organized board structure is generally rewarding for practitioners; alumni in particular welcome the opportunity to give back to educational institutions and the profession. Students and faculty benefit from learning about aging issues from the field.

All agencies, both aging- and non-aging-rich sites, have a responsibility to prepare social workers for the realities of our aging society. Unfortunately, some practicum instructors are not knowledgeable about aging or inter-generational issues, and thus are limited in their ability to supervise students in preparation for practice across generations. In such instances, in-service training for practicum instructors is critical, even in settings that do not traditionally define themselves as aging sites (e.g., schools, mental health centers, drug treatment facilities, child welfare). Field instructors can also be proactive in incorporating contact with elders into the students' learning experiences. For example, they can make sure that students in child welfare or school settings learn about the needs of grandparents who are primary caregivers to grandchildren. All GeroRich projects recognize that the number and quality of aging-based sites needs to be expanded beyond traditional settings such as nursing homes or practice with only frail elders. When new aging-rich settings lack social workers with MSWs and two-years practice experience, faculty or retired practitioners who meet these requirements may be able to provide supervision.

Older adults can support the learning goals of class and practicum in myriad ways. It is not just about an elder sharing his or her perspective on aging in a lecture isolated from the rest of the program. Rather, older adults can enrich every aspect of the social work curriculum–as co-instructors, student learners, observers, and mentors. Emeriti faculty is an underutilized resource for students' learning about aging. Ongoing dialogue and interaction with faculty or students are essential to avoid elders feeling used just for interview assignments.

Deans and directors' support is vital to crosscutting these various strategies to ensure an institutional approach conducive to sustainability, but is not in itself sufficient. Coupling institutional support from the top down with the bottom up strategies involving faculty, students, and practicum instructors enhances the probability of a long-term transformative approach, gerontological pervasiveness, and sustainability.

CONCLUSION

This article highlights some of the lessons learned during the three years of planning, implementation and evaluation of the 67 Geriatric Enrichment projects. Extensive data are available regarding what change processes, strategies and actions are most effective in increasing the number of foundation courses with gerontological content; of students exposed to such content; and faculty who "gerontologized" their course structure, content and pedagogy. Findings based on process evaluations to date underscore the importance of attending to an intensive change process that engages all key stakeholders–faculty, students, practitioners, deans/directors, and older adults–to create and sustain aging rich curricular and organizational changes. This process cannot be done hurriedly, or only by a few faculty members. However, the time invested in a thorough organizational analysis or scan, listening to faculty and students' passions along with sources of resistance, finding the "hooks" to engage them in course development and change, building reciprocity into interactions with key stakeholders, and rewarding change lays the groundwork for sustainability and institutionalization. This process model also has implications for how to infuse/transform other areas of social work curricula in way that creates a synergy across substantive areas, rather than past models of fragmentation or competition by populations or fields of practice. Perhaps most vividly, it increases the likelihood that curricular materials developed by CSWE SAGE SW and individual social work programs will not be filed away, but instead be embraced by faculty, students and practitioners who have been engaged in a process of organizational development and curriculum change.

NOTE

1. The terms GeroRich projects and the GeroRich Program are used throughout this article. The GeroRich Program refers to the overall coordinating program based at the University of Washington; the GeroRich projects refers to the projects funded by Hartford in 67 different social work education programs. The GeroRich Program funding ended June 30, 2004. Currently, Professor Hooyman is co-Principal Investigator and Ms. St. Peter is project co-Director for the CSWE National Center for Gerontological Social Work Education.

REFERENCES

Bogolub, E. B. (1998). Infusing content about discharging legal responsibilities into social work practice classes: The example of mandated maltreatment reporting. *Journal of Teaching in Social Work, 17*(1/2), 185-199.

CSWE SAGE-SW. (2001). Strengthening the impact of social work to improve the quality of life for older adults & their families: A blueprint for the new millennium. Alexandria, VA: *Council on Social Work Education.* Retrieved September 26, 2003, from http://www.cswe.org/sage-sw/resrep/blueprint.pdf.

Cummings, S. M., & Galambos, C. (2003). Predictors of graduate social work students' interest in aging-related work. *Journal of Gerontological Social Work, 39*(3), 77-94.

Cummings, S. M., & Kropf, N. P. (2000). An infusion model for including content on elders with chronic illness in the curriculum. *Advances in Social Work, 1*(1), 93-105.

Cummings, S., Kropf, N. P., & DeWeaver, K. (2000). Knowledge of and attitudes toward aging among non-elders: Gender and race differences. *Journal of Women & Aging, 12*(1), 77-91.

Damron-Rodriguez, J., & Lubben, J. (1997). The 1995 WHCoA: An agenda for social work education and training. *Journal of Gerontological Social Work*, 27(3), 65-77.

Damron-Rodriguez, J., Villa, V., Tseng, H. F., & Lubben, J. E. (1997). Demographic and organizational influences on the development of gerontological social work curriculum. *Gerontology & Geriatrics Education, 17*(3), 3-18.

Dorfman, L. T., Murty, S., Ingram, J. G., & Evans, R. J. (2002). Incorporating intergenerational service learning into an introductory gerontology course. *Journal of Gerontological Social Work, 39*(1/2), 219-240.

Gibelman, M., & Schervish, P. H. (1997). *Who are we: A second look.* Washington, DC: NASW Press.

Gleason Wynn, P. E. (1995). Addressing the educational needs of nursing home social workers. *Gerontology & Geriatrics Education, 16*(2), 31-36.

Greene, R. R. (1988). *Continuing education for gerontological careers.* Washington, DC: Council on Social Work Education.

Hamon, R. R., & Way, C. E. (2001). Integrating intergenerational service-learning into the family science curriculum. *Journal of Teaching in Marriage & Family, 1*(3), 65-83.

Hegeman, C. R. (1999, November). *Service learning in elder care.* Paper presented at the Gerontological Society of America Annual Conference, San Francisco, CA.

Jarrott, S. E. (2001). Service-learning at dementia care programs: A social history project. *Journal of Teaching in Marriage & Family, 1*(4), 1-12.

Kane, M. N. (1999). Factors affecting social work student's willingness to work with elders with Alzheimer's disease. *Journal of Social Work Education, 35*(1), 71-85.

Kosberg, J. I., & Kaufman, A. V. (2002, February 15). Gerontological social work: Issues and imperatives for education and practice. *Electronic Journal of Social Work, 1*(1, Article9). Retrieved September 24, 2003, from http://www.ejsw.net/Issue/Vol1/Num1/Article9.pdf.

Kropf, N. P. (1996). Infusing content on older people with developmental disabilities into the curriculum. *Journal of Social Work Education, 32*(2), 215-226.

Kropf, N. P. (2002). Strategies to increase student interest in aging. *Journal of Gerontological Social Work, 39*(1/2), 57-67.

Kropf, N. P., Schneider, R. L., & Stahlman, S. D. (1993). Status of gerontology in baccalaureate social work education. *Educational Gerontology, 19*(7), 623-634.

Kropf, N. P., & Tracey, M. (2000). *Service learning as a transition to foundation field.* Paper presented at the Annual Program Meeting of the Council on Social Work Education, New York, NY.

Lennon, T. (1999). *Statistics on social work education in the United States: 1998.* Alexandria, VA: Council on Social Work Education.

Lubben, J., Damron-Rodriguez, J., & Beck, J. (1992). A national survey of aging curriculum in schools of social work. *Journal of Gerontological Social Work, 11*(3/4), 157-171.

Meredith, S., & Watt, S. (1994). The Gerontology Development Project: Infusing gerontology into social work curriculum. *Gerontology & Geriatrics Education, 15*(2), 91-100.

Olson, C. J. (2002). A curriculum module enhances students' gerontological practice-related knowledge and attitudes. *Journal of Gerontological Social Work, 39*(1/2), 159-175.

Paton, R. N., Sar, B. K., Barber, G. R., & Holland, B. E. (2001). Working with older persons: Student views and experiences. *Educational Gerontology, 27*(2), 169-183.

Peterson, D. A., & Wendt, P. F. (1990). Employment in the field of aging: A survey of professionals in four fields. *The Gerontologist, 30,* 679-684.

Richardson, V. E. (1999). *Teaching gerontological social work: A compendium of model syllabi.* Alexandria, VA: Council on Social Work Education.

Rosebrook, V., Haley, H., & Larkin, E. (2002). Hand-in-hand we're changing the future of education: Introducing the intergenerational approach and promoting the need for trained professionals. Eric Document 463090. Issue: RIESEP2002.

Rosen, A. L., & Zlotnik, J. L. (2001). Demographics and reality: The "disconnect" in social work education. *Journal of Gerontological Social Work, 36*(3/4), 81-97.

Rosen, A. L., Zlotnik, J. L., & Singer, T. (2002). Basic gerontological competence for all social workers: The need to "gerontologize" social work education. *Journal of Gerontological Social Work, 39*(1/2), 25-36.

Scharlach, A., Damron-Rodriguez, J., Robinson, B., & Feldman, R. (2000). Educating social workers for an aging society: A vision for the 21st century. *Journal of Social Work Education, 36*(3), 521-538.

Scharlach, A., Simon, J., & Dal Santo, T. (2002). Who is providing social services to today's older adults? Implications of a survey of aging services personnel. *Journal of Gerontological Social Work, 38*(4), 5-17.

Schneider, R. (Ed.) (1984). *Gerontology in social work education: Faculty development and continuing education.* Alexandria, VA: Council on Social Work Education.

Schneider, R., Decker, T., Freeman, J., & Syran, C. (1984a). *A curriculum concentration in gerontology for graduate social work education.* Washington, DC: Council on Social Work Education.

Schneider, R., Decker, T., Freeman, J., & Syran, C. (1984b). *The integration of gerontology into social work educational curricula.* Washington, DC: Council on Social Work Education.

Schneider, R. L. (2001). A 20 year retro-history of AGE-SW. *AGE-SW Newsletter, Spring 2001.* Retrieved September 26, 2003, from http://www.agesocialwork.org/spring2001feature.html.

Singer, T. (2000). *Structuring education to promote understanding of issues of aging.* Washington, DC: Council on Social Work Education.

Takamura, J. C. (2001). Towards a new era in aging and social work. *Journal of Gerontological Social Work, 36*(3/4), 1-11.

Tan, P. P., Hawkins, M. J., & Ryan, E. (2001). Baccalaureate social work student attitudes toward older adults. *Journal of Baccalaureate Social Work, 6*(2), 45-56.

Watt, S. (1996). *Final report: Gerontology Development Project.* Hamilton, Ontario: McMaster University, School of Social Work.

Watt, S., & Meredith, S. (1995). Integrating gerontology into social work education programs. *Educational Gerontology, 21,* 55-68.

Weinreich, D. M. (2003). Service-learning at the edge of chaos. *Educational Gerontology, 29*(3), 181-195.

doi: 10.1300/J083v48n01_02

Infusing Gerontology Throughout the BSW Curriculum

Judy L. Singleton, MSW, PhD

SUMMARY. How can social work educators ensure that all of their BSW students have the savvy and "know-how" to deal with the needs of our growing aging population? The development of broad-based, innovative gerontological learning opportunities in a BSW program in a small liberal arts and sciences college is presented in this article. Strategies for actively involving community representatives in curriculum changes and participatory learning experiences with students are shared. Ways to incorporate various disciplines in the BSW education are explored in addition to developing intergenerational projects, direct involvement of older persons in the educational process, and ways to unite field practice with theory. doi: 10.1300/J083v48n01_03 *[Article copies available for a fee from The Haworth Document Delivery Service: 1-800-HAWORTH. E-mail address: <docdelivery@haworthpress.com> Website: <http://www.HaworthPress.com> © 2006 by The Haworth Press, Inc. All rights reserved.]*

This project was funded by a Geriatric Enrichment in Social Work Education grant through the Council on Social Work Education, funded by the John A. Hartford Foundation.

The preliminary activities of this project were presented at the First National Gerontological Social Work Conference in conjunction with the 49th Annual Council on Social Work Education Program Meeting, February 27 - March 2, 2003, Atlanta, GA, and at the 29th Annual Meeting of the Association of Gerontology in Higher Education, March 6-9, 2003, St. Petersburg, FL.

[Haworth co-indexing entry note]: "Infusing Gerontology Throughout the BSW Curriculum." Singleton, Judy L. Co-published simultaneously in *Journal of Gerontological Social Work* (The Haworth Press, Inc.) Vol. 48, No. 1/2, 2006, pp. 31-46; and: *Fostering Social Work Gerontology Competence: A Collection of Papers from the First National Gerontological Social Work Conference* (ed: Catherine J. Tompkins, and Anita L. Rosen) The Haworth Press, Inc., 2007, pp. 31-46. Single or multiple copies of this article are available for a fee from The Haworth Document Delivery Service [1-800-HAWORTH, 9:00 a.m. - 5:00 p.m. (EST). E-mail address: docdelivery@haworthpress.com].

KEYWORDS. BSW program, curriculum changes, gerontology, intergenerational, experiential learning

INTRODUCTION

The time for preparing a new generation of baccalaureate social workers (BSWs) to deal with a growing aging population is here. Although older persons (age 65 and over) represent over 12% of the United States population (U.S. Census Bureau, 2000), only about 16% of BSW members of the National Association of Social Workers (NASW) identify social work with this population as their primary practice (Gibelman & Schervish, 1997). Without an increase in the near future, less than 10% of the National Institute of Aging's (NIA) projected need of 40,000 to 50,000 gerontological social workers will be available in the first part of the twenty-first century (O'Neill, 1999). Moreover, BSWs may confront aging issues in all practice settings, not just gerontological sites.

The Geriatric Enrichment in Social Work Education Project is a venture whose goals are to ensure that gerontology pervades all social work students' learning experiences "throughout the curriculum" and to create "sustainable curricula and organizational changes" http://depts.washington.edu/gerorich/hartford/gerorich.shtml. To that end, the project has funded sixty-seven baccalaureate, masters, and joint undergraduate/masters social work programs. The bachelor of social work program at the College of Mount St. Joseph, a small liberal arts and sciences college, was one of the sixty-seven programs initially funded. As a BSW program, the College of Mount St. Joseph provides a generalist framework for students–that is, we provide the students a social work education in which they can apply "an eclectic knowledge base, professional values, and a wide range of skills to target any size system for change" (Kirst-Ashman & Hull, 2001, p. 7).

This article will explain how this small college infused gerontological content throughout all of the courses in its social work curriculum, while also providing a variety of aging-rich learning experiences for students. It will present how we initially assessed our program, and then developed a curriculum transformation approach targeting five specific areas in our social work department. Finally, it will give an assessment of our outcomes thus far, and discuss the implications for social work practice.

BASELINE ASSESSMENT

Prior to implementing any curriculum changes, we assessed our curriculum in a number of ways. Similar to what Watt and Meredith (1995) did in their Gerontology Development Project, we initially reviewed the type and quantity of gerontological content in the social work curricula. In addition to evaluating syllabi, we analyzed class exercises, assignments, and lecture notes within each course. Previous research has indicated that aging content is typically incorporated in the human behavior and social environment, practice, and policy courses, but much less in the research courses or field placement options (Kropf, Schneider, & Stahlman, 1993). Our program was no different. The research sequences and the field practicums were the two major areas with the least aging content.

In addition to specific curricula assessment, we formed a network among faculty, students, field instructors, and community members for developing ideas for curriculum change and obtaining knowledge and skills to implement such changes. We surveyed (1) community professionals in aging as well as those outside of the traditional aging services, such as staff in schools, parenting organizations, etc.; (2) our field placement instructors; (3) our social work program advisory board; and (4) our social work students, including incoming freshmen.

Community professionals provided us with their vision of what aging competencies (knowledge, skills, and professional practice) BSWs most needed, regardless of the work setting. Their responses mirrored the most frequently ranked aging competencies for all social workers found in the national gerontology competencies survey conducted by the Council on Social Work Education's Strengthening Aging and Gerontology Education for Social Work (CSWE SAGE-SW) project (Rosen et al., 2000). The survey's ten most frequently listed aging competencies may be found in the Appendix. Additionally, these community professionals, our social work program advisory board members, and our field placement instructors defined what they believed to be the challenges and opportunities facing social workers who work with older adults. These varied from funding services, to developing more wellness and "productive aging" programs, to working with grandparents raising grandchildren. The question for us, then, was how to incorporate these issues into our BSW curriculum. We also solicited ideas on how to overcome potential student resistance to working with older adults, which yielded numerous possibilities: sponsor guest lecturers who work in an aging setting; provide shared learning experiences between older adults and college students; create placements where aging is not the traditional population (e.g., schools); arrange tours and classes at various community agencies; bring in older adults to guest lecture; and work to decrease the negative stereotypes of older adults.

We found out from these same three groups–the community professionals, advisory board members, and field placement instructors–that they were interested in having a BSW field placement and/or a service-learning placement at their agency.

Furthermore, we learned of ways in which their agencies might use an "aging in social work" website we planned to develop. All three groups suggested topics for the website, including feature stories on consumer-directed care and funding issues; updates on legal issues facing older adults; and agency highlights. We also individually interviewed seven directors from agencies serving older adults to discuss potential classroom exercises and projects.

Last, we surveyed our social work students, including incoming freshmen, to assess their knowledge and stereotypes related to aging and their future career interests. If they did not give aging as a potential social work career choice, we questioned them as to their reasons. Additionally, we inquired of their interest in completing a field placement providing services to an older adult population. Although a few students indicated an interest in working with older adults, most said they had never considered it. They were not necessarily opposed to the idea; it simply was not a career option they had thought about. Many students indicated they had limited contact with older adults. Some students expressed that gerontological social work appeared "depressing," while others said it would be difficult to work with "death" all of the time. These responses support research that says recruiting students to work in the field of aging can be difficult due to these negative attitudes and stereotypes (Damron-Rodriguez et al., 1997).

OUR APPROACH

We wanted students to perceive aging as a continuum, not as some static element in later life, and we wanted our courses to reflect this. Thus, the approach we took to transforming the social work curriculum entailed an intergenerational focus, with an interdisciplinary presentation. To implement this approach, we focused on five specific areas:

- "connecting" the resources readily available on our campus;
- developing intergenerational experiential learning opportunities;
- networking with faculty from different disciplines, students, field instructors, and community members;
- creating a "capstone seminar" to allow social work students to synthesize their learning experiences in aging; and,
- providing research and professional development opportunities for both students and faculty.

"Connecting" the Resources Readily Available on Our Campus

Just prior to receiving the Geriatric Enrichment in Social Work Education Project funding, the College of Mount St. Joseph had adopted a college-wide core liberal arts and sciences curriculum for all majors, including social work. The goal of this new curriculum is for graduates to possess not only the professional skills necessary for success in the workplace, but also qualities that will allow them to thrive in a complicated and diverse world, such as thinking critically and creatively, communicating effectively, appreciating the complexity of human behavior, and understanding the relationship among various ethical systems. Because of this college-wide transformation, we were confident of the potential for an increase in age-enriched learning experiences in our program. As the college was connecting the disciplines already in place, we decided not to frame our curricular transformation on new courses. Instead, we envisioned pulling together various disciplines to provide an undergraduate social work education.

In a liberal arts and sciences college, BSW students learn about aging from many disciplines. Thus, we recruited faculty from, for example, sociology, psychology, and gerontology, to work with social work faculty in this process of infusing age-enriched learning opportunities for BSW students into the overall education. It is from across these disciplines–not just social work courses–that BSWs learn about family dynamics; normal physical, psychological and social changes in later life; values regarding aging, death, and dying; and the diversity of attitudes toward aging. In fact, the BSW education is built upon a liberal arts foundation (CSWE, 2001). For social work educators, it is invaluable to know how to "connect" all of this learning.

The social work program at the College of Mount St. Joseph is part of the Behavioral Sciences Department, which also includes gerontology, sociology, criminology, psychology, recreational therapy, and paralegal studies. Social work majors have required courses from psychology and sociology and may take electives from these other departmental disciplines. Other disciplines outside of this department provide required courses for social work majors as well, such as biology, economics, communications, and math. We decided initially, however, to focus on connecting our Behavioral Science Department's disciplines in an effort to provide a linkage of aging issues throughout these courses.

Although the social work program did not offer any aging-specific courses, we found a wealth of ways in which aging was a part of discussion topics in both social work and non-social work courses in the department. For example, aging was a discussion topic in various social work courses, including introduction to social work, policy, group approaches, and human behavior and the social environment. Required sociology courses for social work majors presented aging issues in the introductory classes, as well as higher-level courses in minority groups and in families. From psychology, a required course for social work majors covered all aspects of the adult lifespan. And, obviously, the gerontology program provided many aging-specific electives available to social work students.

Yet, the social work program was one of "unconnectedness" in its presentation of aging issues. For example, we were lacking the clearly delineated link that connected aging concerns found in field practicums to issues involving older adults in social policy classes, and from there to research, from there to practice courses, and so on. Although we discussed aging issues within these social work and non-social work courses, we had not yet pulled together the "connection" for students to see aging as a continuum.

To deal with this issue of "unconnectedness," we brought the entire Behavioral Sciences Department faculty together for a brainstorming session and, thereafter, several structured meetings to focus on ways to demonstrate to BSW students that aging is a part of these various disciplines. All departmental faculty responded to this effort–that is, to think about, analyze, and review additional ways in which the social work curriculum can offer learning experiences with specific outcomes related to understanding aging. Although this meant that they might have to change teaching methods in their own discipline-specific courses, we were fortunate that we faced little, if any, resistance in this process. However, the team-building relationships were nurtured with one-on-one meetings and the sharing of resource materials–a time-consuming process, but one that was critically beneficial, as faculty engagement and "buy-in" is crucial to keep aging as a topic throughout the course and not just something added at the end of a semester. All faculty have access to the *Teaching Resource Kit,* an extensive collection of resources and tools to help infuse aging content into the social work curriculum (CSWE SAGE-SW, 2002). We give updates and reviews of courses and teaching approaches at monthly social work meetings and quarterly Behavioral Sciences meetings. As a result, collaborative projects have developed among faculty in the Behavioral Sciences Department to create aging-rich learning experiences. Psychology and social work faculty, along with the college's service-learning coordinator, coordinated a mandated service project for Adult Development and Aging, a required course for social work majors. The Corporation for National and Community Service, Learn & Serve Higher Education, funded the project through a grant to The Association for Gerontology in Higher Education in partnership with Generations Together/University of Pittsburgh.

In addition to efforts in the overall Behavioral Sciences Department, the social work faculty met consistently in the first year of this project. In particular, we focused on varying the teaching techniques by creating aging-rich case studies, oral history projects, reflective journaling, simulation learning, games, and use of videos with discussion/debate. We also looked beyond coursework, to find ways to infuse aging content through field placement settings and other educational experiences, such as volunteer work and student association activities.

Developing Intergenerational Experiential Learning Opportunities

To better understand the sometimes abstract concepts and theories presented in coursework, the "real world," or simulations of it, can become the framework by which students can learn social work applications. Some studies have found that students in service-learning activities, for example, are better able to apply concepts beyond the classroom when compared to their non-participating peers (Rocha, 2000). This concept of experiential learning is not new, however. As early as 1902, John Dewey (1938) advocated that thought and action come together in classroom and real-life settings. To bring thought and action together for our students, we focused on intergenerational service-learning opportunities and social work field placements, and the use of various simulations and exercises in class. Role-play scenarios were developed or replicated from the *Teaching Resource Kit* (CSWE SAGE-SW, 2002) to help students learn how to interview and assess older adults with respect to physical and social issues, as well as simulate group work with older adults. *Eldercare: The Game* (Singleton, ©2000) provided an experiential teaching tool for our BSW students to understand the challenges of balancing work and home concerns among employed elder caregivers.

Experiential learning assignments and exercises have been found to reduce the negative stereotypes and attitudes students have toward working with older adults (Haulotte & McNeil, 1998), and we wanted to see if we could accomplish this with our students. As numerous students noted in our initial survey that they had not been around many "old people" and did not know if they would like working with them, we decided to provide opportunities for students to work with an aging population. We would promote interaction between students and older adults and attempt to enhance communication and understanding between them (Kendall & Associates, 1990).

Service-learning is a means of allowing students to volunteer in the community in a project connected with the academic curriculum. The time commitment and skill level is minimal compared to completing a field placement. Our hope was that emphasizing age-enriched service-learning opportunities in the freshman and sophomore years would increase the interest of students to complete a field placement in an aging setting, and even to work in this field after graduation. Thus, in several of our required courses for social work majors, we mandated a service-learning component in agencies serving older adults. For example, in the required Adult Development and Aging course, we implemented a thirty-hour service-learning component in which students serve and work with memory-impaired older adults, completing a variety of tasks. Students could choose one of three sites: an adult daycare center, a continuing care retirement community, or a nursing home for retired nuns.

At the adult daycare center, students worked with both first-grade students and cognitively impaired older adults, helping them learn or review nursery rhymes in a memory-stimulation project for the adults and a memory-development activity for the children. The culmination was a theatrical production of Mother Goose telling nursery rhymes with both the first graders and the adult daycare participants in attendance. The service-learning students dressed as nursery rhyme characters and participated in the production.

At the other two sites, students conducted reminiscence groups with residents of varying cognitive and/or physical abilities, as well as assisted individuals in making "memory boxes"–symbols of who that older adult had been throughout his or her life. Students also helped the retired nuns complete oral histories. The students audiotaped these and had them packaged as a legacy for the nuns to share with family, friends, and the retirement facility. We held guided reflections in class to synthesize what occurred at all three sites, as well as to relate course content and theory with real experiences with older, cognitively impaired adults.

As with any service-learning project at our college, students completed a contract designating their specific learning objectives. The student, professor, agency representative, and college service-learning coordinator all sign this contract before the project begins and when all hours are completed. Service-learning at the College of Mount St. Joseph gives academic credit for student volunteer work in the community, so each student receives one additional college credit, at no tuition charge, for every thirty hours of service performed, up to a total of three college credits. Our social work majors have been able to "test the waters" in work with aging by completing service-learning hours in coordination with an academic course, while at the same time providing mutually beneficial assistance to the community.

The more intense experiential learning for social work students comes in the form of the field placement. Fieldwork education has been considered the most significant part in preparing students to be social work practitioners (Goldstein, 2000). In this pre-professional experience, students serve the community, use course content, and employ their existing skills and expertise to real-life settings while also learning from the designated field instructor (Marullo, 1996). Before initiating this curriculum transformation, we had few field placements in aging services, whether as a primary or a sub-population. Since our initial surveys informed us that we faced a reluctance by our students to work with older adults and since we wanted students to learn about aging across the lifespan, we developed several new, intergenerational, non-traditional aging fieldwork placements, including settings in public schools and various social service agencies, such as protective services for children. Essentially, these placements were our "hooks" to attract students to work with older adults. These settings provided students an opportunity to experience work with multiple generations, such as custodial grandparents for school-age children. In addition, we wanted students to see "outside the box" and apply their generalist skills, as aging competencies may be needed in any setting in the field of social work.

Neither the service learning experience nor the field placement, however, stops with the hours provided by the student. It has been argued that learning does not merely happen through experiences, but through a reflective process as well (Potter, Caffrey, & Plante, 2003). Student reflection may occur in various forms: journals, written assignments, group work, and oral conversations/discussions. Getting feedback from the various parties is an important part of this reflective process. Students receive feedback from those they serve (agencies and clients), their professors, their field instructors, and their peers (Sax & Astin, 1997; Jacoby & Associates, 1996). The students' reflection then encourages them to synthesize their own understandings, think about how their observations, patterns, and behaviors have developed over the course of the experience, and come to new and hopefully better informed conclusions about their experience (Hollis, 2002).

Reflection is a core component in any of our service-learning activities. A group-guided reflection, led by our college's service-learning coordinator, is held for all students in service projects to allow for cross-education among the various service experiences. Thus, our students are able to share and reflect upon their aging experiences with students in completely different settings. We hold an in-class reflection to share individual insights with all class members and to link the experiences to course content. Finally, we have individual journaling to help students reflect on their reactions to the service they have rendered in relationship to their initial learning objectives.

Our fieldwork education also uses reflection extensively as a learning tool. The required field seminar is a venue for students to share experiences in class with peers and the professor and to reflect not only on their work but the activity they see around them in the field setting. A reflective journal is a requirement of the field seminar.

Networking with Faculty from Different Disciplines, Students, Field Instructors, and Community Members

Networking has helped us offer a mixture of age-enriched learning experiences to our students. Developing new or strengthening already-existing ties has allowed us to enlarge the circle of opportunities by offering double majors in social work and gerontology, minors in gerontology, educational programs for our field instructors, and community-based learning projects for students. Furthermore, networking resulted in the development of a Speaker's Bureau and having social work students teach in LifeLearn, a program for mature learners. Networking with paralegal faculty and local senior centers also led to the creation of a legal clinic for lower-income older adults.

Via educational sessions with our academic advisors in social work and gerontology, we established clear delineations of the courses our students would need to take to either double major in social work and gerontology, or minor in gerontology. With careful use of electives, students can accomplish either of these goals without extending their years in school. For social work students not opting to double major or minor in gerontology, we worked with the gerontology program to highlight which courses would complement a student's field placement. For example, social work students in nursing home field placements would benefit from the gerontology-based course, "Clinical Aspects of Long-Term Care Facilities."

As our field instructors are instrumental in providing a well-rounded education to our students, we brought them into this process of providing aging-rich learning experiences. We have developed and presented seminars on gerontological social work at our regular field instructors' meetings, providing continuing education units for attendance. These seminars were based on data obtained from the gerontological social work skills needs assessment of our current and potential field instructors prior to implementing this project's activities.

We also took advantage of our location, which is in a complex containing two long-term care facilities and an adult daycare program. These are sponsored by the Sisters of Charity, as is the College. By having social work faculty become involved in the "Intercampus Committee on Health and Wellness," we integrated the needs of those facilities with learning experiences for our students. For example, social work students in the "Organizational and Community Development" course conducted a needs assessment on wellness programs for the continuing care retirement community. Students also have prepared a community outreach plan for the adult daycare program.

The establishment of our Speaker's Bureau has provided an opportunity for older adults to come to the classroom to discuss various topics related to aging. Our college Alumni Relations office has assisted us in locating older alumni to participate in the Bureau, and we have enrolled other participants by networking with various community-based facilities (e.g., retirement homes and senior centers). The social work program serves as the clearinghouse for the Bureau, which is available to any campus department.

The LifeLearn program, a college-based program for mature learners, has provided another aging-enriched experience for social work students. This program serves older adults, most of whom come from the nearby community or local retirement centers. By networking with Sisters of Charity staff, as well as various departments at the Mount, social work students have been given the opportunity to team-teach LifeLearn courses in word-processing and other computer skills.

Community-based networking has led also to the creation of a Legal Clinic to provide services to low-income older adults. The paralegal faculty, together with the social work faculty, work with local senior centers to provide these services on site. Although the paralegals cannot provide legal advice to the seniors, they can assist directly with some issues, such as completing forms. Referrals are made to local attorneys or to an agency that provides legal services to seniors at a reduced fee. Social work students have been involved in the initial assessment of the older adults for services and assisting them with any other referrals that could be useful.

Creating a "Capstone Seminar" to Allow Social Work Students to Synthesize Their Learning Experiences in Aging

In conjunction with the senior field seminar, we created a capstone seminar to help students synthesize the aging-enriched learning experiences during their years in the BSW program. This three-hour seminar provides an avenue for students to discuss and integrate aging experiences throughout their coursework (not just social work classes), field placements, and other related activities. In combination with our field seminar, this capstone experience allows us to assess the level of aging knowledge and skills students have developed over the course of their education.

Providing Research and Professional Development Opportunities for Both Students and Faculty

Although aging content now has been infused into our research classes for social work students, we wanted to offer research activities for students beyond the class assignments. Therefore, we have promoted independent studies involving aging research. In some local non-profit organizations serving older adults, for example, students assisted staff in assessing needs, then researched funding sources and wrote grant proposals to help meet those needs.

Additionally, students have been encouraged to present their work at local and state conferences. At the 2003 annual meeting of the Ohio Association for Gerontology Education, one student presented her research on "poverty and the elderly," another student presented her qualitative study on "foster grand-parents," and another student presented her applied research study on the most effective methods of establishing an elementary-school-based group for grandparents raising grandchildren.

Professional development activities were critical also for the faculty. Only one social work faculty member, the project director for the Hartford grant, had worked primarily in aging settings. The other faculty were supportive of the project but had very limited backgrounds in aging issues. To facilitate learning and commitment to this curriculum transformation, the faculty collaboratively prepared and presented the work developed from this grant project at several national conferences, including the 2002 Gerontological Society of America annual meeting, the First National Gerontological Social Work Conference held in conjunction with the 2003 CSWE Annual Program Meeting, and the 2003 state meeting of the Association for Gerontology in Higher Education. The faculty also made a state presentation at the 2003 annual conference of the Ohio Chapter of the National Association of Social Workers. Developing the presentations collaboratively was helpful, but the attendance at the conferences further provided enrichment, as other faculty were able to learn more about aging issues.

IMPLICATIONS FOR SOCIAL WORK PRACTICE

Social work with older adults involves issues that everyone must one day encounter, whether they want to or not. Although social workers may not personally be affected by some social problems (e.g., substance abuse, domestic violence, etc.), none can escape "the experience of aging and death for themselves and their families" (McInnis-Dittrich, 2002, p. 17). As educators, we are challenged to equip our BSW students to have the competencies to confront whatever situations they may face with an aging population.

With an increasing number of older adults in our society, social workers will be working more frequently with this population and their families. Studies predict that more professionals and paraprofessionals will be needed to assist family members in caring for older adults than in the past (Administration on Aging, 2001). Although a large network of long-term care and community services has developed, most eldercare is still provided by family members (Administration on Aging, 2000). Yet the caregiving may be cross-generational as well. In 1997, 3.9 million children under the age of eighteen were living in homes maintained by grandparents (Bryson & Casper, 1999). Social workers may be called upon more often to help the families of older adults as well as to help older adults remain productive, particularly in a society in which ageism (the one universal "ism") is profound. Social workers are needed to advocate for changes in public policy.

Research has indicated that little or no gerontology content has been infused in most BSW programs (Scharlach et al., 2000). In this Geriatric Enrichment in Social Work Education project, we attempted to revise our curriculum so that aging content permeated the courses and overall learning experiences. As a generalist program, our objective was not to have students specialize in aging studies, but rather to make certain that no social work major would graduate without a solid foundation in aging competencies. Thus, he or she would be equipped to work with aging issues at the BSW level, regardless of the employment setting. As said by Anita Rosen, former Director of Special Projects/Special Assistant to the Executive Director at the Council on Social Work Education, "The goal isn't to make every social worker or social work educator a gerontology expert, but to ensure that all social work graduates have basic knowledge and skills to deal with older people" (O'Neill, 2003).

Our goal was to have students be able to relate classroom knowledge to the field, that is, social work practice. By using student-centered, small group-based approaches in foundation courses, we pursued student engagement in learning. Basic aging knowledge was critical, but we also wanted students to leave the classroom with skills they could apply in their social work practice. Our experiential learning methods, with their emphasis on learning by doing—that is, role-plays, simulations and games, service-learning, and field placements—were means to develop these skills.

The reflective process of this experiential learning is critical to understanding social work practice. What is this experience the student has had, and what meaning did it have for him or her? Our goal not only was to provide content to the students, but also to furnish learning opportunities to help them create their own knowledge and understanding (Baskind, 2000).

In transforming the curriculum to infuse aging content and learning experiences, we considered various learning styles, including learning individually, in group situations, visually, and by auditory means (Grasha, 1996). We emphasized these different methods in order to help students model these techniques with clients, as clients learn in different fashions also.

Were we successful in transforming our curriculum? In terms of aging knowledge and attitudes toward older adults, students performed considerably better on post-tests of "What is Your Aging I.Q.?" (CSWE, 2002) and of the Age Group Evaluation and Description (AGED) Inventory (Knox, Gekoski, & Kelly, 1995) at the beginning of year three of this project, as compared to the pre-tests given earlier. Student interest in working with older adults has increased dramatically, as our number of requested field placements in aging settings has quadrupled in the past year. Faculty are maintaining these new objectives in their courses, class assignments, and exercises. Thus, we no longer add aging content as an afterthought at the end of a semester. The social work faculty, other departmental faculty, and the college administration support these efforts. The work is being sustained and shows no indication of going by the wayside.

Only when the future social workers enter the job market and tackle assorted job responsibilities will we know for sure that the competencies have transferred from education to practice. However, to the extent that aging issues are no longer delimited in professional social work education, the knowledge base and ability to work with older adult concerns in any setting will be enhanced.

REFERENCES

Administration on Aging. (2001, May). Family caregivers: 2001. Available: *http://www.aoa.gov/factsheets/family-caregiving.html.*

Administration on Aging. (2000, April 9). A profile of older Americans: 2000. Available: *http://www.aoa.gov/aoa/STATS/statpage.html.*

Baskind, F. (2000). Is foundation content an archaic educational construct? No! *Journal of Social Work Education, 36*(1), 16-22.

Bryson, K., & Casper, L. (1999). Co-resident grandparents and grandchildren. U.S. Department of Commerce, Economics and Statistics Administration, Current Population Reports.

Council on Social Work Education Strengthening Aging and Gerontology Education for Social Work, Faculty Development Institute, Teaching Resource Kit. (2002). Alexandria, VA: Author.

Council on Social Work Education. (2001). *Handbook of Accreditation Standards and Procedures.* Alexandria, VA: Author.

Damron-Rodriquez, J., Villa, V., Tseng, H. F., & Lubben, J. E. (1997). Demographic and organizational influences on the development of gerontological social work curriculum. *Gerontology & Geriatrics Education, 17*(3), 3-18.

Dewey, J. (1938). *Experience and Education.* New York: Collier Books.

Gibelman, M., & Schervish, P. (1997). *Who we are: A second look.* Washington, DC: NASW Press.

Goldstein, H. (2000). Social work at the millennium. *Families in Society, 81*(1), 3-10.

Grasha, T. (1996). *Teaching with style: A practical guide for enhancing learning by understanding teaching and learning styles.* Pittsburgh, PA: Alliance Publishers.

Hartford Geriatric Enrichment in Social Work Education. (2002). Geriatric Enrichment Program. Posted to http://depts.washington.edu/gerorich/hartford/gerorich.shtml.

Haulotte, S., & McNeil, J. (1998). Integrating didactic and experiential aging curricula. *Journal of Gerontological Social Work, 30*(3/4), 43-57.

Hollis, S. (2002). Capturing the experience: Transforming community service into service learning. *Teaching Sociology, 30*, 200-213.

Jacoby, B. & Associates. (1996). *Service learning in higher education: Concepts and practices.* San Francisco, CA: Jossey-Bass.

Kendall, J. C., & Associates. (1990). Principles of Good Practice. In *Combining service and learning: A resource book for community and public service.* Volume 1 (pp. 37-55). Raleigh, NC: National Society for Internships and Experiential Education.

Kirst-Ashman, K. K., & Hull, Jr., G. H. (2001). *Generalist practice with organizations and communities.* United States: Wadsworth.

Knox, V. J., Gekoski, W. L., & Kelly, L. E. (1995). The age group evaluation and description (AGED) inventory: A new instrument for assessing stereotypes of and attitudes toward age groups. *International Journal of Aging and Human Development, 40*(1), 31-55.

Kropf, N. P., Schneider, R. L., & Stahlman, S. D. (1993). The status of gerontology in baccalaureate social work education. *Educational Gerontology, 19*, 623-634.

Marullo, S. (1996). The service learning movement in higher education: An academic response to troubled times. *Sociological Imagination, 33*, 117-137.

McInnis-Dittrich, K. (2002). *Social work with elders: A biopsychosocial approach to assessment and intervention.* Boston, MA: Allyn and Bacon.

O'Neill, J. (2003, April). Educators Focus on Aging. Available: http://www.social workers.org/pubs/news/2003/04/educators.asp.

O'Neill, J. (1999, February). Aging express: Can social work keep up? *NASW News, 44*(2), 3.

Potter, S., Caffrey, E., & Plante, E. (2003). Integrating service learning into the research methods course. *Teaching Sociology, 31*, 38-48.

Rocha, C. J. (2000). Evaluating experiential teaching methods in a policy practice course: The case for service learning to increase political participation. *Journal of Social Work Education, 36*(1), 53-61.

Rosen, A. L., Zlotnik, J. L., Curl, A. L., & Green, R. G. (2000, November). CSWE SAGE-SW National Aging Competencies Survey Report. Survey posted to *http://www.cswe.org/sage-sw/resrep/competenciesrep.htm.*

Sax, L. J., & Astin, A. (1997). The benefits of service evidence from undergraduates. *Educational Record,* Summer/Fall, 25-32.

Scharlach, A., Damron-Rodriquez, J., Robinson, B., & Feldman, R. (2000). Educating social workers for an aging society: A vision for the 21st century. *Journal of Social Work Education, 36*(3), 521-538.

Singleton, J. (2000). *Eldercare: The Game.* Cincinnati, OH: Author.

U.S. Census Bureau (2000). Demographic Profiles. "Table DP-1. Profile of General Demographic Characteristics: 2000." Available: http://censtats.census.gov/data/US/01000.pdf.

Watt, S., & Meredith, S. (1995). Integrating gerontology into social work education programs. *Educational Gerontology, 21*(1), 55-68.

doi: 10.1300/J083v48n01_03

APPENDIX

Top Ten List of Aging Competencies for All Social Workers

Assess one's own values and biases regarding aging, death and dying.

Educate self to dispel the major myths about aging.

Accept, respect, and recognize the right and need of older adults to make their own choices and decisions about their lives within the context of the law and safety concerns.

Normal physical, psychological and social changes in later life.

Respect and address cultural, spiritual, and ethnic needs and beliefs of older adults and family members.

The diversity of attitudes toward aging, mental illness and family roles.

Use social work case management skills (such as brokering, advocacy, monitoring, and discharge planning) to link elders and their families to resources and services.

The influence of aging on family dynamics.

Identify ethical and professional boundary issues that commonly arise in work with older adults and their caregivers, such as client self-determination, end-of-life decisions, family conflicts, and guardianship.

Gather information regarding social history such as: social functioning, primary and secondary social supports, social activity level, social skills, financial status, cultural background and social involvement.

Source: Rosen, A. L., Zlotnik, J. L., Curl, A. L., & Green, R. G. (2000, November). CSWE SAGE-SW National Aging Competencies Survey Report. Available at: http://www.cswe.org/sage-sw/resrep/competenciesrep.htm.

Strengthening Aging Content in the Baccalaureate Social Work Curricula: What Students Have to Say

Cheryl E. Waites, EdD, MSW, ACSW
E. Othelia Lee, PhD, MSW

SUMMARY. Encouraging student's interest and preparing them for social work practice with older adults is increasingly important in view of the demographic changes that are taking place. This article describes a study that engages BSW students in a discussion of best models for promoting gerontological social work curriculum infusion. Using two focus groups, the authors explore barriers to student interest and potential strategies to recruit students for gerontological social work. Fear of their own decline and mortality, lack of exposure to older adults and aging issues emerge as the primary reasons for aversion to working with older adults. Strategies

---

The authors would like to thank the students who participated in the focus groups and the two research assistants, Becky Hornby and Natalya Rice, for their work in organizing the group meetings and transcribing the tapes.

This study was funded by the Hartford Geriatric Enrichment in Social Work Education Initiative.

An earlier version of this paper was presented at the Baccalaureate Program Directors 20th Annual Meeting, October 23-27, Pittsburgh PA and the First National Gerontological Social Work Conference, Atlanta, GA, February 28-March 2.

[Haworth co-indexing entry note]: "Strengthening Aging Content in the Baccalaureate Social Work Curricula: What Students Have to Say." Waites, Cheryl E., and E. Othelia Lee. Co-published simultaneously in *Journal of Gerontological Social Work* (The Haworth Press, Inc.) Vol. 48, No. 1/2, 2006, pp. 47-62; and: *Fostering Social Work Gerontology Competence: A Collection of Papers from the First National Gerontological Social Work Conference* (ed: Catherine J. Tompkins, and Anita L. Rosen) The Haworth Press, Inc., 2007, pp. 47-62. Single or multiple copies of this article are available for a fee from The Haworth Document Delivery Service [1-800-HAWORTH, 9:00 a.m. - 5:00 p.m. (EST). E-mail address: docdelivery@haworthpress.com].

47

to promote student interest, organize curricula, and create an inclusive learning context are discussed. doi:10.1300/J083v48n01_04 *[Article copies available for a fee from The Haworth Document Delivery Service: 1-800-HAWORTH. E-mail address: <docdelivery@haworthpress.com> Website: <http://www.HaworthPress.com> © 2006 by The Haworth Press, Inc. All rights reserved.]*

KEYWORDS. Aging, intergenerational, curricula infusion, Baccalaureate Social Work, social work education

We are in the midst of a dramatic shift in the age distribution: the older adult population is expected to increase. By 2030 more than 20% of Americans will be age 65 or older. This change in demographics will result in greater numbers of persons requiring health care, housing, nutrition, caregiving, intergenerational programs, retirement communities and other services. Over the next few decades all social workers can look forward to working with older clients and their families (Kropf, 2002). In view of this change, social work educators must diligently work to prepare future practitioners to serve the needs of older adults.

The National Institute on Aging (NIA) reports that 60,000 to 70,000 trained full-time social workers are required by 2020 to provide services, advance policy and administer programs for this rapidly growing aging population (NIA, 1987; Nelson, 1988). We can anticipate a rapid job growth for gerontological social workers (Scharlach, Damron-Rodriguez, Robinson, & Feldman, 2000). To adequately meet the rising demand, social work education must increase the number of students receiving specialized training in gerontological social work. This presents a dilemma because students have been reluctant to consider gerontological social work careers, and to develop basic gerontological competency (Rosen, 2002). In addition, there are often insufficient programs and resources to provide specialized learning opportunities. As a result, there is a shortage of practitioners, including BSW generalists, who are prepared for social work practice with older adults. Social work programs are not currently producing the estimated numbers of social workers needed to serve this population (Scharlach et al., 2000).

The BSW curriculum prepares students for generalist practice and graduates are often on the frontlines of service delivery, working with a variety of client populations including older adults. At the very minimum, BSW students need basic competency in the bio-psycho-social aspects of aging, and issues related to family caregiving, grandparents raising grandchildren, and social policy that impacts the aging population. There is a need for BSWs to have some competency in the field of aging yet most do not express interest and have very limited preparation.

Many challenges to increasing students' interest in working with older adults have been identified. Among these difficulties are student reluctance due to lack of exposure to or experience with healthy older adults (Scharlach, 2002) as well as a lack of knowledge and preparation (Cummings, Galambos, & DeCoster, 2003; Greene, 1990; Olson, 2002). Negative attitudes and stereo-types about aging present the most difficult barrier to recruiting students to work with older adults. Tan (2001) investigated the attitudes of baccalaureate social work students toward working with older women and men. Data obtained from 204 students indicate that the majority of students did not take any gerontology classes and were not interested in working with older adults. Overall, student attitudes were neutral but more negative toward the older age categories 75 and above.

In view of the demographic changes that will take place over the next 30 years, the reluctance toward careers in gerontological social work is problematic. The question is how do we inspire and encourage students' interest in gerontological social work and help them develop the necessary competencies. To direct our efforts we turned to students for insight. This paper examines feedback from two focus groups conducted with BSW students. We explored students' interest in developing basic gerontological competencies and pursuing careers in gerontological social work. Students' feedback on how to energize, motivate and recruit students to gerontological social work, and how to infuse gerontological and intergenerational content in the Baccalaureate curricula so that all students will have the basic competencies are discussed.

METHODS

Background

The department of social work is located in a large university in North Carolina and has 120 social work majors. The program was selected to participate in the Hartford Geriatric Enrichment in Social Work Education Initiative (GeroRich Initiative) and has focused on transforming the social work program by infusing aging and intergenerational practice content across the social work curricula. In addition, department faculty were involved in two other major initiatives: child welfare education for students and a family-centered practices training for Social Service practitioners. All three projects encourage intergenerational perspectives on social work practice and, thus, worked together to generate a hospitable environment for the GeroRich initiative.

Prior to the GeroRich Initiative, most students were not actively engaged in pursuing interests in gerontological social work. A course on aging had not been successfully offered in over ten years. The course offered the previous year failed to attract sufficient enrollment. Although several aging field sites were available in nursing homes and day-treatment facilities, most students were not interested in these placements. Those who entered these practicum had limited gerontological preparation. For the most part, students demonstrated little enthusiasm or preparation for social work practice with older adults. It was evident that there was a need to identify strategies to engage students in pursuing careers in gerontological social work and to prepare them for practice with older adults and their families.

The two focus groups were conducted within the first year of the three-year GeroRich Initiative. A special topics course, "Social Work and Aging," was offered during the project's first semester. Aging and intergenerational content, sensitivity exercises, guest speakers and field trips were immediately infused in the introductory, human behavior and practice courses. The focus groups provided a mechanism to obtain information from students who were benefiting from the early infusing efforts. They also informed the planning and implementation processes.

Participants

The first focus group was conducted in April, 2002 in the Social Work and Aging course. The students (n = 16) registered for this course and were about to complete the semester-long course in three weeks. While there is no prerequisite for this particular course, all students who registered for the course were in their junior or senior years. Among them, eleven participants were social work majors, and one was a social work minor. Other majors represented in class included Psychology (n = 1), Communication (n = 1), Criminology (n = 1), and Spanish (n = 1). In terms of their age, most students were in their early twenties. Three students were non-traditional, making a career transition in their middle adulthood.

For the second focus group, we targeted students in their junior year who were social work majors with limited exposure to gerontological social work. Invitations to participate were extended in junior level courses. Out of approximately 40 students who were juniors, only six students volunteered to participate, reflecting a low level of interest in this subject matter.

Questions and Formats for the Focus Group

As faculty members the authors facilitated the focus groups. Careful attention was given to creating a safe environment in which students could express their views. At the beginning of each session, the facilitators addressed the purpose and expectations for the focus group. Participants were asked to read and sign the consents to audiotape the session. Issues of confidentiality were discussed. Students were informed that they could withdraw from participating in the focus group at any time during the discussion. Although the facilitators were actively infusing aging content in selected courses they had no teaching responsibilities for the aging course.

The entire focus group contents were recorded. The tapes were stored in a secure location and then given to the research assistant who then transcribed the tapes. Participant names were not included in the transcription, analysis and reports. The following six questions were discussed during each focus group session: (1) What, if anything, sparked your interest in working with older adults? Are there barriers to you working with older adults? (2) What gerontological social work knowledge and skills are covered in the current BSW curricula? What are the program's strengths in this area? (3) What gerontological social work knowledge and skills should be covered? What are the best methods to cover this content? (4) Are there any gaps between the gerontological social work knowledge and skills that the current BSW curricula covers and those you believe are necessary for more effective social work practice with older adults? If so, how can we address this? (5) Any recommendations for strengthening gerontological content in the BSW curricula? (6) Any suggestion for how to get more students interested in social work practice with older adults as an area of practice?

RESULTS

This section presents student comments for both sessions and is organized around the focus group questions. Six areas are addressed: interest in gerontological social work, barriers to gerontological social work, aging content in the social work curricula, major challenges and gaps in gerontological social work education, the efficacy of the special topics course on aging, and effective teaching strategies for baccalaureate social work education. A summary of suggestions to strengthen aging and intergenerational content in the baccalaureate curricula is also discussed.

Interest in Gerontological Social Work

Overall, the cohort of students in the first focus group–those taking the aging course–reported a stronger interest in aging, as compared to the respondents in the second group. Some students cited their prior experience working with older adults as a strong motivating factor for pursuing a career in geronto-logical social work. One student commented:

> I have been interested in working with the elderly since I was in high school and worked in a nursing home. For the last several years I have been volunteering with hospice and I'm just real comfortable there....

The majority of respondents in both focus groups mentioned that geronto-logical social work was not their initial interest but they wanted to expand their competency beyond the area of children and families.

> I have done a lot of work with children and I want to work with children but I figured I might get tired of that one day so I need to learn about other groups as well and I found this interesting.

While the majority of the participants were in their early twenties and had not assumed significant caregiving roles, anticipating these roles in the future motivated them to develop competency for working with aging families. A student commented:

> My grandparents are getting up into their eighties; my parents are getting into their sixties and fifties. So I know it is something I am going to have to be dealing with ... even if I don't get into this field.

The following student related her personal interest to professional opportu-nities.

> My interest is sort of sparked by just people in my family that are older adults and their needs and I am looking at the sort of population explo-sion that is going to happen and it's a practical thing to look at what opportunities are out there in the field right now. Because it is going to be a big area.

Another stated:

> I want to really focus on families and within families they have old aging parents and so I think it is in my best interest to become at least some-what knowledgeable of them.

The following respondent also recognized intergenerational issues within aging families.

> When I was little while my mom worked, my great grandmother and grandmother took care of me. And so I grew up around my great grand-mother who was in her seventies ... she was placed in a nursing home

and stayed there for nine years and so I went through it with my family like the things that families go through when they have to reach decisions about placement. That definitely sparked my interest to work with families ... the whole family and in just making decisions in the later part of people's lives.

Another participant cited that the positive experiences she has shared with her grandparents motivated her to "help older people enjoy the last parts of their lives." Intergenerational relationships and issues emerged as a consistent theme. Most focus group participants seemed to also be aware of the changing demographics and the need for gerontological social workers. However, they were somewhat unsure about pursuing careers in the area of aging.

Barriers to Gerontological Social Work

Participants articulated their perceived barriers to working with older adults–that is what stands in the way of student interest. A troublesome aspect of working with this population for younger social workers was facing their own physical decline and mortality. They expressed feeling apprehensive and fearful of their own aging process.

... maybe fear of [is a barrier] I mean because you need to understand their disorders, for example, Alzheimer's. They may do and say some pretty off the wall stuff that might kind of scare you.

The following respondent confessed her own discomfort regarding dealing with death and dying.

... people our age, or really any age, dealing with death so much [is a barrier] and when you're dealing with aging you're going to see a lot more. That can be a hard thing for people to deal with especially if it is all coming at once.

Participants noted societal myths and negative stereotypes attached to older adults as a major barrier. For instance, older adults have been portrayed in the mass media in the extremes–as either frail or remarkably healthy.

Well, in class we covered advertisements and things. They tend to show, well, they don't show elderly in the media ... and when they do they portray them as dying ... old people can't drive, and it's little things like that. There is nothing you can say it's just the way it's always been. Or oftentimes [they are] extremely active. There is nothing in between.

A respondent mentioned lack of respect toward older people.

> I've seen that people working with the elderly tend to treat the elderly like children.

According to participants, the age difference between young social workers and older adults is often intimidating and creates some discomfort.

> Someone just out of school, you're trying to help ... you go to someone's house ... you're there as their social worker. I think a lot of times people think you're so young and you might feel that on the other end. You know here is this person ... who has lived three times longer than I have, they know what's going on. So, credibility can maybe be an issue, with an age difference.

Students also commented that working with older adults requires patience.

> Learning new things takes a long time. Sometimes even just understanding what they're saying it requires a lot of patience to work with this group. I think some people run short of it [patience] and just gets frustrated and then both sides get frustrated ... and it doesn't work out too well.

The focus group participants indicted some discomfort with older adults and fears concerning their own aging. Issues related to respect, and concern about how they are perceived in the social work role by adults who were much older then themselves were also concerns. In spite of these barriers, the focus group participants indicated that they wanted to be prepared for effective social work practice with this population.

Aging Content in Current Social Work Curricula

Students reported that aging content was rarely mentioned and seldom promoted as a significant area for practice in the social work curricula (prior to the GeroRich Initiative).

> In my classes we have discussed it ... the professor asks who is interested in working with that population and one person might raise their hand ... No one seems interested in learning about it. ... So we spend ten minutes on it, but people want to talk about other things in the field. And so it's [gerontological social work] not viewed as important to cover as other areas.

The early impact of the GeroRich project was evident in the focus group participants' comments. As noted previously, the initiative had begun prior to the focus group sessions. Participants mentioned how some content was covered in the current curricula.

> In our human behavior class we had three elderly women who came in and talked with us. I think the whole class really liked it.

Challenges and Gaps in Gerontological Social Work Education

The most frequently cited challenge for students in pursuing gerontological social work was overcoming their fear of providing services to older adults due to an earlier negative experience or limited exposure or interaction.

> I went to a nursing home when I was younger and it scared me. I saw this woman screaming because she didn't have a bedpan. That's why I was hesitant in going to the assisted living facility [field trip]. But after I did it I wasn't scared anymore.

Though students indicated that taking the course on aging provided new insights they continued to view aging as a sequence of decline. A focus group participant from the aging course states:

> I'm still young and I come out of the class not looking forward to getting older at all. I think the reason is because we focus more on the diseases that come with aging, more so than the good things. Wish we could cover more of that.

Participants advocated for acquiring more specialized competencies in gerontological social work in such areas as: (1) bio-psycho-social assessments, (2) pharmacology and medical terminology, (3) functioning on a multidisciplinary teams, and (4) health promotion.
Students recognized the need to acquire experience and appropriate skills.

> I guess it's one thing to talk about some of the disorders that the elderly have, and it's another to see it, and learn how to actually deal with someone that has Alzheimer's ...

Students also spoke about their need to learn how to set boundaries in working with older adults. A participant who is working at a retirement center shared her emotional involvement:

> The hardest thing for me is trying to not get too personal. I get too involved and it's my weakness. Because a lot of elderly people don't have other relatives they become a part of my family. And it sometimes stresses me out more because I want to do what I can't.

Participants identified lack of coverage in all courses as well as a focus on physical decline, illness and little information on how to navigate professional boundaries as significant gaps in the curricula. They called for specialized coursework including an aging course and curricula that has an intergenerational, strengths based approach and covers a full spectrum of aging and family issues.

Efficacy of the Special Topics Course on Aging

Most students in the first focus group report favorably about their current aging course. The one semester course on aging was helping them to (1) become less skeptical and apprehensive about gerontological social work, (2) enhance their understanding of key issues in aging, and (3) increase their competency in working with older adults and their families. Most respondents agreed that the course also helped to decrease negative stereotypes of aging. This student seems to appreciate gaining a balanced perspective.

> I think one plus of this class has been that … we focus mainly on the elderly and the aging process but you know we've also brought in depression and some disorders that elderly people get, but so do younger people.

One of two male students in both focus groups commented that he learned more about the variety of career options in gerontological social work.

> When it came to working with older adults I thought of working in a nursing home … that's all I knew before I took this class. So this opened up what other jobs were out there.

Offering an aging course in the BSW curricula affords students an opportunity to learn about gerontology as a field of practice and enhances their knowledge and skills for generalist practice.

Effective Teaching Strategies for Baccalaureate Social Work Education

Most students spoke highly about the efficacy of incorporating experiential components into the learning process. Particularly, they cited the positive impact of simulation exercises and field trips that connected people across generations.

I found it to be less depressing when I actually went out and saw the people, than just reading about stuff in the textbook. I also liked the day we had to walk around with glasses on, with the corn in our shoes and all that stuff. I mean as dumb as I felt walking down the street talking like that it puts it into perspective. That's the kind of stuff that you remember, and those are two things in this class that are going to stick for me.

Learning by doing was a critical component that encouraged students to extend their empathy.

When we were putting the different glasses on, different kinds of diseases, and the gloves on for arthritis that's just like when people talk about arthritis you never think about how bad it actually is, or any type of eye disease you don't know how bad it actually is. When you sit there and you can't pick up anything, can't do anything especially the sewing … you can't do any of it. It's very aggravating … you can kind of relate better when you're actually doing it.

Most students reported after taking the course on aging their fears decreased.

We visited a bunch of assisted living facilities and I found that to be less depressing because the people there seemed to be pretty happy. If I were getting to around sixty I would be looking forward to moving in there. It looked like a nice place. Good community.

Participants asserted their need to encounter older adults in a variety of settings. They discussed field trips to a local senior center, and a retirement community.

I also found that the residents of the places we visited seemed to be really excited to see us they always were 'oh where do you go to school' … it obviously was a two-way street. We learned all about what they do and they just seemed to be so happy to be visited by people.

The following respondent also emphasized the importance of having continued and gradual exposure (exposure over time) to the older adult population.

I think it would be a really good idea to have an assignment to go visit somebody in assisted living or a nursing home or something and just visit with them maybe three or four times, just to see how they are doing and get to know them.

Such gradual exposure can help students assess and integrate all aspects of aging.

> When I was younger I had a great-grandmother that was in a nursing home and we would go see her every week ... sometimes it would be a bad experience, but then sometimes it would be good. So I never was scared of it because I went often, saw the good and bad. In our field trip, we ended up seeing all the people when they were really happy, but we could have gone on a bad day and seen them very upset and then it would have affected us the wrong way. So it might be better if people went and saw it over a period of time or saw the same place a couple of times.

Another student appreciated the safety she felt in sharing these experiences collectively with her classmates.

> We went through the Alzheimer's unit and I found it really interesting to observe, but it would have been a lot harder if I weren't surrounded by a lot of people that I knew. If I went there to volunteer and my first day I got put in there to help somebody out I just would have been so lost and so freaked out. I mean I think that the field trips are a good way of introducing you to the field without just throwing you right into the fire and scaring you into not wanting to go back. I feel like now I could handle it, I could go back in there by myself, and be fine.

Also respondents emphasized the importance of having early exposure in the introductory social work course.

Strengthening Gerontological Content in the Baccalaureate Curricula

One of the major goals in our GeroRich Initiative is to infuse aging and intergenerational content across the curricula, but especially the core courses: social work practice, human behavior, social welfare history, social policy, field work, child welfare, legal aspects, and multicultural social work courses. Students provided several suggestions. First they recommended that a stimulating guest speaker present a gerontological social work topic in the introductory course. In the human behavior and practice classes students recommended visits to assisted living facilities and senior centers and suggested that students conduct a bio-psycho-social assessment. In social work practice, child welfare, and school social work courses intergenerational issues such as grandparents raising grandchildren, interviewing techniques and effective communication skills with older adults were proposed as important topics to study. For our policy and legal aspects courses, covering living wills, guardianships, decision-making processes with regard to nursing homes, Medicare, social security and the Older Americans Act were identified as pertinent. Students also emphasized their need for more information on assessing older adults, understanding medical diagnoses, and working with multidisciplinary teams. Advocacy for the respect for the dignity and worth of older adults was also indicated as a relevant topic for most courses but especially the multicultural (diversity or oppression) course. In addition, students encouraged volunteer work in aging-rich agencies–agencies that provided some services to older adults.

Respondents in the first focus group strongly advocated for establishing a permanent course on aging and offering it at least once a year. To promote the course on aging, and to guarantee higher enrollment, the focus group participants brainstormed and identified the following strategies: (1) Creating an attractive course title, and course description to inform students about the course content and expectations; (2) Introducing students to the course through academic advising, other social work classes, by posting course flyers in visible places; (3) Cross-listing the course to attract some students in related majors; (4) Conducting a survey among students who had taken the aging course and post the results on a listserv or departmental newsletter; (5) Videotaping field trips and make them available to students and faculty. The focus group participants endorsed a curricula infusion approach that includes content on aging and intergenerational practice. They supported a strategy that would enable students to interact with older adults, address myths and stereotypes, and strengthen gerontological knowledge.

DISCUSSION

Participants from both focus groups agreed that BSW students must enhance their competencies in gerontological social work and intergenerational policy and practice. They identified barriers and strategies and three themes emerged.

First, participants reported apprehension and limited exposure and experience with older adults. They suggested that interaction with older adults in a variety of settings could help ease fears as well as resolve self-efficacy concerns. Students indicated tremendous benefit from innovative and reflective experiential learning activities, including field trips, volunteer work, and field practicum. They also reported positive outcomes from taking a course on aging.

Second, aging content is often not infused into the social work curricula and is not sufficiently covered in core courses. Students identified this deficit and specified the importance of the inclusion of aging and intergenerational content throughout the curricula. They endorsed a strengths-based model that included sensitivity to aging issues and dispelling myths.

Finally, students indicated that the full spectrum of aging and intergenerational practice issues was not covered in core courses. As a result, stereotypes about aging and a focus on the frail elderly in nursing homes prevailed. To provide a more complete account of aging issues the curricula must not only focus on pathology and social problems, but also on healthy aging, grandparents raising grandchildren, family caregiving, multigenerational families, policy, and innovative programs.

Strengthening Aging Content

It is evident that BSW programs need to create an aging-rich learning context to meet the goal of attracting students to gerontological social work. This includes a curriculum that weaves aging and intergenerational content and emphasizes self-awareness, sensitivity and the bio-psycho-social aspects of aging.

Addressing the apprehension and fears of students cannot be overlooked. Students' exposure and contact with older adults seemed to alleviate some concerns and skepticism. Employing activities to engage students in exploring their fears and self-efficacy issues, facilitating more contact with older adults, and connecting intergenerational practice and advocacy to dispel ageism and stereotyping can aid this process.

Intergenerational themes, in particular, enrich child welfare, as well as generalist practice courses. The authors found that having initiatives in child welfare and family-centered practice were beneficial. The faculty were able to connect with aging content by using an intergenerational perspective that linked older adults as integral members of families and communities.

The insights gained from the focus group participants helped shape our GeroRich Initiative's infusion strategy. Student comments confirmed the challenges. They also made clear that incorporating an aging and intergenerational practice framework was a good method to engage students. Our plan to regularly offer an undergraduate course on aging was also validated as a good approach to building interest and competency in gerontological social work. We also discovered that infusing aging content was not enough; it is necessary to create an aging-rich learning environment.

Field practicum and volunteer placements opportunities play a pivotal role in creating an aging-rich learning context. Expanding field placements options beyond local nursing homes, assisted living facilities and day-treatment programs is indicated. The authors have engaged in identifying intergenerational programs that promote strength-based perspectives in working with older adults. Another strategy for building competence and an aging-rich environment is to encourage faculty and students to attend professional conferences that address aging issues. The GeroRich project provided a small stipend for students attending professional conferences on aging.

Finally, we advocate that cultivating an aging-rich learning environment must include activities outside the classroom. In order to gain the attention of BSW students it is important to be creative and incorporate both educational and social components. To this end, we have sponsored annual aging colloquium, a campus-wide event to raise the awareness, and visibility of gerontological social work.

The authors are in the process of conducting a student survey to evaluate the process and outcomes of our intervention of gerontological enrichment. The preliminary results indicated that the GeroRich project positively impacted students' levels of gerontological knowledge, skills, and competency.

CONCLUSIONS

As we move into an era where older adults make up a larger segment of society, social workers must be competent in providing services to this population. Social work educators must employ innovative methods to inspire and prepare future professionals for work with older adults and their families. This is an area where BSW graduates may find themselves employed, as there will be a need for effective and skilled generalists who can work with families around issues of aging, retirement, health care, housing, and caregiving. The study indicates that this is not an impossible goal. An aging-rich environment and an intergenerational framework, where students are exposed to older adults in a variety of settings, is an important step. Innovative experiential learning activities and being proactive in securing field placements that are representative of gerontological programs enrich the curricula. Pulling in community resources and providing access to cutting edge research, professional meetings, conferences and workshops are also important. Employing these strategies to infuse aging content and to enrich the social work learning context will help the social work profession prepare the next generation of social workers for practice with older adults.

REFERENCES

Cummings, S., Galambos, C., & DeCoster, V. A., (2003). *Educational Gerontology*, *29*, 295-312.

Greene, R. R. (1990). Exploring the needs of social workers for continuing education in the field of aging. *Journal of Continuing Social Work Education, 5* (2), 21-26.

Kropf, N. (2002). Strategies to increase student interest in aging. *Journal of Gerontological Social Work, 39* (1-2), 57-67.

National Institute on Aging. (1987). *Personnel for health needs of the elderly through the year 2020.* Bethesda, MD: Department of Health and Human Services, Public Health Services.

Nelson, G. M. (1988). Personnel and training needs in geriatric social work. *Educational Gerontological, 14,* 95-106.

Olson, C. J. (2002). A curriculum module enhances students' gerontological practice-related knowledge and attitudes. *Journal of Gerontological Social Work, 39,* (1-2), 159-175.

Rosen, A., Zlotnik, J. L., & Singer, T. (2002). Basic Gerontological competence for all social workers: The need to "Gerontologize" social work education. *Journal of Gerontological Social Work, 39* (1-2), 25-36.

Scharlach, A., Damron-Rodriguez, J., Robinson, B., & Feldman, R. (2000). Educating social workers for an aging society: A vision for the 21st century. *Journal of Social Work Education, 36* (3), 521-538.

Tan, P., Hawkins, M. J., & Ryan, E. (2001). Baccalaureate social work student attitudes toward older adults. *Journal of Baccalaureate Social Work, 6* (2), 45-56.

doi: 10.1300/J083v48n01_04

Geriatric Enrichment:
Guaranteeing a Place for Aging
in the Curriculum

Barbara W. Shank, PhD
W. Randolph Herman, EdD

SUMMARY. Two years ago, the School of Social Work embarked upon a new and challenging initiative to create sustainable structural changes that enrich gerontological learning experiences for all our BSW and MSW students, faculty, fieldwork instructors and community practitioners. We envisioned that participation in this initiative would enable us to expand and embed geriatric content in the undergraduate and graduate curriculum, to increase our geriatric fieldwork placement opportunities, to evaluate and enhance our teaching and learning resources on aging, and to develop two new aging specific courses.

Having reached our third year of operation, we find ourselves reflecting on what have been our successes, what could we have done differently, and where do we go in the future. This article will describe our process of developing a model of curriculum change that will guarantee a place for aging in both our undergraduate and graduate curricula. doi: 10.1300/J083v48n01_05 *[Article copies available for a fee from The Haworth Document Delivery Service: 1-800-HAWORTH. E-mail address: <docdelivery@haworthpress.com> Website: <http://www.HaworthPress.com> © 2006 by The Haworth Press, Inc. All rights reserved.]*

[Haworth co-indexing entry note]: "Geriatric Enrichment: Guaranteeing a Place for Aging in the Curriculum." Shank, Barbara W., and W. Randolph Herman. Co-published simultaneously in *Journal of Gerontological Social Work* (The Haworth Press, Inc.) Vol. 48, No. 1/2, 2006, pp. 63-81; and: *Fostering Social Work Gerontology Competence: A Collection of Papers from the First National Gerontological Social Work Conference* (ed: Catherine J. Tompkins, and Anita L. Rosen) The Haworth Press, Inc., 2007, pp. 63-81. Single or multiple copies of this article are available for a fee from The Haworth Document Delivery Service [1-800-HAWORTH, 9:00 a.m. - 5:00 p.m. (EST). E-mail address: docdelivery@haworthpress.com].

KEYWORDS. Gerontology, curriculum, fieldwork, social work, education

INTRODUCTION

Aging is no accident. It is necessary to the human condition, intended by the soul. Aging is built into our psychology; yet, to our puzzlement, human life extends long beyond fertility and outlasts muscular usefulness and sensory acuteness. For this reason we need imaginative ideas that can grace aging and speak to it with the intelligence it deserves.

–James Hillman

Two years ago, the School of Social Work embarked upon a new and challenging initiative to create sustainable structural changes that enrich gerontological learning experiences for all our BSW and MSW students, faculty, fieldwork instructors and community practitioners. We envisioned that participation in this initiative would enable us to expand and embed geriatric content in the undergraduate and graduate curriculum, to increase our geriatric fieldwork placement opportunities, to evaluate and enhance our teaching and learning resources on aging, and to develop two new aging specific courses.

Having reached our third year of operation, we find ourselves reflecting on what have been our successes, what could we have done differently, and where do we go in the future. This article will describe our process of developing a model of curriculum change that will guarantee a place for aging in both our undergraduate and graduate curricula.

BACKGROUND

Knowledge is proud that he has learn'd so much;
Wisdom is humble that he knows no more.

–William Cowper

How Did We Get Into This?

We started this process asking, "Why is a geriatric enriched curricula important for social work?" The timing of this project aligned with the current state and national demographics on aging and their increasing challenge to the social work profession. Between 1908 and 2000, the populations over age 65 grew by 36%; the number of people 85 and older doubled and the number of people over 100 tripled (*A Profile of Older Americans: 2000*). In the next 20 years the populations over 65 is expected to grow by 54% (Dill, 2001). This growth in the older populations is accompanied by another demographic trend. As the aging population is growing in the United States, younger populations are shrinking. According to the U.S. Census Bureau, by 2025, the number of people age sixty to sixty-nine will be expanding at a faster rate than the number of people age 20 to 29 (U.S. Bureau of Census, 1996).

These rising numbers in the aging population, who are also living longer, against the backdrop of shrinking numbers of family caregivers, creates what Drucker calls the most dominant aspect of the "Next Society" (Drucker, 2001). These demographics will "challenge our nation's financial and human resources and enrich traditional notions of old age. They will require more elder qualified health professionals and force our nation to reshape and improve health care delivery to meet the needs of the elderly" (*John A. Hartford Foundation Goals*, 2002).

The state of Minnesota through the 2030 Aging Initiative has identified the demographic changes that will occur over the next fifty years. Today twelve percent of the population, one out of eight Minnesotans, is over 65 years of age. By the year 2030, it is estimated that 24% of the populations, one out of four Minnesotans will be over the age of 65. The 2030 report projects that between 2000 and 2030 the population of Minnesotans over the age of 65 will double from 600,000 to 1.2 million and that between 2000 and 2050 the population over 85 will nearly triple from 90,000 to 250,000. These predictions recognize that this demographic growth will affect both gender and ethnic groups. In 2030, there will be 130,000 more women than men and 2050 there will be 160,000 more women than men. Culturally and ethnically diverse populations will grow from 10,316 persons, 1.5% in 2000 to 50,8000 persons and 4.5% in 2030. These aging and diverse populations will be facing the challenges of aging and functional impairments with many having limited incomes and/or access to services (*Aging Initiative: Project 2030*, MN Department of Human Services, p. 9). They will need health care, long-term care and supportive environments. The new millennium presents the largest aging cohort ever to exist and with a variety of challenges to local, national and global development.

> As societies age they require transformations in existing mind-sets in the areas of cultural attitudes, social practice (e.g., work and retirement patterns), economics, living arrangements and housing, health-care and social-service delivery, and the general scientific and medical research agenda, among other things. (Maddox, 1995, p. 387)

This challenge has been coming for many years and various proactive and reactive responses have already occurred. In the profession of social work as early as 1970, Brody (1970) urged social work educators to overcome the disparities of what is "known and taught" in the field of geriatric social work and to address the shortage of social workers without special knowledge to meet the eventual needs of the elderly. Greene, Vourlekis, Gelfand, and Lewis (1990) gave the same warning: "A significant proportion of social work practitioners are unlikely to have received the depth of information and the specialized skills required to work with the aged and their families during their formal education" (p. 39). In fact, Lubben (1992), after conducting a national survey of curriculum on aging in schools of social work, made an even stronger plea to address the current paucity of courses and concentrations addressing the needs of the elderly:

> Failure of schools of social work to expand gerontological curriculum will mean that schools of social work will have missed a momentous opportunity to train social workers for jobs in an arena of rapid growth and that the social work profession will continue to be inadequately prepared to meet the needs of the rapidly aging population. (p. 170)

Lubben's survey of curriculum revealed statistics that were alarming, considering the growing awareness of the changing demographics of the aged. In 1992, Lubben found that a majority of the undergraduate social work programs taught a generalist curriculum without concentrations in specific areas such as aging. Nine percent stated that they had a concentration on aging and 11% offered one or more courses focusing specifically on growing old. Eighty percent offered no courses on aging. Most programs indicated that they did have information on aging distributed throughout their core curriculum, but Lubben's statistic highlighted the difficulty in ascertaining exactly how much material was dedicated to aging. These findings were troubling since most social workers working in nursing homes have a BSW (p. 159).

At the graduate level, seventy-one percent of the 100 master's in social work degree programs (MSW) indicated that they taught a generalist curriculum, and 34% noted having a concentration in aging. The number of MSW programs with a concentration in aging had dropped from 50% to 34% since 1984 in sharp contrast to the rising demographics of aging.

Although 97% of the surveyed programs ranked training in working with the aging as important to very important, fewer than 15% of the programs planned to develop more in the curriculum in the next five years (p. 164). They stated the barriers to expanding content on aging were an already over-full curriculum, lack of trained faculty (80% of the BSW programs were without geriatric research experience), and the resistance of students to working with and studying aging. There was some evidence of an increase in student interest in aging in those schools that had a clear concentration or link to gerontological center on campus (p. 168). Thus, it seemed that existing schools with a clear commitment to geriatric social work were emerging as potential mentors to other programs looking to develop a more specialized curriculum (Greene, 1989).

Since Lubben's 1992 survey the data shows that little has changed. The majority of BSW and MSW educational programs provide little or no direct infused gerontological content (Scharlach, Damron-Rodriquez, Robinson, & Feldman, 2000) and only 2.7% (938) of the nearly 35,000 students pursuing social work degrees select an aging concentration (Lennon, 1999). These demographics present a significant challenge to our profession. In the next ten years the projected need for social workers will require a 30% increase in graduates (*Bureau of Labor Statistics*, 2002). It is clear that not only do we need trained social workers to meet general needs, but we desperately need those who are knowledgeable and skilled in working with the elderly. As a profession we have identified and recognize the problem, however, we have not individually or collectively developed the necessary strategies to address these challenges effectively. The overwhelming evidence supports the need for more comprehensive planning, community building, curriculum development and research on aging (*A Blueprint for the New Millennium*, CSWE/SAGE, 2000).

John A. Hartford Foundation:
Geriatric Enrichment in Social Work Education

> ... by the way in which a society behaves toward its old people it uncovers the naked, and often carefully hidden truths, about its real principles and aims.
>
> –Simone De Beauvior

The John A. Hartford Foundation, recognizing these needs and truths, provided a major grant to the University of Washington, School of Social Work, to coordinate a joint effort between the Foundation and the Council on Social Work Education entitled "Geriatric Enrichment in Social Work Education." Planning and implementation grants were available to both baccalaureate and masters social work programs nationwide who would commit themselves to increase aging-rich learning opportunities for students in their programs.

The opportunity to receive funding for 'geriatric enrichment' was a strong incentive for making a commitment to engage this process of structural change while in the midst of our reaffirmation process for both our BSW and MSW programs. We knew we did not have the internal resources, both emotional and financial, to take on this additional work without external funding. Furthermore, in dialogue with all full-time faculty, we learned that they understood the predicted demographic changes and their far-reaching implications for social work practitioners, they recognized the need to more explicitly include geriatric content in their courses as a principle of best-practices and many were anxious about teaching aging content. An award of a geriatric enrichment grant would serve as encouragement, reinforcement and support.

THE CSC/UST GERIATRIC ENRICHMENT MODEL

How far you go in life depends on your being tender to the young, compassionate with the aged, sympathetic with the striving and tolerant of the weak and strong. Because someday in life you'll have been all of these.

–George Washington Carver

Curriculum Review and Assessment

From vision to evaluation, Drs. Randy Herman and Barbara Shank have shared the responsibility of project development and implementation. Six assumptions emerged, which serve as the guiding principles for this GeroRich Model:

- to obtain 'buy-in' from all faculty is essential to initial change, sustainability and project success;
- to engage all key constituencies in the project is essential to increase visibility and secure commitment;
- to address intergenerational practice using multi-methods and formats as learning styles differ among key constituencies;
- to integrate content on intergenerational practice throughout the BSW and MSW curricula to ensure that it is an integral part of the required curricula;
- to ensure that all BSW and MSW students are exposed to issues of working with older adults and their families as this area of practice will increasingly be a significant area of practice for all social work professionals; and

- to design inter-professional components of the project as partnering and collaboration with other professions is a reality of professional practice.

Prior to beginning the project, a comprehensive review to determine how and where content on aging was addressed in the BSW and MSW curricula was completed. We realized the importance of documenting the gaps in the curricula as well as establishing a baseline of the current geriatric material in each content area. Not surprisingly, our review documented minimal content on aging addressed at either level. Review of syllabi and required readings, identified some attention to ageism, elder abuse, late adulthood as part of the life cycle, and social security. It was clear to us that we were not adequately preparing our students with the knowledge and skills needed to practice competently with older adults and their families.

From our alumni base, we were able to identify individuals who had expressed a commitment to practice with older adults. They confirmed that their coursework, both class and field, contained little or no information regarding the elderly. The respondents offered five recommendations: (1) to acknowledge and develop a response to the expected exponential growth in the elderly populations, (2) to integrate content on elderly throughout the core curriculum, (3) to develop specific content mental health strategies and services, (4) to develop electives (foundation and clinical) on aging, and (5) to enhance field placement opportunities to work with the elderly.

Both our curriculum review and the response of our alumni, guided our thinking in developing our goals and objectives for our grant application. In January 2001, we were notified that we were among the 15 combined programs out of 67 BSW and MSW programs that had been awarded planning grants. Needless to say, we were grateful for the funding and the flexibility of the grant which would enable us to develop a model for making a major change in the curricula.

Goals and Objectives

The GeroRich Grant allowed us to simultaneously engage in four areas of program development relating to practice with older adults and their families, intergenerational practice. These areas encompass curriculum, faculty, students and community development. We believe that our two overarching project goals provide support for our work in these four areas. Our project goals are:

- To create sustainable structural changes that enrich gerontological learning experiences for all BSW and MSW social work students by integrating geriatric content into the BSW and MSW curriculum.

- To expand gerontological learning experiences for faculty, fieldwork instructors and community practitioners, creating inclusive and collaborative processes for learning.

From these goals six project objectives were established:

- To enhance the quantity and quality of geriatric content in the classroom based core curriculum of the BSW and MSW programs;
- To enhance the quantity and quality of geriatric content in the field-based curriculum of the BSW and MSW program;
- To increase the number of BSW and MSW graduates who are committed to providing services to older adults and their families;
- To increase the presence of minority social work practitioners in the field of aging;
- To strengthen faculty competence to effectively teach content on practice with older adults and their families; and
- To create a shared vision among key constituents (faculty, students fieldwork instructors and community practitioners) that supports our purpose to create sustainable structural changes that enrich geriatric learning experiences for all social work students.

Based on our goals and objectives, we developed an assessment plan and procedures for evaluating the outcomes of our objectives, and for using the results of the evaluation, to expand geriatric learning experiences and sustain structural curriculum change. As planned, the third year of the grant focuses on evaluation and dissemination of results. We are currently involved in the process of compiling evaluations, analyzing data and disseminating results.

Curriculum Enrichment

As noted above, the analysis of the undergraduate and graduate core curricula clearly identified minimal attention to content on aging. Syllabi, required readings and handouts for fourteen BSW courses and fifteen MSW courses were reviewed to reveal minimal and inconsistent attention to aging and intergenerational material. To remedy this situation required full faculty involvement. But a major challenge in accomplishing these changes was how to engage the faculty. This was a potential problem as many of the faculty were feeling ambivalent due to various competing demands in curriculum development.

In the spring of the planning year, all full-time faculty participated in a three hour meeting and a full day retreat where we explored our personal and professional beliefs and feelings about 'getting old'. The majority of the faculty are approaching late middle age and the personal impact of aging was as important to explore as the professional requirements for the students. The retreat day was structured to include presentations, small and large group discussion, activities with a geriatric music therapist, and video-conference with a graduate faculty aging specialist.

The core purposes of the retreat was to confirm total faculty 'buy-in' for curricular structural change, increasing faculty comfort level with aging content, and determining responsibilities for integration of aging content in each core BSW and MSW course. After viewing the video 'Big Mama' a faculty member brainstormed with the group ways to use the video in his undergraduate senior practice course highlighting intergenerational practice, and issues around diversity, professional ethics, social justice, advocacy, systems change and policy. Faculty were divided into BSW and MSW content area groups and at the end of the working session, each faculty member volunteered to take leadership for coordinating input from all faculty teaching a particular course and then integrate content on intergenerational practice into the course description, objectives, content outline, required readings, and assignments. All faculty were awarded a stipend when they completed the course revisions. The course revisions were completed for Fall, 2002.

For the past several years, the School Advisory Committee has reviewed the baccalaureate and graduate curricula to provide an external analysis regarding the integration of the eight curriculum content areas. During 2002-2003, the advisory committee focused on the integration of aging content throughout the curriculum, serving as validity check. Members of the advisory committee were asked to serve due to their expertise in aging. Advisory committee members reviewed syllabi, required readings, met with faculty and students, and attended classes and content area meetings. We were relieved when their findings confirmed that each course was infused with content on aging, intergenerational practice, appropriate for the level and focus of the course.

In addition to enrichment of content in all core courses, another strategy for curricular transformation was the development of two aging specific electives. At the foundation level, cross-listed between undergraduate and foundation graduate, we reinstituted an elective titled 'Social Work Practice with Older Adults and Their Families'. This elective was offered fall semester 2002 with twelve students enrolling. The course introduced students to social work knowledge, values and skills for practice with older adults and their families as well as examining theories and attitudes toward aging, the nature and limitations of gerontological social work, forces shaping delivery systems, major bio-psychological dimensions of practice and different models of intervention. Most of the students enrolling in this elective were concurrently doing their field placement in a geriatric-focused setting. For our clinical students, we developed a 'Clinical Practice with Elderly' course. The course examined the interaction of the biological, psychological, emotional, spiritual and so-cial/economic factors, focusing on assessment, diagnosis, treatment and eval-uation of clinical practice with older adults. Based on a strengths perspective, the role of the clinical social worker was examined in various settings and agencies serving aged populations. Eighteen clinical students enrolled. The course was co-taught by three geriatric social work practitioners with the GeroRich project director serving as resource person and facilitator.

Faculty Enrichment

We believed that increasing faculty comfort with and knowledge about ag-ing content was a critical element for this project to succeed. Faculty had been open about sharing their concerns and desire to do this well. Many had never practiced in settings where they worked directly with older adults, and some had negative experiences working with elderly clients when they were begin-ning professionals. All but two faculty members are closer to sixty than thirty, so issues of aging took on a personal dimension that some had not expected.

To decrease anxiety, faculty were provided with easy access to GeroRich and CSWE/SAGE-SW curriculum development materials including copies of the resource discs. The project directors were available any time for consulta-tion. Faculty received lists of all new library and audio-visual acquisitions and newly added journal subscriptions to enhance course bibliographies and for reference. Five faculty participated in the faculty development workshops sponsored by CSWE/SAGE-SW in Washington, Seattle, Pittsburgh and Nash-ville. Funding was available for faculty to attend local workshops on aging and several took advantage of these opportunities.

A proposal was submitted and accepted to feature geriatric enrichment as the theme for the Fall, 2002 Minnesota Conference on Social Work Education. Fourteen of the sixteen undergraduate social work programs in Minnesota sent faculty to engage with aging content. Drs. Catherine Tompkins and Virginia Richardson from CSWE/SAGE-SW presented on 'Integrating Gerontology Material into the Curriculum with a Focus on Addressing Issues Across the Life Span'. The fourteen schools that were represented all received the CSWE/SAGE gerontological notebooks on disc. Opportunities for collabora-tion and coordinated sharing of resources were outcomes of this forum.

Faculty development is a continuing part of our monthly faculty work together. One half of each full-time faculty meeting is dedicated to faculty development. The focus of our sessions during 2002-2003 were on six issues of aging. Outside speakers were engaged to present the workshops so that all faculty had the opportunity to be learners rather than teachers. The topics covered were resiliency and aging: quality of life and psychological well-being, controversial issues for providers and consumers of services for older people, Hmong elders, kinship care and the role of grandparents in African American families, a model for end of life planning and GLBT aging. One very specific outcome from these sessions was the development and marketing of 'Elder Issues' by one of our BSW alums, Gretchen Scheffel and her associate Deb Seaberg. They provide geriatric consultation and case management services for older adults and their families. For their presentation they created a board game. Faculty were so enthusiastic about their experience that they encouraged Gretchen and Deb to copyright and market their game for use in the classroom with students/or in the community with professionals.

Student-Field Enrichment

Field education encompasses several areas including faculty, students, and agency based community practitioners. Our fall fieldwork instructor training workshop, a collaboration between the field programs at our school, Augsburg College and the University of Minnesota, brought in Dr. Ed Canda to speak on 'Encountering Spirituality in Field Supervision' with an emphasis on supervision in agencies working with older adults. Fifty fieldwork instructors and fifteen faculty attended that workshop. The focus of our spring field training workshop presented by Ted Bowman was on 'Addressing Grief and Loss as a Family Ages'. One hundred and twenty field instructors, students and faculty attended.

Field Directors, Marla Hanley and Barb Berger worked with field faculty on design of a cross-listed (senior BSW and foundation MSW) Hartford field seminar and a clinical Hartford seminar. Six senior social work students and eight foundation graduate students enrolled in the Hartford foundation seminar. These students had a variety of placements in nursing homes, adult day care, assisted living, department on aging, a Parkinson's center, and the Alzheimer's Association. Structuring field seminars for two levels and based on only one area of practice was a pilot for our field program. Meeting the needs of both undergraduate and graduate students, even though each student indicated a commitment to working with older adults and was placed in a geriatric setting, proved to be challenging.

Of the two pilot seminars, feedback from the students was most positive from the clinical group who appreciated the specialized emphasis on aging and indicated that they often felt most students were not interested in working with the elderly and their issues got shortchanged in seminar by students working with other, 'more exciting,' client groups. They appreciated the mutual support and peer consultation. Nine clinical students enrolled in the Hartford clinical seminar representing placements in mental health, aging services, hospital social work, hospice care, and aging crisis care.

Students who were enrolled in both a geriatric focused elective course and Hartford field seminar, were designated Hartford Scholars and received a $500 stipend upon successful completion of their field placement. The Hartford Scholars openly stated that they appreciated the stipend support and they viewed it as recognition of their commitment to practice with older adults. Several students indicated that they would not have considered accepting a placement with older adults without the stipend, but found that they very much liked working with the elderly and were excited about looking for a job in geriatric social work practice.

As was available for faculty, funding for attending professional workshops on aging was also available for students. Several students requested funding to attend half-day workshops sponsored by the Senior Federation and Catholic Eldercare. To stimulate additional student interest, two Hartford awards of $50.00 each were given to students at the 5th Annual Student Social Work State Conference for presentations on practice with elderly. Both of these presentations were well attended.

One area of our grant proposal that had not been received favorably by the grant reviewers was our attention to interdisciplinary practice. It was made clear that the focus of this project was to be social work curriculum enrichment. Holding to our belief of the importance of collaboration and team-building, we developed a health care team-building workshop for undergraduate and graduate students in nutrition, nursing, occupational therapy, physical therapy and social work. Students were divided into interdisciplinary teams, working through a case study of Helen, an 82-year-old woman admitted to the hospital from the Emergency Department with a fractured right hip. In addition to determining a care plan for Helen, students identified the theoretical, philosophical or ethical similarities and differences between the disciplines and the unique contributions of each member of the interdisciplinary team. Over two hundred students and faculty participated in the workshop. A highlight of the workshop was the panel by three nuns, two at 100 years, who were Nun Study Participants. One student noted, "It is really important to have a multi-professional approach to case management to aid in a holistic approach for care. It is really critical to have many different perspectives to helping an older adult and their family."

Clinical Research Enrichment

To graduate from our program, MSW students must complete a year long clinical research paper. Students develop a research question, design and carry out the study, complete a thesis length document and present their findings at the end of the year at the annual Clinical Research Symposium attended by students, field instructors and community practitioners. The symposium serves as a means to disseminate research findings and to provide ongoing dialogue among students, faculty and agencies. Between 1992 (the first graduating class) and 2000, ten MSW students completed their clinical research on topics addressing clinical social work practice with the elderly. In Fall, 2002, the number increased to ten in one year designing projects addressing areas of aging. Their research topics covered:

Loss Experience of Caregivers of Person with Memory Loss;

Benefits of Support Group Attendance for People with Early Stage Alzheimer's Disease;

Minnesota Nursing Home Social Workers' Intervention with Their Alcoholic Residents;

The Nature of Spiritual Assessment with Hospice Patients;

How Baby Boomers Experience Their Parents Aging;

Family vs. Professional Caregivers in Late Life: Baby Boomer Experience;

Coping Strategies Utilized by Older Adults and Their Perceived Efficacy;

Volunteer Involvement in Respite Care: Serving Caregivers of the Older Adult;

A Process Evaluation of a Community-Based Chemical Dependency Aftercare Program for Older Adults; and

The Strengths and Challenges Reported by Older Transgender Adults

Students who were designated Hartford Scholars (completing elective coursework and field practicum in aging) and completed their clinical research on an aging topic, received a $500 stipend to assist with research expenses. In a note from a recent alum, she related that she has been asked to publish the results of her research on the use of ethical wills by nursing home and hospital social workers. We are pleased that our students are contributing to fill the gap for more research on aging.

PROJECT EVALUATION

> Be satisfied with success in even the smallest matter, and think that even such a result is not trifle.

> –Marcus Aurelius Antonius

The old adage that 'success is in the pudding' belies the difficult in actually measuring the success of a multifaceted model to enrich aging content in a BSW and MSW core curricula. Our evaluation plan includes both internal and external curriculum assessment, participant evaluation of all workshops, student evaluation of field seminars, mid-year focus group of Hartford fieldwork instructors, and pre and post tests of students using the Aging Semantic Differential and Palmore Facts on Aging Quiz. Also, we tracked and compared the number of clinical research projects completed on aging for the first eleven years of the MSW program, to others completed since the first year of he GeroRich project. As we are currently in the middle of evaluation of this project, we only have preliminary results to report.

As noted above, the Community Advisory Committee provided an assessment of our efforts to integrate content on intergenerational practice into all of our core BSW and MSW courses. Although they found some unevenness in the breadth and depth of content covered in each content area, overall their findings were positive and their analysis supported our plan that every BSW and MSW core course would include content on social work practice with older adults.

A written evaluation was completed addressing expectations met or unmet and knowledge gained, as well as suggested topics for future workshops following every field instructor or student workshop. Fieldwork instructors stated that their major area of concern was in working at the macro level but appreciated the focus on one area throughout the year so they could have a more in-depth understanding of geriatric social work. Even those fieldwork instructors who worked directly with the aged, stated they had little or no education on working with the elderly when studying social work. Students rated the Interdisciplinary Health Care Workshop at a nine on a scale of ten. They commented that this was the first time they had really had to think about working with other professionals and learned a great deal about how each professional group viewed their role working together on an intergenerational case situation. At the annual curriculum review workshop, faculty completed an evaluation of the six faculty development workshops that had focused on aging topics. Faculty rated the workshops as excellent, stating that the diverse topics were helpful in expanding their understanding of issues unique to aging and those shared throughout the lifespan.

Currently we have three major tools to track student satisfaction and outcome: (1) a senior BSW satisfaction survey that asks questions about core curriculum and field classroom learning, (2) a two-year BSW/MSW outcome study that provides data on career choices and information about alumni working with the aged and their families, and (3) an annual BSW alumni survey that provides data on licensure and employment. The last two instruments provide data to assist the project directors and field faculty to evaluate trends in employment in aging services. Seniors stated that they appreciated the faculty's energy in creating new learning opportunities and that they wished stipends could be an ongoing incentive for pursuing certain areas of interest. Results of the BSW employment survey for last year's graduates have not yet been completed.

All students in field placement complete an end of semester evaluation. Student ratings of the dedicated Hartford field seminars will be compared to rating of students in mixed focused seminars to measure positive and negative outcomes.

Students, rating both the instructor and the course, evaluate every course in the curriculum at the end of the semester. On a scale of one to five with five being the highest, students rated the foundation social work practice course with older adults at 4.2. Students in the clinical practice course with elderly rated the course at 3.9. Students stated that they felt some of the material was repetitive from the foundation course although the majority of the students felt they had learned a great deal from the team of three teachers who represented the clinical, community and research components of intergenerational practice.

At the beginning of the Fall, 2001 semester, all junior undergraduate students and all foundation MSW students were asked to complete the Aging Semantic Differential and the Palmore Facts on Aging Quiz. All graduating BSW and clinical MSW students were given the same two measures in the Spring semester, 2003. These two measures will help us assess the impact of infusion of geriatric content in all core courses. The results of both administrations of these measures are being entered in SPSS for data analysis. It is planned that this data will be shared with Dr. Zvi Gelles, from the University of Maryland, as he has used the same measures with his students. The Social Work with Aging Skill Competency Scale (Hartford Practicum Partnership Program) was used as a pre and post-test in the clinical MSW elective. Comparison of the pre and post scores identifies that students scored significantly higher after the course demonstrating major learning in the field of aging.

Finally, comparing the number of clinical research papers completed with a focus on aging prior to the initiation of this project to those completed during the three years of the project will give us an indication of student interest in aging. Prior to the GeroRich project, we had only one aging related research paper a year and since the beginning of the project, we have had 11 projects over two years, an amazing increase. MSW students present their research findings in the spring at the Clinical Research Symposium attended by students, faculty, field instructors, and community practitioners. This symposium is one vehicle to disseminate findings on aging, and provide ongoing dialogue among students, faculty and agencies on issues facing the older adults and their families.

We believe the preliminary outcomes from the various forms of evaluation demonstrate the success of our project and achievement of our goals and objectives. Future analysis of data will help us determine what strategies we will need to employ to ensure that we can sustain our level of commitment.

Sustainability

In implementing change that is pervasive as well as sustainable, any organization must address what Margaret J. Wheatley (1994) states is a paradox of self-organizing systems to change, remain stable and yet be open to renewal. Faculty have clearly demonstrated that they are open to change and renewal as concrete changes are evident in syllabi goals, objectives, content and assignments. Only continual monitoring and critical dialogue will ensure that these changes will be sustained.

An area that we have not been successful in is securing additional funding resources. In collaboration with our University Office of Institutional Advancement, we have submitted fourteen grant proposals to foundations who have indicated that addressing issues of older adults is within the priorities. To date, we had negative responses from all but one of the foundations. With external support, we believe that we could sustain a cohort of students annually who would focus on practice with aging, much like the Title IV-E funding has done for child welfare. Without external support, our ability to interest students and to provide opportunities and resources for faculty development in this challenging area of practice is less likely.

CONCLUSION

The common stock of intellectual enjoyment should not be difficult to access because of the economic position of him who would approach it.

–Jane Addams

Funding from the John A. Hartford Foundation allowed us to commit ourselves to increase aging-rich classroom and field-learning opportunities for students and faculty in our programs. We have been inspired and challenged by this experience. The past two years have taught us numerous lessons.

The first lesson learned is that faculty 'buy-in' is essential for establishing a working agreement is essential for an honest assessment of challenges and barriers to the project and critical to establishing and moving faculty to a deeper level of commitment. Without 'buy-in' and full participation, change is limited and minimal. Even with faculty 'buy-in' curriculum change is slow and challenging. Faculty anxiety about teaching aging content is lessened with additional training, but not totally alleviated.

We also learned that field instructors lacked knowledge about aging and about intergenerational practice. This was especially true in meeting the goals of macro practice. The supervisors stated they lacked the necessary skills to work at the agency, community and governmental level. Resources and networking were also identified as being difficult to access when practice was primarily focused at the micro level.

Providing multiple venues and varied offerings addressing aging is critical to increase comfort, tap into various interests and learning styles for faculty, field instructors and community practitioners. For the project to succeed, program leadership must be actively supportive. It takes more than an enthusiastic project director to move this project forward. Active, not passive, support needs to come from the Dean, Faculty and Field Directors.

A fourth lesson learned is that providing stipends for students and faculty is an effective incentive for increasing interest and commitment to the field of aging; students view stipends as recognition of the importance of aging practice. If child welfare students receive stipends, why shouldn't gerontology students? We have also learned that faculty view stipends as a recognition of additional effort. But we are also aware that a stipend does not guarantee working in the area of intergenerational social work once out of the educational process.

In considering how to integrate another practice area into an already full curriculum, faculty concluded that focusing on intergenerational practice was the most positive approach, as it focuses attention on the need to address the aged client but does not exclude their families and the larger community.

Finally, the most difficult lesson learned is that locating additional funding to support this project and ensure its sustainability, is proving to be more challenging than ever anticipated. The Hartford Grant enabled us to stimulate change on an individual and on a programmatic level that could have not been done otherwise. Although the grant was not large, the competition for ongoing funds is a major challenge.

We remain committed to our goals of creating sustainable structural changes and expanding gerontological learning experiences. In retrospect the amount of work required during the planning period was much greater than anticipated. The planning period was constricted so that it was a challenge to complete all that was required in seven months. It was also painful to identify gaps in our existing program and to honestly set goals to address them. We can say with some pride, the faculty truly extended themselves in preparing to implement curricular change. Our field directors actively recruited and supported the development of the Hartford field track while maintaining an already demanding field program. The synergy that resulted has been most energizing to a faculty already committed to diverse interests.

Our School of Social Work is unique in that it is jointly offered by two institutions, resulting in faculty being on a variety of schedules, teaching sites and times. The Hartford project has provided the resources to take time to reflect on curriculum in a way that is both professionally and personally rewarding. Probably the most profound lesson learned is an old one: Open dialogue–between people, programs and funding sources–can result in change.

Our GeroRich experience has presented new opportunities and challenged old ways of thinking. We encourage all schools who have not engaged in this process to get involved to reduce the gaps in training that remain for many graduates. If estimates are true, we will need 70,000 professionally trained social workers to work with the elderly by the year 2020 (Solomon, 1992, p. 177). Thanks to the John A. Hartford Foundation, the work has begun!

REFERENCES

De Beauvoir, S. (1972). *The Coming of Age.* New York: G.P. Putnam's Sons.

Dill, M. (2001). The aging of America: Implications for the health workforce. Center for Health Workforce Studies, University of Albany, School of Public Health, NY.

Drucker, P. (2001). The next society. *The Economist,* Vol. 361 (8246), 1-20.

Greene, R., Barusch, A., & Connelly, R. (1989). *Social Work and Gerontology: An Update.* Washington DC: Final Report to the Administration on Aging and the Association for Gerontology in Higher Education.

Greene, R., Gueres, R., Vourlekis, B., Gelfand, D., & Lewis, J. (1992). Current realities: Practice and education needs for social workers in nursing homes. *Journal of Gerontological Social Work, 18,* (3/4), 39-54.

John A. Hartford Foundation (2002). John A. Hartford Foundation Goals.

Lennon, T. (1999). Statistics on Social Work Education in the United States: 1998. Alexandria, Virginia, Council on Social Work Education.

Lubbens, J., Damron-Rodriquez, J., & Beck, A. (1992). A national survey of aging curriculum in schools of social work. *Journal of Gerontological Social Work, 18,* (3/4), 157-171.

Maddox, G. (1994). Social and behavioral research on aging: An agenda for the United States. *Aging and Society. 14,* 97-107.

Minnesota Department of Human Services. (2000). *Aging Initiative: Project 2030.* St. Paul: Minnesota: Department of Human Services.

Scharlach, A., Damron-Rodriquez, J., Robinson, B., & Feldman, R. (2000). Educating social workers for an aging society: A vision for the 21st century. *Journal of Social Work Education, 36* (3), 521-538.

U.S. Bureau of the Census (1996).

U.S. Bureau of Labor Statistics (2002).

doi: 10.1300/J083v48n01_05

Building on the Life-Span Perspective:
A Model for Infusing Geriatric Social Work

Molly Ranney, PhD, LCSW
Catherine C. Goodman, DSW
Philip Tan, PhD
Agathi Glezakos, PhD, ACSW

SUMMARY. The growth in the older adult population and the demand for better trained geriatric social workers challenge the existing curricula of social work programs. The Geriatric Enrichment Grant funded by the John A. Hartford foundation has provided financial support for curricular reform. Curriculum reform is a challenging undertaking at any level. Each program and educational institution experiences the process of curriculum reform in unique ways. This paper describes one program's experience of curriculum reform for the purpose of infusing geriatric content. doi: 10.1300/J083v48n01_06 *[Article copies available for a fee from The Haworth Document Delivery Service: 1-800-HAWORTH. E-mail address: <docdelivery@haworthpress.com> Website: <http://www.HaworthPress.com> © 2006 by The Haworth Press, Inc. All rights reserved.]*

KEYWORDS. Geriatric social work, gerontology, social work education, curriculum modules, curricular change

---

[Haworth co-indexing entry note]: "Building on the Life-Span Perspective: A Model for Infusing Geriatric Social Work." Ranney, Molly et al. Co-published simultaneously in *Journal of Gerontological Social Work* (The Haworth Press, Inc.) Vol. 48, No. 1/2, 2006, pp. 83-96; and: *Fostering Social Work Gerontology Competence: A Collection of Papers from the First National Gerontological Social Work Conference* (ed: Catherine J. Tompkins, and Anita L. Rosen) The Haworth Press, Inc., 2007, pp. 83-96. Single or multiple copies of this article are available for a fee from The Haworth Document Delivery Service [1-800-HAWORTH, 9:00 a.m. - 5:00 p.m. (EST). E-mail address: docdelivery@haworthpress.com].

Available online at http://jgsw.haworthpress.com
doi:10.1300/J083v48n01_06

BACKGROUND

Throughout the past decade there has been accumulating evidence suggesting that social work educators were not doing enough to prepare students to work with the growing number of older adults (Berkman, Dobrof, Harry, & Damron-Rodriguez, 1997; Damron-Rodriguez, Villa, Tseng, & Lubben, 1997; Lubben, Damron-Rodriguez, & Beck, 1992; Netting & Williams, 1998; Scharlach, Damron-Rodriguez, Robinson, & Feldman, 2000). For example, Lubben et al. (1992) conducted a national survey of the accredited Bachelor of Social Work (BSW) and Master's of Social Work (MSW) programs in an attempt to understand the status of gerontological social work. They concluded that only 1% of BSW and 4% of MSW students took an aging class. Lubben et al. also found that only 34% of MSW offered concentrations in aging. The main reason reported as to why the schools were unable to address aging was because the curriculum were already "too full" (p. 164).

Damron-Rodriguez et al. (1997) examined the status of gerontological curriculum development at the BSW and MSW level between 1988-1993. The researchers used Damron-Rodriguez and Lubben's (1994) basic versus substantial criteria for evaluation of aging curriculum. In 1993, Damron-Rodriquez et al. (1997) found that 45% of the schools surveyed met the criteria for substantial aging curriculum–an increase from the 34% found in 1988. Approximately 24% met none of the criteria, which was a decrease from the 33% found in 1988.

The Department of Social Work at California State University, Long Beach (CSULB) has consistently met Damron-Rodriguez and Lubben's (1994) criteria for substantial geronotological curriculum and has been on the forefront of graduating geriatric social workers. Since the inception of the MSW program at CSULB in 1985, the two concentrations offered were an Older Adult and Families (OAF) and a Children, Youth and Families (CYF) concentration. In spite of this achievement, the projected growth in the older adult population has mandated an expansion of the geriatric curriculum. Whereas the existing curriculum was unique to each concentration, a paradigm shift involved adopting the philosophy that *all* students needed education on practice with older adults.

In January 2002, the Department was awarded a Geriatric Enrichment Grant by the John A. Hartford Foundation which provided financial support for curricular change. This paper describes the planning phase of the Geriatric Enrichment Grant and how the life-span perspective is being used as a broad conceptual framework for infusing of gerontological social work content across the entire curriculum.

AGING ENRICHMENT PROJECT

Setting

The Department of Social Work at CSULB serves the Los Angeles region, which includes five counties (Los Angeles, San Bernardino, Ventura, Riverside, and Orange). This area is one of the most ethnically and culturally diverse regions in the United States (Waldinger & Bozorgmehr, 1996). This metropolitan area encompasses over 33,000 square miles, almost twice the size of New York city or San Francisco. Los Angeles County was home to over 9.5 million people in 2000 and approximately 16.3 million for the five county areas. Of the five county areas, persons over the age of 65 made up 10.0% of the population (U.S. Census, 2000).

The Department has full and part time models at both the BSW and MSW level, with a statewide Distance Education program that offers an MSW program at rural sites in California. The goal of the program is to graduate entry level, generalist BSW and MSW social workers, who can work with all sized systems and with diverse client populations across the life-span. The students are ethnically diverse, with approximately two-thirds being other than Non-Hispanic White. During the planning phase of the Geriatric Enrichment Grant, there were 111 students enrolled in the BSW and 756 in the MSW program.

Project Goals

The long-term goals of the project were to institutionalize a curriculum infused with gerontological content and increase the number of students interested in geriatric social work. The objectives of the planning phase were: (1) to establish partnerships with key geriatric social work leaders; (2) to assess geriatric social work gaps in BSW and MSW curriculum; (3) to establish needs assessment data on interests in geriatric social work among BSW and MSW students; and (4) to develop curricular modules to address the gaps in curriculum.

Conceptual Framework

The life-span perspective was selected because it has been the conceptual basis for the CYF and OAF concentrations at the MSW level. Berkman, Doborf, Harry, and Damron-Rodriquez (1997) describe the life-span perspective as providing "positive goals for social work interventions, focusing on practice on factors that affect successful aging and normal growth and development in the course of living" (p. 223). By choosing to build on the existing conceptual model of the Department, it was determined that the faculty as a whole would be more likely to buy-in to adopting an infusion based approach.

Key Components

1. *Advisory Board*: An Advisory Board comprised of sixteen representatives from all key constituencies (i.e., students, faculty, field instructors, alumni, and leaders in the field of geriatric social work) met quarterly during the planning phase of the grant. Building on existing relationships, support was obtained by the leaders of several aging community agencies who served on the Aging Enrichment Project (AEP) Advisory Board and in any other capacity necessary to support the Department's efforts to strengthen the geriatric curriculum.

2. *Gap Analysis of the Curriculum*: A gap analysis of the existing curriculum was conducted using a procedure developed by Academic Geriatric Resource Center (AGRP) at the University of California, Los Angeles (UCLA) (Zuckerman, 2002). Zuckerman developed the UCLA/AGRP instrument based on the list of competencies developed by the Geriatric Social Work Education Consortium (GSWEC), supported by the Hartford and Archstone foundations. Specifically, the standardized course syllabi were analyzed to assess for strengths and weaknesses in regards to aging content in the BSW (n = 9) and MSW (n = 6) foundation courses. The field seminars were not included as part of the analysis because they were not lecture-based classes.

To create the evaluation tool to assess the syllabi, the UCLA/AGRP instrument was used as a starting point to create of a list of aging terms. Additional terms were added to fully reflect the curriculum at CSULB. To assess for content validity, the final list of aging terms was checked by four gerontologists. The aging terms were categorized into the following: general (e.g., old, elderly, late-life), values (e.g., ageism), ethical (e.g., elder abuse/neglect), legal (e.g., advance directives), policy (e.g., Older Americans Act, Omnibus Reconciliation Act), human behavior/mental health (e.g., depression, aging process), biology/medical (e.g., dementia, stroke), practice/intervention (e.g., life review, case management), services (e.g., Area Agency on Aging, Adult Protective Services), theory (e.g., life course, life-span), and research/assessment (e.g., Geriatric Depression Scale). For the complete instrument, see website: http://www.csulb.edu/depts/socialwk/.

The syllabi were evaluated by having a research assistant (R.A.) read through each syllabus highlighting each aging term. The R.A. marked each occurrence of the aging term on the evaluation tool. A second reader followed the same process to make sure all of the aging terms were identified.

The gap analysis revealed that all of the foundation courses had some aging content but the amount and type of content varied greatly. As indicated on Table 1, the BSW and MSW courses that had most aging content were the human behavior

TABLE 1. Results of Gap Analysis (N = 15)

BSW Foundation Classes	General Aging Terms	Values	Ethical	Legal/ Policy	Mental Health/ Behavior	Biology/ Medical/ Health	Interven- tions/ Practice	Service System	Assess- ment/ Research	Theory	Total Count
Intro. to Social Welfare	4			1		4	3	1		1	16
HBSE (1st half lifespan)	1	1				3				18	23
Social Policy: Law & Court Decisions	3			1		2	11				17
HBSE (2nd half of lifespan)	26	6	3	1	8	14	30			19	107
Intro. Generalist Practice	1					3				18	22
Social Policy: Formulation and Analysis	1		3	3		1	4	1			13
Generalist Practice with Groups	1					1	7			1	10
Generalist Practice Individuals & Families	1						20			1	22
Research Methods	1						3		1		5
MSW Foundation Classes											
Intro. Generic Cross Cultural Practice	1						8				9
Cross Cultural HBSE (1st half lifespan)	1				1		14			6	22
Cross Cultural HBSE (2nd half of lifespan)	38	3	9	2	6	19	23			1	101
Social Policy: Oppressed Groups	3		4			2	2	1		1	13
Research Methods	1								1		5
Computers/Statistics	5		1				1		1		7

Note: To simplify the reporting, the aging content was collapsed into each category. The total count equals the number of occurrences of the terms by category of an aging content.

classes, and the research courses had the least. The amount of aging content was less than expected for the practice courses. Based on the results, it was determined that all of the foundation classes could benefit from curriculum modules. Since all courses had some aging content, the AEP team decided to build and expand on the content that was already in the syllabi.

3. *Needs Assessment*: During the planning phase, data were collected about BSW and MSW student interest in gerontology, exposure to gerontology content in the foundation courses, and aging knowledge level. Interest questions were adapted from the CSWE/SAGE-SW student survey (with permission from Anita Rosen), and the knowledge and attitude questions are Palmore's (1998) *Facts on Aging Quiz: Part 2* (pp. 15-24). All BSW and MSW students who were in the final weeks of completing their foundation courses were surveyed. A convenience method of sampling was used whereby instructors distributed the survey to students present in their classes. A total of 50 BSW and 152 MSW students responded to the AEP Survey. The research methods classes, at the undergraduate and graduate level, were selected to be surveyed because they represent the last of the foundation classes for both BSW and MSW (CYF and OAF) students.

As illustrated on Table 2, students from the three groups did not significantly differ by gender, ethnic, or age. Female students (comprising over 85%

TABLE 2. Demographics by Type of Educational Program (N = 202)

| | Type of Educational Program | | | | |
Demographics	BSW (n = 49) %	MSW (CYF) (n = 112) %	MSW (OAF) (n = 41) %	x^2	p
Gender				.15	.93
Male	12.2	12.5	14.6		
Female	87.8	87.5	85.4		
Ethnicity				9.84	.28
African American	14.9	12.5	7.3		
Asian	10.6	8.9	12.2		
European American	12.8	33.9	31.7		
Hispanic/Latino	57.4	38.4	43.9		
Other	4.3	6.3	4.9		
Age				3.98	.41
20-29	79.2	69.4	60.0		
30-39	14.6	21.6	30.0		
40 and older	6.2	9.0	10.0		

Note: For program type, CYF stands for the Children, Youth and Families Concentration and OAF stands for the Older Adults and Families Concentration.

of respondents) outnumbered male students in all the programs. There was considerable ethnicity diversity represented by African American, Asian Pacific Islander, European American, and Hispanic/Latino students across the three programs. With the exception of Latinos (comprising of 57.4% in the BSW program), no group represented more than 50% of the respondents, and with the exception of Asians in the MSW (CYF) program (comprising 8.9%) and African Americans in the MSW (OAF) program (comprising 7.3%), no group was represented by less than 10% of the respondents. The modal age range was between 20-29 (comprising of 60% or more of respondents). Students were between 30-39 years of age (up to 30%) and to a lesser degree those 40 years and over (up to 10%).

In order to identify the perception of exposure to aging, students were asked to rate the amount of aging content in their foundation (i.e., behavior, policy, practice, and research) classes using a four-point Likert-type of response set. The responses included: 1 = aging not included, 2 = limited amount of aging content, 3 = moderate amount of aging content, and 4 = substantial amount of aging content. As indicated on Table 3, the three groups significantly differed on exposure to

TABLE 3. Exposure to Aging Content in Foundation Classes (N = 201)

Variable	n	M	SD	df	F	p
HUMAN BEHAVIOR				2	13.30	.000***
BSW[a]	49	3.22	.74			
MSW (CYF)[b]	111	2.59	.76			
MSW (OAF)[a]	41	2.98	.76			
POLICY				2	1.662	.192
BSW[a]	49	2.18	.81			
MSW (CYF)[a]	111	2.12	.72			
MSW (OAF)[a]	41	2.37	.73			
PRACTICE				2	54.29	.000***
BSW[a]	49	2.51	1.04			
MSW (CYF)[b]	110	1.83	.71			
MSW (OAF)[c]	41	3.14	.73			
RESEARCH				2	9.79	.000***
BSW[a]	49	1.96	.83			
MSW (CYF)[a]	110	1.90	.91			
MSW (OAF)[b]	41	2.56	.79			

Notes: For program type, CYF stands for the Children, Youth and Families Concentration, and OAF stands for the Older Adults and Families Concentration.
One-Way ANOVA tests were used. Means with a different letter are significantly different. Means with the same letter are not significantly different from each other.
*p < .05, **p < .01, ***p < .001

aging content in the behavior ($F = 13.30$, $df = 2$, $p = .0001$), practice ($F = 54.29$, $df = 2$, $p = .0001$), and research ($F = 9.29$, $df = 2$, $p = .0001$) classes. In term of the behavior classes, the OAF and BSW students reported a moderate level of exposure that was significantly higher than the CYF students, who were less than moderate. All three groups differed significantly on exposure to content in the practice classes, with OAF students reporting a moderate level, BSW students less than moderate, and CYF students only limited aging content. The OAF students reported a moderate level of exposure in the research classes which was significantly different than the limited amount of aging content reported by the BSW and CYF students. All three groups reported a limited amount of exposure to aging content in the policy classes.

Students were next asked to rate their overall experience working with older adults to establish student attitudes towards geriatric social work during the planning phase. A five-point Likert-type of response set was used for the overall experience with older adults questions ranging from 1 = not very positive to 5 = very positive. As indicated on Table 4, the average experience for BSW and CYF was positive. The OAF students scored in the positive to very positive range which was significantly higher than BSW and CYF students ($F = 8.75$, $df = 2$, $p = .0001$).

TABLE 4. Amount of Experience Working with Older Adults, Willingness to Accept Job Working with Older Adults After Graduation, and Palmore's Facts on Aging Quiz 2

Variable	n	M	SD	df	F	p
EXPERIENCE				2	8.75	.000***
BSW[a]	50	4.30	.76			
MSW (CYF)[a]	111	4.00	.85			
MSW (OAF)[b]	40	4.60	.71			
ACCEPT JOB				2	53.90	.000***
BSW[a]	50	3.80	1.20			
MSW (CYF)[b]	110	2.57	.92			
MSW (OAF)[a]	41	4.24	.89			
FACTS ON AGING SCORE				2	2.28	.105
BSW	45	13.66	2.25			
MSW (CYF)	104	13.69	1.99			
MSW (OAF)	40	14.51	2.41			

Notes: For program type, CYF stands for the Children, Youth and Families Concentration, and OAF stands for the Older Adults and Families Concentration.
One-Way ANOVA tests were used. Means with a different letter are significantly different. Means with the same letter are not significantly different from each other.
*p < .05, **p < .01, ***p < .001

The students were also asked about willingness to accept a job after graduation working with older adults. A five-point Likert-type response set was used which ranged from 1 = strongly disagree to 5 = strongly agree. The OAF and BSW students indicated a significantly higher level of their willingness to accept a job compared to the CYF students ($F = 53.90$, $df = 2$, $p = .0001$).

Palmore's (1998) twenty-five items from Quiz 2 of the *Facts on Aging* were used to assess knowledge. These items have a true/false response set. Correct answers were given a score of "1" and incorrect answers "0." The correct answers were summated, with the possible range being 0-25. Example items included: (1) a person's height tends to decline in old age; (2) more older persons (65 or older) have chronic illnesses that limit their activity than do younger persons; and (3) older persons have more acute (short-term) illnesses than do younger persons. As indicated on Table 4, the three student groups scored just above the mid-point of Palmore's Quiz 2 which suggested a moderate level of knowledge of aging.

4. *Curriculum Modules*: Consistent with Scharlach et al.'s (2000) call for the development of curriculum to infuse aging content into foundation class, the main focus of the project was on modular development. Specifically, a financial-based incentive program was used to promote interest in developing modules to strengthen the gerontology curriculum by bringing bridging concepts and topics to CYF and BSW students. The use of incentives is consistent with Rosen, Zlotnik, and Singer's (2002) assertion that curriculum change does not occur unless faculty perceive "substantive incentives for effecting curricular change" (p. 33). Faculty, field instructors, members of the advisor board, and alumni were invited to submit proposals to develop curriculum modules. The goal of using this approach is to work collaboratively with key constituencies who have expertise in geriatric social work to strengthen the curriculum.

The results of the gap analysis were used to determine topics of the modules. The life-span perspective was used as the guiding framework to ensure that the topics were relevant for OAF and CYF students. A standardized template (http://www.csulb.edu/depts/socialwk/) for the modules was developed. The dollar amount given for the module was based on the breadth of the topic. A module prototype (practice module on "Grandparents Raising Grandchildren") was created and given to potential participants to help let them know what was expected of them. The prototype consisted of a comprehensive lecture outline, handouts, overheads, and a supplementary bibliography.

After reviewing the requirements,14 faculty and advisory board members agreed to develop 19 curriculum modules (see Table 5). The project director matched the interest of the potential participant to curriculum needs identified in the gap analysis. For example, the gap analysis revealed the MSW foundation

TABLE 5. Modules Developed During Planning Phase

Title of Module	Type	Target Group
Diversity and Aging	Practice	MSW
Death and Dying	Practice	Two separate modules developed for BSW and MSW classes.
Gay and Lesbian Aging	Human Behavior/ Practice	BSW/MSW[1]
Grandparents Raising Grandchildren	Practice	Two separate modules developed for BSW and MSW classes.
Social Security Act	Policy	Two separate modules developed for BSW and MSW classes.
Older Americans Act	Policy	BSW
The Elder Immigration Experience	Human Behavior/ Practice	MSW
Overview of Older Adult Mental Health	Human Behavior/ Practice	BSW/MSW[1]
Differentiating the Three D's: Dementia, Delirium, & Depression	Human Behavior	MSW
Transference and Countertransference	Practice	MSW
Measurement and Ethics Research Module	Research	BSW
Operationalization and Measurement	Research	MSW
Instrumentation Research Module	Research	MSW
Social Work Administration: Social Capital to Serve the Aging	Practice	MSW
Spiritually Sensitive Social Work	Practice	BSW/MSW[1]
Assessing Family Caregiver Stress and Burden: Interventions and Resources	Practice	BSW/MSW[1]

[1] *Note*: Module developed so that it could be used either for BSW and MSW classes.

practice class had some content related to age as diversity. Therefore, the project director worked with faculty member responsible for this course on a module titled "Aging and Diversity" to expand on the gerontological content across all key areas (e.g., values, ethics, interviewing and assessment skills) of the course. All modules were completed by the start of the implementation year.

DISCUSSION

The use of a conceptual framework consistent with the mission of Department was critical to the success of the planning phase. This discovery is consistent with Rosen, Zlotnik, and Singer's (2002) assertion that widespread curricular change can not occur unless administrators and faculty are able to see the link between aging content and the departmental mission. For the AEP, the life-span perspective provided both a conceptual framework for how to begin the infusion process and the rationale for doing it. Since faculty were already committed to the importance of the life-span perspective, it was not difficult to convince them of the need to introduce more aging content in the curriculum. Expanding on the aging content that was already present in the foundation classes also made the infusion process less threatening to faculty.

The use of an advisory board proved to be a very important component of the AEP on many levels. Involving representatives from all the key constituencies in the aging network, raised the visibility of geriatric social work at CSULB and fostered new collaborative partnerships. The benefits of this collaborative approach occurred early in the project when an advisory board member approached the Department about working together on an interdisciplinary geriatric training grant. This grant opportunity provided further evidence to university administrators of the value of geriatric social work which, in turn, helped foster the investment in the curriculum reform process. Rosen, Zlotnik, and Singer (2002) described the competing interests as a potential barrier to curricular reform that social work educators must face when they attempt to raise the visibility of aging in the curriculum. The ideas and resources generated by the advisory board members kept the Department's attention on geriatric social work which helped the AEP overcome the challenge of competing interests.

The gap analysis was an important step in the infusion process. Singer (2000) described the infusion process as requiring aging content to be in every aspect of the curriculum. Conducting an assessment of the existing curriculum was the first logical step in the infusion process. Prior to the AEP, it was unknown to what degree aging content was already in the foundation classes. The UCLA/AGRP model provided a useful method for objectively assessing the status of the curriculum. Gaining a better understanding of what type of aging content was present or absent enabled the AEP team to better determine what curriculum modules were needed. Also, using the gap analysis approach helped the infusion process more accurately target the curriculum needs which, in turn, made the modules useful to faculty. As a result, the modules were accepted with gratitude by the faculty because they addressed an unmet need in the curriculum.

The data gathered from the student assessment were also helpful to the infusion process. For example, the student perspective on the presence of aging content in the curriculum closely paralled the findings of the gap analysis. Specifically, the gap analysis and the student assessment revealed that the exposure to aging content was the greatest in the human behavior classes and the lowest in research. This confirmatory information helped the AEP team proceed with more confidence on the modular development.

As expected, the OAF students reported having positive to very positive experiences with older adults, but it was unexpected that BSW and CYF students would also rate their experiences as positive. While social desirability bias could have played a role in how students responded (i.e., it may be difficult for social work students to ever report a negative experience with a particular client group), the fact that attitudes were more positive than expected provided hope for increasing interest in geriatric social work at CSULB. Similarly, interest in accepting a job working with older adults was higher than expected for CYF and BSW students. The results of Palmore's (1998) *Facts on Aging: Quiz 2* revealed that the three student groups could benefit from additional exposure to aging content. This finding justified the need to infuse all foundation courses.

The main accomplishment of the planning phase was the development of curriculum modules for the BSW and MSW foundation courses. The use of a life-span perspective as a guide to the modular development helped OAF and CYF faculty feel equally qualified to participate, which increased the numbers of faculty involved in curriculum reform. The use of the financial incentives generated interest in the modular development and helped faculty experience a direct benefit for their involvement. The use of a template as a guide in the module development ensured that modules were easy to use, which created good will among faculty members towards using the modules in their teaching.

The use of bridging approach (i.e., linked gerontology to child welfare and other topics relevant to the curriculum) for the topics and the life-span perspective provided a mechanism and conceptual framework to ensure that the modules were relevant for OAF and CYF students. This approach enabled faculty to think "out of the box" regarding the aging topics. As a result, the topics of the modules were far more creative and relevant to the curriculum than was expected. For example, the module on the "Elder Immigrant Experience" was pertinent to issues students encounter in the field because of the diversity of the Los Angeles Region and the high number of immigrants living in this area. The focus on immigration was also consistent with the mission of the Department to prepare students to work within a multicultural society. Similarly, the topic of "Gay and Lesbian Aging" was a good fit with the curriculum because of the emphasis on diversity issues. Expanding the students' knowledge on this topic was perceived as relevant because Long Beach area is home to a large gay population. It is interesting to note that many of the faculty and advisory board members became so interested in the topic of the module that they applied and were accepted to present on it at professional meetings.

IMPLICATIONS

The growth in the older adult population and the demand for better trained geriatric social workers challenge the existing curricula of social work programs at both the BSW and MSW levels. This awareness and the availability of funds has provided the impetus for a philosophical shift from a specialization only to an infusion-based approach in geriatric social work education at CSULB. This shift is congruent with the expressed aspirations of visionary social work educators who dared to think "out of the box" on how to prepare more students for competent practice with older adults (Berkman et al., 1997; Damron-Rodriguez et al., 1997; Lubben, Damron-Rodriguez, & Beck, 1992; Netting & Williams, 1998; Scharlach et al., 2000). Their efforts led to the funding opportunities made possible by the John A. Hartford Foundation, which has created a national movement to infuse aging content throughout the BSW and MSW curriculum.

Curriculum reform is a challenging undertaking at any level. Each program and educational institution experiences the process of curriculum reform in unique ways. This paper describes one program's experience of curriculum reform for the purpose of infusing geriatric content. The process has proven effective and it is hoped that it can serve as a guide to other social work programs that contemplate curricular changes with a similar objective.

REFERENCES

Berkman, B., Dobrof, R., Harry, L., & Damron-Rodriguez, J. (1997). White paper: Social work. In S. M. Klein (Ed.), *A national agenda for geriatric education: White papers* (pp. 53-85). New York: Springer.

Damron-Rodriguez, J., Villa, V., Tseng, H., & Lubben, J. (1997). Demographic and organizational influences on the development of gerontological social work curriculum. *Gerontology & Geriatrics Education, 17*(3), 3-18.

Lubben, J., Damron-Rodriguez, J., & Beck, J. (1992). A national survey of aging curriculum in schools of social work. *Journal of Gerontological Social Work, 18*(3/4), 157-171.

Netting, F. & Williams, F. (1998). Can we prepare geriatric social workers to collaborate in primary care practices? *Journal of Social Work Education, 34*(2), 195-210.

Palmore, E. (1998). *The Facts on Aging Quiz: Second Edition*. New York: Springer Publishing Company.

Rosen, A., Zlotnick, J., & Singer, T. (2002). Basic gerontological competence for all social workers: The need to "geronotologize." In M. Mellor and J. Irvy (Eds.), *Advancing Gerontological Social Work*, pp. 25-36. New York: The Haworth Press.

Scharlach, A., Damron-Rodriguez, J., Robinson, B. & Feldman, R. (2000). Educating social workers for an aging society: A vision for the 21st century. *Journal of Social Work Education, 36*(3), 521-538.

Singer, T. L. (2000). Structuring education to promote understanding of issues of aging. Retrieved July 28, 2003, from http://www.cswe.org/sage-sw/resrep/understandaging.htm.

U.S. Bureau of the Census. (1996). Current populations reports, Special Studies, pp. 23-190, 65 + in the United States. Washington, D.C.: U.S. Government Printing Office.

U.S. Bureau of the Census. (2000). *Current Population Report*. Washington D.C.: U.S. Department of Commerce.

Waldinger, R., & Bozorgmehr, M. (Eds.). (1996). *Ethnic Los Angeles*. New York: Russell Sage Foundation.

Zuckerman, R. (2002). UCLA/AGRP Curriculum Review. Unpublished Report. Los Angeles: University of California, Los Angeles.

doi: 10.1300/J083v48n01_06

Increasing Aging Content
in Social Work Curriculum:
Perceptions of Key Constituents

Stacey R. Kolomer, PhD
Terri Lewinson, LMSW
Nancy P. Kropf, PhD
Scott E. Wilks, LMSW

SUMMARY. This mixed methodology study examines the perceptions of key constituents regarding methods for effectively integrating aging content into the foundation curriculum of the BSW and MSW program at the University of Georgia School of Social Work. Students were asked to complete a survey to determine their perception of geriatric content that existed within the foundation coursework. Following an analysis of the survey results, eight semi-structured focus group discussions were conducted with a purposeful sample of students, faculty, field instructors, social work alumni, older adults from the community, and representatives from aging agencies. The intention of these focus groups was to find out what aging content should be infused within the curriculum. The focus

---

This project was made possible via a grant from the Geriatric Enrichment in Social Work Education (GeroRich) Program, funded by the John A. Hartford Foundation through the Council on Social Work Education.

[Haworth co-indexing entry note]: "Increasing Aging Content in Social Work Curriculum: Perceptions of Key Constituents." Kolomer, Stacey R. et al. Co-published simultaneously in *Journal of Gerontological Social Work* (The Haworth Press, Inc.) Vol. 48, No. 1/2, 2006, pp. 97-110; and: *Fostering Social Work Gerontology Competence: A Collection of Papers from the First National Gerontological Social Work Conference* (ed: Catherine J. Tompkins, and Anita L. Rosen) The Haworth Press, Inc., 2007, pp. 97-110. Single or multiple copies of this article are available for a fee from The Haworth Document Delivery Service [1-800-HAWORTH, 9:00 a.m. - 5:00 p.m. (EST). E-mail address: docdelivery@haworthpress.com].

group meetings were held in various locations throughout Northeast Georgia and in one remote location in South Georgia. Participants were interviewed about the necessary skills and knowledge for social workers practicing with an aging population in the areas of: essential intervention skills, program policies and regulations, critical information needed to develop client service plans, strategies for addressing service delivery fragmentation, and community collaboration to support intergenerational family needs. The results of this study will be discussed to provide suggestions on how existing foundation courses can integrate aging content. doi:

10.1300/J083v48n01_07 *[Article copies available for a fee from The Haworth Document Delivery Service: 1-800-HAWORTH. E-mail address: <docdelivery @haworthpress.com> Website: <http://www.HaworthPress.com>* © *2006 by The Haworth Press, Inc. All rights reserved.]*

KEYWORDS. Aging content, focus groups, key informants, infusion

The Administration on Aging ([AoA], 2000) has reported that by 2030 over 70 million persons living in the U.S. will be over age 65. In addition, the fastest growing age cohort is individuals over the age of 85 (Council on Social Work Education/Strengthening Aging in Gerontology Education for Social Work, 2001). With advances in medical technology, the influx of immigrant groups, and the baby boomer cohort on the verge of turning 60, in the future there will be a larger and more diverse group of older adults. Therefore, all human service professions are being challenged to reconsider how students are being prepared to work with older adults. Programs have to consider how to enhance training and increase exposure in and out of the classroom to issues affecting older adults. Social Work has been identified as a profession that will have a shortage of professionals skilled to provide services to a geriatric population. By 2010, it is estimated that there will be a need for 60,000-70,000 social workers to work specifically with older adults (CSWE SAGE-SW, 2001). Over the past 10 years, social work programs nationally have been increasing aging content within the curriculum. These initiatives were a response to demographic changes within the population, as well as opportunities and resources (e.g., John A. Hartford Foundation funding) to help schools increase content and capacity in aging (Kropf, 2001). In 2001, The John A. Hartford Foundation responded to the need to include aging knowledge in the social work curriculum by funding the Hartford Geriatric Social Work Initiative. One of the HGSWI projects, The Geriatric Enrichment in Social Work Education, provided funding to 67 programs to infuse additional aging content into the curriculum. This transformation was intended to be pervasive and sustainable (Hooyman, 2001).

While social workers are central to developing home and community-based services for our aging population, they often lack current gerontological knowledge and skills. Social workers have relevant foundation practice and policy content that includes a strengths-based emphasis on empowerment, capacity building, and health promotion. They are able to work with individuals, families, groups, communities, organizations, and in public policy arenas. Yet, most social workers lack adequate gerontological knowledge and skills that can enhance older people's opportunities and quality of life (The John A. Hartford Foundation, 2002).

Recognizing this inadequate preparation, the field of social work must be proactive in planning for current and future needs in assisting persons who are aging. Scharlach, Damron-Rodriguez, Robinson, and Feldman (2000) assert that the social work profession is not yet prepared for this growing demographic. Longevity creates a complex web of intergenerational kin relationships of four or five vertical generations in a family system. In addition, life longevity is related to an increase of various chronic illnesses and social workers will need to work in this realm of practice to provide long-term healthcare assistance. Social workers must also expand knowledge about subsets of the aging population (e.g., adults with developmental disabilities or persons who are incarcerated), so that specialized assessment and intervention methods can be appropriately designed and used with diverse segments of the aging population.

Understanding gender and ethnicity will be important, as differences exist between the life expectancy of females and males within various cultural communities (CSWE SAGE-SW, 2001; US Census, 2000). Another challenge for social workers is the need to be well informed about the mental and emotional functioning of the aged. For example, being able to recognize differences between dementia and depression is critical for solid assessments. Further, it is essential that social workers are familiar with policies that affect seniors. Practitioners not well versed in policies, service delivery, and resources for seniors are putting their clients at a disadvantage.

Scharlach and colleagues (2000) point out that the field of social work will be challenged because of the shortage of gerontological social workers, the lack of gerontological competence, negative attitudes toward older adults, inadequate social work curriculum in aging, lack of gerontological expertise among social work faculty, a cut-back in federal resources to train social workers in aging, and a lack of compensation for aging positions. Given this disturbing lack of preparation in the field of social work amidst the rising trend of elderly citizens and non-citizens, social work education must begin to increase the numbers of social work professionals who are competent to work with older adults and lead research in this national trend.

Researchers have identified several components necessary for preparing social work students including enhancing gerontology content (Lubben, Damron-Rodriguez, & Beck, 1992; Scharlach et al., 2000), training faculty (Kropf, Schneider, & Stahlman, 1993; Scharlach et al., 2000), building student interest in this area (Kosberg & Kaufman, 2002; Gorelik, Damron-Rodriguez, Funderburk, & Solomon, 2000; Scharlach et al., 2000), evaluative research (Scharlach et al., 2000), and improving prospects of vocational success in the field of aging (Peterson, 1990). Based on the findings of previous studies, it seemed the next logical step at the University of Georgia School of Social Work was to assess how to transform the learning experiences and strengthen the competence of both students and faculty via incorporation of aging content.

METHOD

In this study both quantitative and qualitative approaches were used. In the first phase of the study Bachelor of Social Work (BSW) and Master of Social Work (MSW) students were asked to complete a brief survey evaluating gerontological content from their foundation social work courses. There were several reasons for conducting this survey. First, surveying first year students allowed the researchers to capture those who may not have sought out gerontological knowledge and therefore may not have noticed if it was lacking in their studies. Secondly, as current students had recently taken the foundation courses, they had a fresher perspective on what was currently happening within the school, as opposed to what may have happened in years past. Finally, the initial survey served as a baseline for the future evaluation of the gerontological content inclusion in the school.

In the second phase of the study key informants of the School of Social Work were asked to participate in focus group meetings. The purpose of this phase of the study was to explore what specific subject matter, skills, and material were needed to increase the aging content within the foundation curriculum.

Data Collection

A sample of first year MSW and BSW students were asked to voluntarily complete the questionnaire in their research classes. Second year students were excluded because the survey was only inquiring about the foundation year courses. Second year students might not have accurate recall of their experiences in foundation courses taken a year before. The instrument asked for demographic information including age, gender, race, year in the program, status in the program (part time or full time), and desired area of future employment. No self-identifying information such as name or contact information was required. The BSW and MSW students were then asked to report how much geriatric content was included in their foundation courses (e.g., Human Behavior in the Social Environment, Policy, and Practice).

Results

A total of 96 surveys were completed out of a possible 107. Sixty-three of the students were in the MSW program and 33 of the students were in the BSW program. The mean age of the students who completed the survey was 26 years old ($SD = 6.8$). The youngest student was 21 years old and the oldest student was 75 years old. Of 10 male students only five completed the survey. Eighty-four percent of the students identified themselves as Caucasian, 10% as African American, 2% as Asian, 3% as Hispanic, and 1% as other.

The students answered eight questions about their experiences with aging issues in their classes. Table 1 illustrates how frequently aging content was the focus in foundation courses based on students' experiences in those classes.

TABLE 1. Geriatric Content in Social Work Courses as Reported by BSW (n = 33) and MSW (n = 63) Students

Course	Not discussed	Discussed very little	Discussed as much as other topics	**Most discussed topic**
BSW				
Human Behavior in the Social Environment	30%	67%	3%	0%
Research	52%	33%	12%	3%
Policy	6%	58%	33%	3%
Direct Practice	21%	52%	21%	6%
MSW				
Human Behavior in the Social Environment	5%	63%	30%	2%
Research				
Policy	32%	56%	13%	0%
Direct Practice	**50%**	**29%**	**9%**	**12%**

Overwhelmingly students reported that aging content was lacking across all foundation classes.

Qualitative Phase

Based on the results of the survey the researchers moved forward with exploring what specific aging and lifespan content should be included within the foundation courses, with the goal to increase students' exposure and awareness of the geriatric population. Information was also being sought about the types of resources needed to prepare students for working with older adults and which resources might be useful for faculty to use in their classes. Research questions included (1) what are the essential practice skills social workers need to acquire to work with older adults? (2) how can the curriculum be enhanced to address the social needs of older adults? and (3) in what way can the UGA School of Social Work participate in serving the needs of older adults in the community?

METHOD

Subjects

A critical component in considering how to change the curriculum in the School of Social Work was the inclusion of key informants in the process. For any proposed change to be successful it is important to recognize that all constituencies must support the idea of increasing the aging knowledge base of the school. By including representatives from both within the school and outside in the community, the direction can be more reflective of what changes are needed at the school from the perspective of all invested parties.

Participants in this study included students, faculty, field instructors, social work alumni, professionals from local aging agencies, and older adults from the community. The students were recruited from one BSW, one MSW, and one MSW part-time class. Community representatives included administrators from local senior centers, home health agencies, hospitals, and resources centers, School of Social Work alumni, and older adults who have an affiliation with the local senior center. The participants from the community were given an honorarium for their participation, but students were not.

Data Collection

Eight focus groups were conducted and facilitated by the researchers in classrooms and conference rooms. Each focus group had eight to twelve participants, with the exception of one group of 22 part-time students. Faculty and student group participants were first given a brief description of the project before being asked to participate. Those who volunteered to participate signed a consent form and received a copy of the questions to be discussed during the focus group. The researchers facilitated the semi-structured focus group meetings with the written questions guiding the open discussion among participants. The focus group meetings each lasted approximately one and a half to two hours. This process was also used with the community focus groups, except that participants were also asked to introduce themselves and the organizations represented.

The focus group questionnaire consisted of six questions covering the areas of practice knowledge and skills for working with older adults, as well as community strategies for improving services to this population. The questions can be found in Table 2.

Sufficient time was allocated to each question to allow participants to become immersed in the discussion and to think through responses. Through this method, a level of saturation was met as participants built off of each other's comments, confirming emerging ideas and perspectives until comments became repetitious. After the group progressed through the written questions, researchers asked participants if there were areas not addressed that pertained to the study as a means of obtaining any additional information that the questions may not have captured.

Responses were recorded for each focus group by use of microphones, tape recorders, and hand-written notes. Recorded data were transcribed. Hand-written notes were documented inside the transcribed reports.

TABLE 2. Interview Questions for Key Informant Focus Groups

1) When considering the expansion of aging content as a priority in the foundation curriculum at the University of Georgia School of Social Work, what are important themes and ideas that must be included?
2) What are the essential practice skills social workers need to acquire to work with older adults?
3) What knowledge of policies, regulations, and programs for older adults living in Northeast Georgia are necessary for social workers to have to be effective when working with this population?
4) What information is critical for social workers to know about developing service plans that address the needs of older adults and their families?
5) What are some strategies the School of Social Work can develop to address the fragmentation and barriers within the aging service delivery system in Northeast Georgia?
6) As CSWE/SAGE-SW have identified integenerational approaches as a priority to addressing the needs and strengths of older adults, their families and loved ones, how can the School of Social Work utilize the community to accomplish this goal?

Data Analysis

Transcribed data were analyzed for each focus group and across all focus groups to delineate major categories of response types. After major categories were found for each focus group, these categories were then compared across all focus group. Those categories that were found over two or more focus groups were reported as major categories in this study's findings. Emerging themes inside these categories were also identified and reported.

Findings

During data analysis, three major categories were identified: resources, curriculum content, and community partnerships. The resources category contained responses that pertained to the materials needed to facilitate the process of increasing aging content in the current social work curriculum. The themes for this category were faculty materials, student funding, and practicum placements.

RESOURCES

Faculty Materials. Respondents reported that existing faculty has had little preparation in teaching in depth aging topics. Content regarding older adults are the last chapters in textbooks and therefore are generally covered at the end of the semester. Faculty without expertise in the area often find themselves using guest speakers, either gerontologists or older adults from the community. A major theme that came from the groups was the need of faculty for need support in preparing their course plans to incorporate aging content. Faculty without a research interest in gerontology felt that they were at a great disadvantage when preparing lectures and discussions in this area. Specific requests included packages of classroom reading materials, video recommendations and activities that would facilitate discussions among students. Also, speakers and media presentations that would engage students in the dynamics of the older adult lifestyle are important. In addition, faculty reported needing assignments and classroom techniques in delivering the material using interesting methods.

Faculty members responded:

> Since I started teaching, when I hear from students what they wanted to do and who they want to work with, they are not interested in working with the aging population...And how do we present the material in a way that will interest students and not really scare them?

> Somebody should analyze if there are certain (aging) chapters, or can be such coursework and the idea of having modules to be able to make sure we are integrating it in would be very helpful.

Students pointed to other resource possibilities:

> In working with older adults there's a couple of things that we need to learn how to do and one of them is to give out...mini mental status and then there's an Alzheimer's assessment. And I know, I'm aware that we can't learn this in the classroom but even show a video or something just to give us some kind of idea of how these assessments are done and what they involve; assessments for dementia and a few of the tests that we are going to need to know how to do.

> I think that certain professors like _____ brought in the Council on Aging to talk to our class...the little bit I learned, it, it, has me wanting to know more about that population because I mean, like he said, it's inevitable we are going to be that population...And I would like to know more about that, um...but yeah, I think the professor has to be comfortable with it first.

A frequent concern regarding available teaching material about aging was the focus tended to be on disease, disability, and death. Participants felt that students are only exposed to the negative consequences of aging and therefore see it as a depressing time. Limited attention is paid to healthy and active aging. One older adult commented:

> Old age is not a disease. You need to get rid of the stereotypes. Older people are sexually active. Students should have a mandatory assignment of reading an article about sexuality and the older adult. Older adults are thriving people. (community participant)

Student Funding. Another resource identified was funding for students as an incentive for them to learn and participate more in the aging field. Respondents expressed that financial incentives have generally sparked interests in other neglected fields like child welfare and substance abuse. As funding in aging placements is limited, potential students are drawn to other areas of interest. With funded placements in agencies servicing older adults, it is likely that students will begin to recognize this field as a viable career option. Participants pointed out:

> ... the only reason there are so many students involved in child welfare right now is we're paying their tuition; ... money is a great motivator... reward people for doing it. (Faculty member)

And think of that as a connection [to] the first job that they get out of graduating from the BSW, MSW program. It might set their career for the rest of their lives. So, perhaps the notion of, of perhaps getting some stipend money to attract them into the aging areas. (Faculty member)

Practicum Placements. Focus group respondents reported a need for better promotion of existing practicum placements to students, as well as improved selection of students for community placements. The experience has been that placements for working with older adults are often turned down or selected last because of students' disinterest in working with this population. Also, there is at times a mismatch between the student selected and the placement because of the student's discomfort, lack of knowledge, and inexperience in working with older adults. Or, the problem may rest in the practicum supervisor having to invest an extended amount of time orientating and training the student on basic intervention methods because of the student's lack of practice readiness with this population.

… Students have a great concern about what to say to the clients. They become too focused in what they have to say rather than listening to the clients… (Service provider)

Exposure/Contact. Personal contact with older adults was a priority for many of the groups. The general feeling was that students who have living grandparents are more comfortable around older adults. Getting students connected with older people in the community may increase their interest in this population. Some tips on how to do this included guest panels, life reviews with seniors from local agencies, and site visits of local facilities.

Curriculum Content

Biophysical/Pharmaceutical. There was great concern among the student, faculty, and agency groups that students are not familiar with commonly prescribed medications for seniors. Students were concerned that without this knowledge they would have difficulty with licensing exams and securing positions in health care facilities. One graduate student commented,

I think it might be helpful to know what they (clients) are taking and what kind of symptoms they are going through, especially if they are taking pills and if they are having some type of reactions to the medications…

Another student commented on the different medications that the older adults in her agency were prescribed and expressed her frustration about not knowing what the medications were for.

> Some (clients) are on 15 medications where I work...It's incredible.... you wonder how you even talk to them because you do not know whether what they are exhibiting (behaviors) is due to the medications or due to some problem that they are having. You have no clue.

Ageism. Understanding discrimination against seniors and how it impacts their quality of life was reported by all groups as essential information for future social workers to receive. The faculty was honest about their own misconceptions about aging. In addition, the importance of acknowledging cultural and gender differences among older adults was noted. Making assumptions that all people over 65 are alike discounts unique cultural experiences that contribute to how a person functions as an older adult. As one older adult commented,

> Need to get rid of stereotypes about being older.
> More people rust out than wear out.

Intergenerational Family Support. There was concern in all of the groups that by separating older adults from other content areas, there is a lack of awareness that older people are a vital part of families. How families are defined needs to be broad and inclusive. In addition, recommendations were made to include curricular content on alternative family lifestyles, such as grandparents raising grandchildren, intergenerational households, gay/lesbian families, and single parents families.

COMMUNITY PARTNERSHIPS

Service Learning Projects. A common theme in the groups was the lack of exposure to aging agency settings. Unless a student's field placement was at an organization that served older adults, there was very little opportunity to visit such agencies. One recommendation was to incorporate service learning projects in aging agencies into foundation courses. Service learning connects life experiences with scholastic learning, personal growth, and civic responsibility. Creating partnerships between the school and area aging agencies would be a means of building linkages within the community. The agency representatives who participated in the focus group reported a willingness to have students come and volunteer at their agencies for service learning projects.

Incorporating activities and assignments in foundation courses where students are expected to contribute their time would provide additional exposure to work opportunities and local aging resources.

DISCUSSION

Developing Curriculum: Considerations

From the results of this study, it is clear that increasing aging content in the BSW and MSW curricula is essential for preparing effective and competent social work practitioners. At the time of the survey it was evident that students perceived that there was very little content focused on older adults in the social work foundation curricula. The greatest concern noted in the focus group discussions was the need to ensure that students in the social work programs are exposed to content on aging. In addition, the exposure must be adequately incorporated in generalist theoretical paradigms and infused in practice skills classes. Further, classes on community development and policy analysis must incorporate the issues relevant to the elderly, such as housing options, social security, and Medicaid/Medicare procedures, for students to learn effective intervention strategies in working with older clients and their families.

Students can also gain exposure to members of this demographic by the in-class pedagogical use of elder speakers, personal kinship assignments, service learning projects and examination of later adulthood stages earlier in the life cycle presentations. Training materials for educators should be developed to provide innovative methods to include aging content in subject area lectures. Web-based course modules would also increase the likelihood of instructors including aging material in their course preparation. Faculty buy-in is critical to the success of the infusion of aging and lifespan content so materials must be designed with faculty in mind.

Community agencies and representatives would like to see practicum students and graduated professionals come into their agency settings with practical knowledge and skills that enhance interventions with elderly populations. The social work curriculum must prepare students for competency in filling out patient chart paperwork, common pharmacology usage, interpersonal communication and assessment with elderly clients. In addition, students must overcome fears of working with older people and become confident and comfortable in agency settings with these clients. Students need to acquire more hands-on skills both in the classroom and in their agencies.

Finally, students and faculty must be aware of and dispel common misconceptions and stereotypes about the aging population. They must recognize that all elderly citizens do not age exactly alike. Therefore, assessment of life situations (e.g., physical health, income, sufficiency, sexual orientation and activity, mental health, subjective well-being) must be conducted on a case-by-case basis. Students should also be sensitive to the impact of ageism, policy decisions, and family relationships on the emotional and social health of an aging client.

For Schools of Social Work to successfully integrate aging content throughout the curriculum it is essential that all of the stakeholders have a voice in how the knowledge and skills are transferred to students. Just as older adults are diverse, so are Schools of Social Work. Each organization has its own culture and structure. Having buy-in from the constituents of the school increases the likelihood that products developed to infuse aging content across the curriculum will be utilized and sustainable. It is also essential to remember that change is a slow process. Not all of the stakeholders will immediately embrace transformation of the curriculum. Regardless of the resistance to change, it is imperative that Schools of Social Work ensure that future professionals are prepared to meet the needs of society's aging population.

REFERENCES

Administration on Aging. (2000). *A profile of older Americans 2000.* Available: www.aoa.dhhs.gov

Ashford, J., Lecroy, C., & Lortie, K. (2001). *Human behavior in the social environment.* Stamford, CT: Wadsworth.

Barusch, A., Greene, R., & Connelly, J. (1990). *Strategies for increasing gerontology content in social work education.* Washington, D.C.: Association for Gerontology in Higher Education.

Council on Social Work Education/SAGE-SW. (2001). *Strengthening the impact of social work to improve the quality of life for older adults & their families: A blueprint for the new millennium.* Washington, D.C.: Council on Social Work Education.

Damron-Rodriguez, J., Villa, V., Tseng, H., & Lubben, J. (1997). Demographic and organizational influences on the development of gerontological social work curriculum. *Gerontology & Geriatrics Education, 17*(3), 3-18.

Gorelik, Y., Damron-Rodriguez, J., Funderburk, B., & Solomon, D. (2000). Undergraduate interest in aging: Is it affected by contact with older adults? *Educational Gerontology, 26,* 623-638.

John A. Hartford Foundation (2004). Programs. Retrieved October 1, 2003. http://www.jhartfound.org/grants/grants.asp.

Kosberg, J., & Kaufman, A. (2002). Gerontology social work: Issues and imperatives for education and practice. *Electronic Journal of Social Work. 1*(1), 1-15.

Kropf, N. P. (2002). Strategies to increase student interest in aging. *Journal of Gerontological Social Work, (39)* 1/2, 57-67.

Kropf, N. P., Schneider, R. L., & Stahlman, S. D. (1993). Status of gerontology in baccalaureate social work education. *Educational Gerontology, 19*(7), 623-634.

Lubben, J., Damron-Rodriguez, J., & Beck, J. (1992). National survey of aging curriculum in schools of social work. *Journal of Gerontological Social Work, 18*(3-4), 157-171.

Peterson, D. (1990). Personnel to serve the aging in the field of social work: Implications for educating professionals. *Social Work, 35*(5), 412-415.

Scharlach, A., Damron-Rodriguez, J., Robinson, B., & Feldman, R. (2000). Educating social workers for an aging society: A vision for the 21st century. *Journal of Social Work Education, 36*(3), 521-538.

United States Census (2004). *Your Gateway to Census 2000.* Retrieved October 20, 2004 from http://factfinder.census.gov/servlet/.

doi: 10.1300/J083v48n01_07

A Competency Approach
to Curriculum Building:
A Social Work Mission

Colleen Galambos, MSW, DSW
Roberta R. Greene, PhD

SUMMARY. This article discusses The John A. Hartford Foundation CSWE SAGE-SW Project through an historical reflection of curriculum development within the profession. The project's relationship to several curriculum building models is also explored. A curriculum development tool for combining the Hartford Competencies with the CSWE EPAS requirements is provided. doi: 10.1300/J083v48n01_08 *[Article copies available for a fee from The Haworth Document Delivery Service: 1-800-HAWORTH. E-mail address: <docdelivery@haworthpress.com> Website: <http://www.HaworthPress.com> © 2006 by The Haworth Press, Inc. All rights reserved.]*

KEYWORDS. Gerontological competencies, social work competencies, curriculum development, competency based education

The aging of America is a significant trend that will continue to have an impact on our society. Today, elders make up 13% of the population and it is predicted that one out of every five persons in this country will be 65 years of age

[Haworth co-indexing entry note]: "A Competency Approach to Curriculum Building: A Social Work Mission." Galambos, Colleen, and Roberta R. Greene. Co-published simultaneously in *Journal of Gerontological Social Work* (The Haworth Press, Inc.) Vol. 48, No. 1/2, 2006, pp. 111-126; and: *Fostering Social Work Gerontology Competence: A Collection of Papers from the First National Gerontological Social Work Conference* (ed: Catherine J. Tompkins, and Anita L. Rosen) The Haworth Press, Inc., 2007, pp. 111-126. Single or multiple copies of this article are available for a fee from The Haworth Document Delivery Service [1-800-HAWORTH, 9:00 a.m. - 5:00 p.m. (EST). E-mail address: docdelivery@haworthpress.com].

or older by 2030 (AoA, 2000). In response to this unprecedented growth in the aging population and in acknowledgment of the need for an increase in social workers trained in gerontology, the John A. Hartford Foundation of New York City committed their resources to developing a sustained, focused, and centralized effort to strengthen the social work profession's response to the growing aging population (CSWE SAGE-SW, 2001).

The Hartford Foundation Geriatric Social Work Initiative's (HGSWI) major objective is to expand the depth of gerontological content in schools of social work, ultimately producing graduates who are better prepared to serve older adults. The initiative encompasses activities to support research scholars, establish innovative field units, and develop schools of social work curriculum resource centers. In 1999, the Hartford Foundation funded the CSWE SAGE-SW Project to establish what content is necessary to geriatric social work practice. The Project began with a survey that included sixty-five well-researched items specific to geriatric social work related to three domains: (1) knowledge about elderly people and their families, (2) professional skills, and (3) professional practice. The survey was mailed to 2,400 social work practitioners and academics, with and without aging interest. The outcome was a list of 65 competencies deemed necessary for practice at various educational levels. Since their development, the competencies have been used to establish student field units, to design faculty development institutes, and to build curriculum.

Similarly, in 2002, the Council on Social Work Education (CSWE) issued the profession's revised Educational Policy and Accreditation Standards (EPAS) (CSWE, 2002). EPAS "sets forth the basic requirements for curricular content and educational context that were thought necessary to prepare students for professional social work practice" (p. 3). Specifically, the standards define the foundation content–knowledge, values, and skills–that lead to "competent social work practice" (p. 6). Furthermore, the standards mandate that "students gain the knowledge and skills necessary to serve diverse constituencies, addressing clients' age, class, color, culture, disability, ethnicity, family structure, gender, marital status, national origin, race, religion, sex, and sexual orientation" (ibid). As with SAGE-SW Competencies, EPAS serves as a guide in establishing educational program objectives. How do these two initiatives support and complement each other? In what ways can they enhance content in gerontology?

The profession has not always had a clearly codified foundation, nor has it had a broad view of diversity or multicultural populations (De Anda, 1997; Hooyman, 1996). Rather, the history of social work suggests that the profession has been troubled with the number and nature of specializations (Frumkin & Lloyd, 1995). This lack of clarity continues today with far ranging choices of specializations including a focus on method, field of practice, problem areas, population groups, methodological function, geographic areas, size of target, specific treatment modalities, and advanced generalist (Popple, 1995). Thus, faculty who call for the inclusion of gerontological content in social work curriculum face many of the same hurdles as advocates for other specializations or population groups.

Inclusion of content on diversity in schools of social work curricula has had a similar, somewhat turbulent history. Attention to populations-at-risk has evolved over time, becoming increasingly broad and inclusive (Hooyman, 1996; Tully, 1994). This inclusiveness reflects the tumultuous political changes of the 1960s that began with the mandate that content on women and people of color be incorporated in curriculum content. Therefore, it is necessary to understand the CSWE SAGE-SW competencies and their relationship to EPAS within this historical context. This context encompasses four areas of professional concern discussed in this article: (1) recognizing competency-based education; (2) unifying the curriculum; (3) establishing a generalist base; and (4) expanding the parameter of cultural diversity within our professional accrediting body. The article also explores suggestions for infusing content on aging in the foundation areas.

RECOGNIZING COMPETENCY-BASED EDUCATION

Competency-based education concerns itself with what common body of knowledge, skills, and attitudes is considered so essential that every student should master them before leaving the educational environment. That is, what are the core concepts that are considered the cornerstone of formal education for a particular field? (Wendt, Peterson, & Douglass, 1993). Competence-based learning moves beyond simple knowledge acquisition and into application and skill development. It is concerned with both the obtainment of content and the application of this knowledge to the professional arena (Everwijn, Bomers, & Knubben, 1993).

Faculty may find some guidance for how one achieves competence based learning in the contrasting, but complementary, curriculum building models of Tyler and Schon (1969). Tyler espouses a method of curriculum building that begins with a definition of purpose and a clear conception of goals. He suggested that curriculum should always be planned and be considered a process involving continuous improvement. A basic curriculum plan would outline content, develop instructional procedures, test, and then evaluate these procedures regularly.

Tyler (1969) believed that education was intended to change behavior and norms, with teachers keeping in mind their conception of the standard or norm they want to achieve in the curriculum development process. Furthermore, for curriculum objectives to be relevant, they would meet contemporary needs with practitioners and educators determining the function and content. Philosophical beliefs would also drive a curriculum, and the development of curriculum objectives. Moreover, curriculum developers would be mindful about eliminating contradictory objectives that may be adopted due to philosophical differences. The major objective in curriculum building is to achieve a unified whole. Therefore, objectives should be integrated, coherent, and reinforce one another. Continuity, sequence, and integration, are key components in the development of a strong curriculum (Tyler, 1969).

Shon's (1983, 1987) approach to curriculum can be described as an epistemology of reflective practice. He believed that knowledge used in practice involved three competencies: Knowing in action, reflection in action, and reflection about action. The type of learning espoused by this model is dependent on the use of a problem-based curriculum and the development of mental schema. The paradigm shift as expressed by Shon suggests that professional education is characterized by competing values from different universes. Practice learning must address problems that are complex, unique, and lacking in certainty. Shon's model centers around four important questions:

- What is the nature of professional practice?
- What knowledge and competencies are needed and how are they acquired?
- What possibilities exist for articulating and codifying professional practice?
- What modes of initiation are appropriate for professional practice?

As with most professions, social work curriculum development began with the delineation of general areas of study. For example, in 1944, the American Association of Schools of Social Work (AASSW), one of the precursor organizations to CSWE, required the so-called basic eight curriculum: social casework, public welfare, social group work, community organization, administration, research, medical information, and psychiatric information (Frumkin & Lloyd,1995); while the National Association of Schools of Administration had a different list of study areas focused on macro-level aspects of practice. At the time of their merger as CSWE in 1950, the two associations had issued 32 conflicting standards.

Social work educators have gradually become advocates for a competency-based curriculum. For example, competencies for child welfare practice were established in the 1990s and federal funds were provided to increase the number of social work graduates competent in this field. It was not until 1992 that CSWE standards linked what a student is taught and what he or she was able to do–*a competency*. Namely, the need for schools to demonstrate that they had defined measurable learning objectives and an assessment plan to determine outcomes was added to the standards. This approach to learning encourages the development of skills for which knowledge acquisition is the foundation. The use of competencies provides a mechanism for monitoring and evaluating student performance and behavior as well as faculty performance. Evaluative mechanisms such as exam questions, capstone experiences, evaluation of student field placement performance, or paper requirements may also integrate the competencies.

A competence approach to social work practice is currently reflected in the profession's most important documents. For example, EPAS language directs educators to pay attention to the preparation of competent and effective professionals. The EPAS specifically states that the educational process is a mechanism for the integration of knowledge and skills to achieve effectiveness within the professional practice arena. It specifies that, "social work education enables students to integrate the knowledge, values, and skills of the social work profession for competent practice" (EPAS, p. 6). The National Association of Social Workers' Code of Ethics also grounds the mission of the profession in a set of core values including competence. The Code indicates that competence is an ethical obligation and mandates that, "Social workers practice within their areas of competence and develop and enhance their professional expertise" (p. 1).

UNIFYING THE CURRICULUM

Historically, social work education has searched for a conceptual definition of practice and struggled with the development of knowledge, values, and skills to support methods consistent with the purpose of the profession. Yet, the lack of unity and multiplicity of programs, services, and people served present a challenge to the development of this definition (Austin, 1986; Bartlett, 1970; Greene, 1994). Key milestones in the movement toward a common social work framework have included the 1923 through 1927 Milford Conferences that convened practitioners and educators who developed a single model for social work practice and the 1951 Hollis-Taylor study which recommended that professional social work education be represented by a single combined organization, rather than the seven existing specialty associations, inspiring the creation of CSWE.

The achievement of a unified knowledge base was greatly advanced by the Boehm (1959) curriculum study. With the suggestion that social work adopt person-in-environment as an overarching perspective, the Boehm CSWE–sponsored curriculum study became a turning point in the unity of the profession. The outcome of that work was the solidification of the professional goal of enhancing an individual's social functioning. Social work was thus defined as

> a profession concerned with the restoration, maintenance and enhancement of social functioning. It contributes, with other professions and disciplines, to the prevention, treatment and control of problems in social functioning of individuals, groups and communities. (Boehm, 1959, p. 1)

The study also concluded that curriculum should remain broad enough to encompass work in all settings; use of all practice methods, research, ethics and values; and field education. The profession has since struggled with this challenge.

ESTABLISHING A GENERALIST BASE

The Boehm initiative also began to define a generalist base that would support advanced specializations. Defining the priorities for the professional foundation has continued throughout the past decades (CSWE, 1984, 1992, 2002). During the 1980s, studies conducted among undergraduate program directors and deans and directors of masters degree programs revealed a high degree of consensus about the content of professional foundation at both educational levels (Eure, Griffin & Atherton, 1987; Griffin & Eure, 1986).

Various curriculum policy statements have continued the explication of the professional foundation (CSWE, 1984). More recently, EPAS has mandated content for the foundation courses (CSWE, 2002). The social work curriculum is structured in such a way that students are first exposed to a broad knowledge base that is germane to any type of professional practice. This broad knowledge base is referred to as generalist practice and can be defined as "the application of an eclectic knowledge base, professional values, and a wide range of skills to target systems of any size" (Kirst-Ashman & Hull, 1999, p. 5). Within the generalist framework, curriculum is organized around student's attainment of knowledge, values, and skills for each curriculum content area.

Knowledge refers to information needed to develop an accurate understanding of the client's life experiences and life patterns. It involves both an understanding of situational dynamics and the recognition of the type of skills necessary to address the situation. *Values* refer to what is considered important, worthy and valuable, and judgments about these factors. *Skills* refer to the approaches and activities necessary to plan and implement the change process. Social workers should obtain a solid base of skills for working at the micro, mezzo, and macro levels of practice (Kirst-Ashman & Hull, 1999).

As already stated, this broad knowledge base is one in which students should be able to demonstrate competency upon graduation. The generalist model is infused throughout the baccalaureate curriculum, and within the foundation courses at the graduate level. The second component of graduate level education includes emphasis on a specialization.

Given the agreement about what might constitute foundation program objectives, it was possible for the authors to develop an infusion curriculum model for integrating CSWE/SAGE-SW competencies with the CSWE EPAS (Greene & Galambos, 2002). This earlier publication meshed the CSWE SAGE-SW competencies with the eight learning areas (except field) described in EPAS.

The CSWE-SAGE-SW competencies provides the profession with a set of identified competencies that can be applied to generalist social work practice, as well as specialized social work practice in aging. Survey respondents were asked to indicate which competencies *all* social workers needed to know about gerontology and which constituted *specialized* knowledge for advanced practitioners. In the data analysis of geriatric social work competencies, the level of specialization needed was assessed through mean scores, with those closer to "1" being a competency for all social workers, and those near "2" or higher for those with more advanced or specialized education. Using the mean scores as a guide, these competencies may be applied to the generalist practice model. Competencies close to the "1" range are ones that should be included in baccalaureate or MSW foundation curriculum (Table 1).

As can be observed from Table 1, 20 out of the 65 SAGE-SW Competencies received a mean score of 1.50 or lower. These items are most appropriate for matching with the EPAS foundation objectives. Those SAGE-SW competencies with a mean score closer to 2 are most appropriate for integrating within specialization curricula.

Course objectives within the generalist curriculum content areas may be written to incorporate these competencies. Table 2 illustrates the placement of specific competencies from the CSWE SAGE-SW Project into EPAS foundation program objectives. The inclusion of aging competencies within accreditation standards will serve as a guideline for how specific aging related topics may be infused into the foundation curriculum. These competencies may help shape lecture content, reading assignments, and in-class exercises to promote student exposure to aging content.

The integration of the competencies within social work foundation courses will provide community agencies with information on what they can expect

TABLE 1. Knowledge Competencies

#	Knowledge Competencies	Mean
	Knowledge Competencies	
#	Knowledge Items	Mean
1	Normal physical, psychological and social changes in later life.	1.15
2	The diversity of attitudes toward aging, mental illness and family roles.	1.29
3	The influence of aging on family dynamics.	1.30
4	The diversity of elders' attitudes toward the acceptance of help.	1.43
5	The diversity of successful adaptations to life transitions of aging.	1.45
6	The availability of resources and resource systems for the elderly and their families.	1.48
7	Theoretical models of biological and social aging.	1.50
8	The relation of diversity to variations in the aging process (e.g., gender, race, culture, economic status, ethnicity and sexual orientation).	1.58
9	Wellness and prevention concepts for older persons.	1.67
10	The effect of generational experiences (e.g., the Depression, WWII, Vietnam War) on the values of older adults.	1.72
11	Love, intimacy and sexuality among older persons.	1.74
12	The impact of aging policy and services on minority group members.	1.78
13	The impact of aging policy and services on women.	1.79
14	The impact of policies, regulations, and programs on direct practice with older adults.	1.94
15	Managed care policies concerning older persons and adults with disabilities.	1.98
16	Policies, regulations and programs for older adults in health, mental health and long-term care.	2.01
17	Basic pharmacology and the interaction of medications affecting the elderly.	2.31
	Skill Competencies	
#	Skill Items	Mean
18	Use social work case management skills (such as brokering, advocacy, monitoring, and discharge planning) to link elders and their families to resources and services.	1.33

#	Skill Items	Mean
19	Gather information regarding social history such as: social functioning, primary and secondary social supports, social activity level, social skills, financial status, cultural background and social involvement.	1.34
20	Collaborate with other health, mental health and allied health professionals in delivering services to older adults.	1.42
21	Engage family caregivers in maintaining their own mental and physical health.	1.45
22	Assist individuals and families in recognizing and dealing with issues of grief, loss and mourning.	1.49
23	Assist families that are in crisis situations regarding older adult family members.	1.50
24	Recognize and identify family, agency, community, and societal factors that contribute to and support the greatest possible independence of the older client.	1.50
25	Enhance the coping capacities of older persons.	1.56
26	Incorporate knowledge of elder abuse (physical, sexual, emotional and financial) in conducting assessments and intervention with clients and their families.	1.56
27	Assess psychosocial factors that have an effect on the physical health of older persons.	1.61
28	Use empathetic and caring interventions such as reminiscence or life review, support groups, and bereavement counseling.	1.63
29	Demonstrate awareness of sensory, language and cognitive limitations of clients when interviewing older adults.	1.65
30	Gather information regarding mental status, history of any past or current psychopathology, life satisfaction, coping abilities, affect and spirituality.	1.68
31	Develop service plans that incorporate appropriate living arrangements and psychosocial supports for older persons.	1.70
32	Assist older persons with transitions to and from institutional settings.	1.73
33	Develop service plans that include intergenerational approaches to the needs and strengths of older persons, their families or significant others.	1.73
34	Gather information regarding physical status such as: disabilities, chronic or acute illness, nutrition status, sensory impairment, medications, mobility, and activities of daily living (ADLs) and independent activities of daily living (IADLs).	1.78

TABLE 1 (continued)

#	Skill Items	Mean
35	Provide information to family caregivers to assist them in caregiving roles, such as information about the stages and behaviors of Alzheimer's disease and other dementias.	1.83
36	Conduct a comprehensive biopsychosocial assessment of an older person.	1.89
37	Set realistic and measurable objectives based on functional status, life goals, symptom management, and financial and social supports of older adults and their families.	1.92
38	Reevaluate service or care plans for older adults on a continuing basis, incorporating physical, social and cognitive changes and adjusting plans as needed.	1.93
39	Assess and intervene with alcohol and substance abuse problems in older adults.	1.94
40	Assess organizational effectiveness in meeting needs of older adults and their caregivers.	1.98
41	Conduct long-term care planning with older persons and their families to address financial, legal, housing, medical, and social needs.	2.01
42	Identify mental disorders and mental health needs in older adults.	2.04
43	Demonstrate knowledge and ability to use relevant diagnostic classifications such as the DSM-IV for use with older persons.	2.12
44	Identify legal issues for older adults, including: advanced directives, living wills, powers-of-attorney, wills, guardianship, and Do-Not-Resuscitate (DNR) orders.	2.12
45	Adapt psychoeducational approaches to work with older adults.	2.14
46	Assess short-term memory, coping history, changes in socialization patterns, behavior, and appropriateness of mood and affect in relation to life-events of those who are aging.	2.14
47	Adapt assessment protocols and intervention techniques so that they are appropriate for older, vulnerable adults.	2.17
48	Assess for dementia, delirium and depression in older adults.	2.33
49	Conduct clinical interventions for mental health and cognitive impairment issues in older adults.	2.36
	Professional Practice Competencies	
#	Professional Practice Items	Mean
50	Assess one's own values and biases regarding aging, death and dying.	1.08

# ·	Professional Practice Items	Mean
51	Educate self to dispel the major myths about aging.	1.08
52	Accept, respect, and recognize the right and need of older adults to make their own choices and decisions about their lives within the context of the law and safety concerns.	1.10
53	Respect and address cultural, spiritual, and ethnic needs and beliefs of older adults and family members.	1.24
54	Identify ethical and professional boundary issues that commonly arise in work with older adults and their caregivers, such as client self-determination, end-of-life decisions, family conflicts, and guardianship.	1.36
55	Evaluate safety issues and degree of risk for self and older clients.	1.46
56	Apply knowledge of outreach techniques with older adults and their families.	1.57
57	Ensure clarity of social work roles in providing services to older clients, their caregivers, other professionals, and the community.	1.64
58	Engage and work with older adults of varying stages of functional need within the home, community-based settings, and institutions.	1.71
59	Advocate for the employment and retention of professionally educated social workers in the aging network and service delivery system.	1.72
60	Keep informed of changes in theory, research, policy, and practice in social work services to older persons.	1.79
61	Educate the public, other agencies and professional staffs on the needs and issues of a growing aging population.	1.85
62	Engage and mediate with angry, hostile and resistant older adults and family members.	1.88
63	Develop strategies to address age discrimination in relation to health, housing, employment, and transportation.	1.89
64	Creatively use organizational policy, procedures and resources to facilitate and maximize the provision of services to older adults and their family caregivers.	1.98
65	Develop strategies to address service fragmentation and barriers within the aging services delivery system.	2.10

TABLE 2. CSWE EPAS and the CSWE SAGE-SW Competencies

CSWE Foundation Program Objectives
and

The CSWE/SAGE-SW Gerontology Competencies

The professional foundation, which is essential to the practice of any social worker, includes, but is not limited to, the following program objectives: (EPAS, p. 9).

The CSWE/SAGE-SW knowledge, skills, and professional practice competencies considered necessary for all social workers: (CSWE/SAGE-SW, 2000).

Graduates demonstrate the ability to:

1. Apply critical thinking skills within the context of professional social work practice. *(Skills Competencies)*

- *Recognize and identify family, agency, community, and societal factors that contribute to and support the greatest independence of the older client.*
- *Incorporate knowledge of elder abuse (physical, sexual, emotional, and financial) in conducting assessments and interventions with clients and their families.*
- *Assess psychosocial factors that have an effect on the physical health of older persons.*
- *Demonstrate awareness of sensory, language, and cognitive limitations of clients when interviewing older adults.*
- *Conduct a comprehensive biopsychosocial assessment of an older person.*
- *Set realistic and measurable objectives based on functional status, life goals, symptom management, and financial and social supports of older adults and their families.*

2. Understand the value base of the profession and its ethical standards and principles, and practice accordingly. (*Values Competencies*)

- *Assess one's own values and biases regarding aging, death and dying.*
- *Educate self to dispel the major myths of aging.*
- *Accept, respect, and recognize the right and need of older adults to make their own choices and decisions about their lives within the context of the law and safety concerns.*
- *Identify ethical and professional boundary issues that commonly arise in work with older adults and their caregivers, such as client self determination, end-of-life decisions, family conflict, and guardianship.*
- *Evaluate safety issues and degree of risk for self and older clients.*

3. Practice without discrimination and with respect, knowledge, and skills related to clients' age, class, color, culture, disability, ethnicity, family structure, gender, marital status, national origin, race, religion, sex, and sexual orientation. (*Knowledge and Values Competencies*)

- *Understand the diversity of elders' attitudes toward the acceptance of help.*
- *Comprehend the diversity of attitudes toward aging, mental illness and family roles.*
- *Appreciate the diversity of successful adaptations to life transitions.*

4. Understand the forms and mechanisms of oppression and discrimination and apply strategies of advocacy and social change that advance social and economic justice. (*Knowledge and Skills Competencies*)

- *Respect and address cultural, spiritual, and ethnic needs and beliefs of older adults and family members.*
- *Develop strategies to address age discrimination in relation to health, housing, employment, and transportation.*

5. Understand and interpret the history of the social work profession and its contemporary structures and issues. (*Knowledge and Skills Competencies*)

- *The impact of aging policy and services on minority group members.*
- *The impact of aging policy and services on women.*
- *The impact of policies, regulations, and programs on direct practice with older adults.*
- *Policies, regulations, and programs for older adults in health, mental health, and long term care.*

6. Apply the knowledge and skills of a generalist social work perspective to practice with systems of all sizes. (*Knowledge and Skills Competencies*)

- *Use social work case management skills (such as brokering, advocacy, monitoring, and discharge planning) to link elders and their families to resources and services.*
- *Recognize and identify family, agency, community, and societal factors that contribute to and support the greatest possible independence of the older client.*
- *Understand the availability of resources and resource systems for the elderly and their families.*

7. Use theoretical frameworks supported by empirical evidence to understand individual development and behavior across the life span and the interactions among individuals and between individuals and families, groups, organizations, and communities. (*Knowledge Competencies*)

- *Gather information regarding social history such as: social functioning, primary and secondary social supports, social activity level, social skills, financial status, cultural background and social environment.*
- *Understand the theoretical models of biological and social aging.*
- *Comprehend normal physical, psychological and social changes in later life.*
- *Understand the influence of aging on family dynamics.*

8. Analyze, formulate, and influence social policies. (*Skills Competencies*)

- *Develop strategies to address age discrimination in relation to health, housing, employment, and transportation.*
- *Creatively use organizational policy, procedures, and resources to facilitate and maximize the provisions of services to older adults and their family caregivers.*
- *Advocate for the employment and retention of professionally educated social workers in the aging network and service delivery system.*

TABLE 2 (continued)

9. Evaluate research studies, apply research findings to practice, and evaluate their own practice interventions. *(Skills Competencies)*

- *Assess organizational effectiveness in meeting needs of older adults and their caregivers.*
- *Set realistic and measurable objectives based on functional status, life goals, symptom management, and financial and social supports of older adults and their families.*
- *Reevaluate service or care plans for older adults on a continuous basis, incorporating physical, social, and cognitive changes, and adjusting plans as needed.*

10. Use communication skills differentially across client populations, colleagues, and communities. *(Skills Competencies)*

- *Collaborate with other health, mental health and allied health professionals in delivering services to older adults.*
- *Engage family caregivers in maintaining their own mental and physical health.*
- *Assist individuals and families in recognizing and dealing with issues of grief, loss and mourning.*
- *Assist families that are in crisis situations regarding older adult family members.*

11. Use supervision and consultation appropriate to social work practice. *(Skills Competencies)*

- *Ensure clarity of social work roles in providing services to older clients, their caregivers, other professionals, and the community.*
- *Creatively use organizational policy, procedures, and resources to facilitate and maximize the provisions of services to older adults and their family caregivers.*
- *Collaborate with other health, mental health, and allied health professionals in delivering services to older adults.*

12. Function within the structure of organizations and service delivery systems and seek necessary organizational change. *(Skills Competencies)*

- *Assess organizational effectiveness in meeting the needs of older adults and their caregivers.*
- *Creatively use organizational policy, procedures, and resources to facilitate and maximize the provisions of services to older adults and their family caregivers.*
- *Collaborate with other health, mental health, and allied health professionals in delivering services to older adults.*

social work graduates to know about aging and older adults. Given the expected growth of the aging population, social work programs will increasingly be asked to meet the demands of these demographic changes. Providing clear guidelines in this area will assist in meeting the future demands of organizations and society.

CONCLUSION: EXPANDING THE PARAMETERS

The profession is challenged to continue to expand the parameters related to populations-at-risk and our expectation to provide services that are culturally and population sensitive (Tully & Greene, 1994; Galambos, 2003). To help achieve this goal, this article provided a discussion of various curriculum building models. It explored the development of social work competencies through an historical reflection of curriculum development within the profession. The authors illustrated how the Hartford Project provides the profession with identified competencies for generalist social work practice and social work practice in the specialized area of aging. Therefore, this information can serve as a guideline for curriculum development in both foundation and concentration courses. A discussion of how the John A. Hartford Foundation CSWE SAGE-SW Competencies inform curriculum building supported combining these competencies with the CSWE EPAS requirements.

The integration of the competencies within social work foundation courses will provide community agencies with information on what they may expect every social work graduate to know about aging and older adults. Given the expected growth of the aging population, social work programs will increasingly be asked to meet the demands resulting from these demographic changes. Providing clear guidelines in this arena will assist in meeting the future demands of organizations and society. Now is the time for these changes to occur within professional social work curriculum.

REFERENCES

Administration on Aging. (2000). A profile of older Americans: 2000. [On-line]. Available: www.aoa.dhhs.gov/aoa/stats/profile2000.

Austin, D. (1986). A history of social work education. *Social Work Education Monograph Series*. Austin, TX: University of Texas Press.

Bartlett, H. (1970). *The common base of social work practice*. New York: NASW Press.

Boehm, W.W. (1959). *Social work curriculum study*. New York: Council on Social Work Education.

Council on Social Work Education. (2002). *Educational policy and accreditation standards*. Alexandria, VA:Author.

Council on Social Work Education/SAGE-SW (2001). *Strengthening the impact of social work to improve the quality of life for older adults and their families: A blue print for the new millennium*. Alexandria. VA: Author.

Council on Social Work Education (1992). *Curriculum policy statement for master's degree programs in social work education*. Alexandria, VA: Author.

Council on Social Work Education (1991-1992). *Handbook of accreditation standards and procedures*. New York: Author.

Council on Social Work Education (1984). *Handbook of accreditation standards and procedures*. New York: Author.

DeAnda, D. (1997). *Controversial issues in multiculturalism*. Needham Heights, MA: Allyn & Bacon.

Eure, G.K., Griffin, J.E., & Atherton, C.R. (1987). Priorities for the professional foundation: Differences by program level. *Journal of Social Work Education, 21 (1),* 19-29.

Everwijn, S., Bomers, G., & Knubben, J. (1993). Ability or competence-based education: Bridging the gap between knowledge acquisition and ability to apply. *Higher Education, 25,* 425-438.

Frumkin, M., & Lloyd, G.A. (1995). Social work education. In R.L. Edwards (Editor-in-Chief), *Encyclopedia of Social Work* (vol. 3, 19th edition, pp. 2238-2247). Washington D.C.: NASW Press.

Galambos, C. (2003). Moving cultural diversity toward cultural competence in health Care. *Health and Social Work, 28 (1),* 3-7.

Greene, R.R. (Ed.) (1994). *Human behavior: A diversity framework*. New York: Aldine De Gruyter.

Greene, R.R. & Galambos, C. (2002). Social work's pursuit of a common professional framework: Have we reached a milestone? *Journal of Gerontological Social Work, 39 (½),* 7-23.

Griffin, J.E. & Eure, G.K. (1985). Defining the professional foundation in social work education. *Journal of Social Work Education, 21 (1),* 73-91.

Hooyman, N. (1996). Curriculum and teaching: Today and tomorrow. In *White paper on social work education–today and tomorrow* (pp. 11-24). Cleveland: Case Western Reserve University Press.

Popple, P. (1995). Social work profession: History. In R.L. Edwards (Editor-in-Chief), *Encyclopedia of Social Work* (vol. 2, 19th edition, pp. 2282-2292). Washington, D.C.: NASW Press.

Schon, D.A. (1983). *The reflective practitioner: How professionals think in action*. New York: Basic Books.

Schon, D.A. (1987). *Educating the reflective practitioner: Toward a new design for teaching and learning in the professions*. San Francisco: Jossey-Bass.

Tully, C.T. (1994). Epilogue: Power and the social work profession. In R.R. Greene (Ed.), *Human behavior: A diversity framework* (pp. 235-243). New York: Aldine De Gruyter.

Tully, C. & Greene, R. R. (1993). Cultural diversity defined: Twenty-one years of journal publications. *Arete, 19* (1), 37-45.

Tyler, R. W. (1969). *Basic Principles of curriculum and instruction* 2nd edition. Chicago: University of Chicago Press.

Wendt, P., Peterson, D.A. & Douglas, E.B. (1993). *Core principles and outcomes of gerontology, geriatrics, and aging studies instruction*. Washington, D.C.: Association for Gerontology in Higher Education.

doi: 10.1300/J083v48n01_08

Transforming the Curriculum
Through the Intergenerational Lens

Mildred C. Joyner, PhD
Eli DeHope, PhD

SUMMARY. Our society is aging at a rapid rate and with this trend comes many of the social and economic demands that the profession of Social Work addresses. A key dilemma of the profession is how to interest and educate undergraduate social work students in aging and gerontology so that the needs of elderly can be supported. Social Work students notoriously are primarily interested in working with children and adolescents. With the support of the John A. Hartford Foundation's *Geriatric Enrichment in Social Work Education* grant, the authors developed a *Spiral Perspective* to infuse intergenerational content into the curriculum of their department and to give students exposure to geriatric content throughout their educational experience. doi: 10.1300/J083v48n01_09 *[Article copies available for a fee from The Haworth Document Delivery Service: 1-800-HAWORTH. E-mail address: <docdelivery@haworthpress.com> Website: <http://www.HaworthPress.com> © 2006 by The Haworth Press, Inc. All rights reserved.]*

KEYWORDS. Aging, elderly, intergenerational, social work education, spiral perspective

The United States is aging. In 1900, the average person in the United States lived 47 years; by 2000 life expectancy had increased to 76 years (United States Census,

[Haworth co-indexing entry note]: "Transforming the Curriculum Through the Intergenerational Lens." Joyner, Mildred C., and Eli DeHope. Co-published simultaneously in *Journal of Gerontological Social Work* (The Haworth Press, Inc.) Vol. 48, No. 1/2, 2006, pp. 127-137; and: *Fostering Social Work Gerontology Competence: A Collection of Papers from the First National Gerontological Social Work Conference* (ed: Catherine J. Tompkins, and Anita L. Rosen) The Haworth Press, Inc., 2007, pp. 127-137. Single or multiple copies of this article are available for a fee from The Haworth Document Delivery Service [1-800-HAWORTH, 9:00 a.m. - 5:00 p.m. (EST). E-mail address: docdelivery@haworthpress.com].

2000). Not only is the population of the United States aging, there are more elderly people than ever before. Today there are 35 million individuals over 65. By 2040, the number is expected to grow to 78 million. Not only is the elderly population growing in size, but the older population, those 85 years and over, showed the highest percentage increase, making up 12 percent of the elderly. Women comprise the largest portion of elderly. In 2000, there were 20.6 million women over the age of 65, and 14.4 million men in that same category (United States Census, 2000).

The aging of our society has many implications for social and personal economic conditions, health care provisions, care-giving issues and family relations. What is clear is that younger people entering the social work profession need to understand the elderly and the implications of this growing population for all areas of social work practice. Beginning social work students appear to prefer working with children and adolescents, often expressing fear when considering work with older adults.

As a result of the projected increase of elderly in our society, the John A. Hartford Foundation awarded grant monies to 67 social work programs at universities and colleges throughout the United States to promote infusion of geriatric content and experiences in social work education. The major focus of the grant was to infuse and sustain geriatric content in the curriculum of social work education (John A. Hartford Foundation Geriatric Social Work Initiative, 2001). The grant proposed to do this in three broad categories: (1) the education of the faculty about aging; (2) the infusion of geriatric content into coursework; and (3) the exposure of students to aging.

SURVEY OF STUDENTS

Shortly after receiving the grant, our department surveyed the undergraduate social work students to see what interest there was in working with the elderly. Survey results showed that the majority of students expressed an interest in working with children or adolescents. In fact, only 16% of the students demonstrated a preference for practice with adults or the elderly (Table 1). Only 7% identified a desire to practice with the elderly.

TABLE 1. Survey of Students–Prior to Implementation of Grant–Practice Area Interest

Interest in Children	62%
Interest in Adolescents	22%
Interest in Adults	9%
Interest in Elderly	7%

Scharlach, Damron-Rodriguez, Robinson and Feldman (2000) noted that more social workers are needed to serve the elderly than those that are currently trained. "Gerontological social work ranked fifth behind mental health, child welfare, health and family service" (p. 54). It is clear that more social workers will need to be trained in order to meet the needs of an aging society. Peterson and Wendt (1990) noted that over half (62%) of NASW members reported a need for knowledge of the elderly in their professional positions. Yet, most students in baccalaureate social work (BSW) level education programs are not exposed to gerontology; BSW programs lack gerontology courses, gerontology specializations, aging content reflected in core courses or a large number of students in aging field placements (Scharlach et al., 2000).

A departmental survey of the student perspectives and myths of aging was also conducted prior to implementation of the grant. One of the more interesting results of this survey was that the majority of students identified "being old" as meaning people over the age of 50 (Table 2). In the survey, students saw older individuals in a negative way, expressing a view that the elderly are always complaining and usually sick. Students also expressed a fear of working with older adults, sensing their own inadequacy for dealing with death and illness.

"Ageism is similar to racism and sexism in that it involves discrimination, placing older people in a marginal social position. Ageism in the social work profession can lead to making treatment judgments and policy decisions based upon stereotypes" (Scharlach et al., 2000, p. 84).

TABLE 2. Summary of Pertinent Questions on a Survey of Students–Prior to Implementation of Grant–Perspectives of Aging

"Being Old" means...	Over age 50	74%
	Over age 60	23%
	Over age 65	01%
	Over age 70	02%
Elderly people are...	Always Complaining	82%
	Usually sick	88%
	Don't have sex	94%
Students expressed...	Fear of death	79%
	Fear of dealing w/death	93%
	Fear of aging	53%
	Fear of health issues	89%

SURVEY OF FACULTY AND CURRICULUM

Faculty, too, were surveyed for their expertise in aging. Of the six full-time faculty members, only one (and one of the co-project directors of the grant) had expertise in gerontology through education and practice. Coursework also lacked geriatric content (Table 3). Only one foundation course included geriatric content at the onset of the grant. Damron-Rodriguez et al. (1997) point out that a significant reason why gerontology is not infused into the curriculum of social work education programs is due to the lack of faculty who have been trained in aging.

Upon receiving the grant, it became apparent that the faculty of the Department, while supportive and willing, were concerned about the exclusive focus of gerontology. A major part of BSW education, in fact, is to teach *generalist practice*. As a result, it quickly became apparent that geriatrics alone could not be addressed when changing coursework. The faculty agreed to use an *intergenerational approach* when changing curriculum and teaching their courses.

THE SPIRAL PERSPECTIVE

The generalist intervention model (GIM) is characterized by four major features. First, the model is based on a foundation of knowledge, skills, and values which reflect the unique nature of social work. Second, GIM is oriented toward solving problems, which involve not only individuals, but also groups, organizations, and even major social policies. In other words, the model involves micro, mezzo, and macro systems as targets of change. Third, the model's generalist approach means that virtually any problem may be analyzed and addressed from a

TABLE 3. Faculty Survey of Teaching and Curriculum

	Prior to start of grant	After grant implementation
Faculty teaching foundation/required courses who have made structural changes to their syllabi and in their teaching		
Full Time Faculty	1	6
Number of foundation/ required courses including geriatric content	1	10

wide range of perspectives. Fourth, GIM uses a specific problem-solving method which is infinitely flexible in its application (Kirst-Ashman & Hull, 1993, p. 9).

Currently the field of social work and social work educators teach relevant course content that helps students integrate and infuse curriculum content so that students can work with a diverse group of people. Many baccalaureate and some master social work programs teach course content in a linear approach, beginning, middle and end. In fact, the interactional model states a focus on the "dynamic interaction with many important social systems (e.g., family, school, hospital)" (Shulman, 1999, p. 9). This assumes that there are "essential symbiotic relationship between people and their social surroundings ... this mutual need is systematically blocked by obstacles ...[and] the social worker must always assume and reach for the client's (and system's) strengths for change" (p. 9).

This linear approach may suggest to students that problems, no matter how complex, can and must be solved. This problem solving method often confuses new social work practitioners. Students often offer simplistic solutions to complex issues that clients face day to day. Social work students often utilize a problem solving method by offering concrete needs and services to clients, rather than exploring the issues from a client perspective. It is often hard for students to learn that people will have problems. Perhaps social work educators are to blame for students' naiveté. "Human behavior in the social environment (HBSE) focuses on the Systems Impact Model (SIM) propose that social work practitioners work not only with clients to solve client problems but with many other systems with which the client is involved" (Kirst-Ashman & Zastrow, 2001, p. 25).

The course content, nevertheless, is generally taught from life cycle development stages: birth to aging; beginning to end; alpha to omega. Students begin the HBSE sequence learning about birth and the issues that come with raising a family. Social work students often conclude the HBSE sequence focusing on aging and death. No wonder most students who enter social work state they would like to work with children. How has the social work profession helped students to learn about the complexity of working with families? "Families are made up of people who have a common history, experience a degree of emotional bonding, and engage in shared goals and activities. Family issues and concerns may include physical survival, social protection, education, and development" (Thomlinson, 2002, p. 4). Very rarely does the student engage in learning the *spiral perspective*, which includes all of the challenges that families will face on a micro, mezzo, and macro level. By focusing on the *spiral perspective*, an array of theories and methods can be utilized, and the challenges and opportunities that families face on all levels of practice will be the foci of the students' work with clients.

Intergenerational family issues engage students and by exposing them early to older people who are also a part of families, this may assist students to love the field of gerontology. Teaching from an intergenerational approach for social work courses seemed to be a viable and valid idea, but one that appeared to lack some of the dynamics of real life. As a result, a *Spiral Perspective* was created and applied with the intergenerational concept. The main focus of this perspective was for the process of aging to be seen simultaneously within various stages of the life cycle. This premise supposes that students are exposed to the theoretical and realities of aging through direct interactions with people of all age groups. Within the *Spiral Perspective*, students are given a framework to understand that people will always have problems; that these problems are dynamic, integrative and interdependent with other problems that people have experienced; and that social workers need to manage the critically significant issues without assuming the problems have totally been solved. The *Spiral Perspective* with the intergenerational lens holds three major goals:

- Each of the core courses in a BSW educational program should reflect the understanding that aging is fluid and can be seen from all ages' perspectives;
- Students in a BSW educational program should work closely with older people, using task-centered approaches to assist with solving problems; and
- The values of students in a BSW educational program need to be targeted in order to promote a receptivity and understanding of elders.

The core courses in a BSW educational program can reflect that aging is fluid by teaching the students from the perspective of where they are at in the life cycle. Typically social work educators focus on the multiple linear problems of clients rather than the complex *spiral perspective* that is their lives. Social work educators do a disservice to their students by teaching mainly toward the presenting problem. Even social services are based on this linear, one issue concept (i.e., "child welfare," "mental health," "aging"). Clients have multiple issues and professionals know that multiple tasks within a complex process are the norm; students need to understand this concept. Assessment of clients should be taught by looking at the client's complex spiral and using the problem-solving method based on this interconnected, multi-layered approach. Students need to be pushed to become aware that each professional experience demands an analysis of the layers of issues affecting the client and those people in the client's life.

One of the key lessons that students could learn from the *spiral perspective* is that everyone from all age groups has problems or issues. At times, these problems or issues may interface with each other and influence multiple generations at the same time. Problem solving, therefore, needs to occur through an analysis of the complex *spiral perspective.*

Students can also be taught ways to confront current issues using an inter-generational lens. One of the important aspects of the *spiral perspective* is to create ways for students to understand issues from various generational perspectives. Family therapists already understand the need to approach therapy with an intergenerational lens (Framo, 1992; Gehart & Tuttle, 2003). Further, many suggest that the "Baby Boom" generation will seek a more integrative role in society and demand ongoing interaction with those of all ages (Freedman, 2000).

The intergenerational *spiral perspective* can also be introduced to students utilizing the Task Centered Approach (Reid, 1992). Within this model, social workers can see that problems occur within the context of the interaction of the individual, family and environmental systems. A practical example when teaching the Task Centered Approach using the intergenerational *spiral perspective* would be for students to negotiate contracts with their clients by including the various generations in the family that may be affected by the presenting problem.

TEACHING THROUGH THE INTERGENERATIONAL SPIRAL PERSPECTIVE

Introducing new BSW students to aging. At the introductory level, students in a BSW educational program can be introduced to elders through service learning projects in the beginning courses. Bringing students and elders together early in the student's educational process may promote understanding and create interest in working with older adults. For example, students can interview a volunteer elder from the community three times over the course of a semester. Within this experience, the student can work with the interviewed elder to develop a resource book for them. To develop interviewing and assessment skills, the student can put together a biographical timeline of the elder's life and events. They can create a genogram of the elder's family in order to understand intergenerational relationships and perspectives. In addition, the student can compile a medical timeline for the elder as well to be used by the older adult during medical appointments. The book can also include community resources that the elder can use.

Infusing aging into the curriculum. Two key strategies to move aging into all areas of the curriculum are: (1) through a comprehensive review of all courses and (2) by training faculty in aging and use of the *Intergenerational Spiral Perspective.*

As students progress through the educational process, students can be exposed to elders through the BEST Club (Bringing Elders and Students

Together). Older individuals from the community are brought into classrooms as speakers about a variety of subjects. Elder volunteers who are part of the BEST Club assist beginning social work students in mock interviews that can be video taped for review. Topics for the mock interviews can include intergenerational issues that reflect real family experiences.

Service learning throughout the student's educational process is a great vehicle to expose students to elders and intergenerational aging issues. In the policy class, for example, students complete a community-based project in which they advocate for older adults. Students in our department hosted a *Town Meeting* which brought together key stakeholders from various agencies that worked with older adults, including the Social Security Administration, Area Agency on Aging, and Senior Centers. Another policy class produced a conference on intergenerational care giving, which brought elders, caregivers, professionals and politicians together.

Diversity can also be taught through the *spiral perspective*. In a class that focuses on understanding diversity, for example, a course requirement could be for the student to interview the eldest member of their family regarding a specific family event or just to understand their family dynamics and history.

In HBSE, students can be taught the development of the life cycle by moving from the student's stage of life, which they currently experience. The student can explore all individuals who are important to them, including those from other generations, when looking at human behavior in the social environment.

In the practice class, students can discuss a topic or issue by moving from the student's stage of life and understanding what other people of different ages may experience on the topic as well.

The *spiral perspective* through the intergenerational approach can be accomplished in a number of other ways, including the use of videos in classes that reflect the intergenerational perspective of life; use of internet links that reflect organizations which deal with all ages; use of articles that reflect all age group issues; viewing the life-cycle from all perspectives when presenting a case in class and using speakers of all ages.

RESULTS OF TEACHING THROUGH THE SPIRAL PERSPECTIVE

Students were again surveyed on their interest in areas of practice after the intergenerational spiral model was implemented in our Department with support of the grant. Using the spiral perspective, students were provided ongoing interactions with elders and taught to consider all generations and how they are affected by the presenting problem when making an assessment.

The results were remarkable. The number of students interested in working with the elderly after graduation went from 7% to 15% (Table 4). Students reported a sense of "understanding" older adults more than before their experiences. In fact, some students were impressed with the elders they met and began to reevaluate their ideas of aging. A key change with the students who were exposed to elders and their families was the increased understanding that issues affect all generations of the family. Almost all of the students (92%) gained perspective on intergenerational links when confronting an issue.

The student's belief in the myths of aging also showed signs of change. Students who formerly perceived "being old" as anyone over age 50 moved that age upwards. In addition, students' perceptions of elderly people moved toward a more positive sense of the older age group (Table 5). Many students

TABLE 4. Survey of Students–After Implementation of Grant–Practice Area Interest

	Prior	After
Interest in Children	62%	57%
Interest in Adolescents	22%	20%
Interest in Adults	9%	8%
Interest in Elderly	7%	15%
Do you think that issues that affect one generation of a family affect all generations in that family, including the elders?		92%

TABLE 5. Summary of Pertinent Questions on a Survey of Students–Prior to Implementation of Grant–Perspectives and Myths of Aging

	Prior	After
"Being Old" means...	Over age 50: 74% Over age 60: 23% Over age 65: 01% Over age 70: 02%	Over age 50: 23% Over age 60: 20% Over age 65: 20% Over age 70: 37%
Elderly people are...	Always Complaining: 82% Usually sick: 88% Don't have sex: 94% Are healthy: 12%	Always Complaining: 65% Usually sick: 62% Don't have sex: 56% Are healthy: 48%
Students expressed...	Fear of death: 79% Fear of dealing w/death: 93% Fear of aging: 53% Fear of health issues: 89%	Fear of death: 72% Fear of dealing w/death: 88% Fear of aging: 45% Fear of health issues: 63%

reported that they did not associate individuals known to them with the age group they thought as "old." For example, many saw their grandparents or well-known actors and musicians as young and vital. When they realized their age, their perception of "old" appeared to change. In addition, meeting elders through service learning projects or classroom speakers influenced students into reevaluating the concept of "age."

CONCLUSION

Social work students need to develop knowledge, values and skills to work with the elderly. Traditionally, students do not readily choose to work with older adults; rather preferring children and adolescents. Without exposure to issues of aging and elderly individuals, students may not receive sufficient experiences that would prepare them to work with people of all generations. Social Work educators, too, struggle with their own knowledge and skills in gerontology. It is clear that social work departments need to infuse aging into their curriculum and experiences for students to benefit in an aging society.

Through assessing intergenerational issues and critically reflecting on their own events and situations, students learn the *spiral perspective*, an intergenerational model which promotes an understanding of clients' problems through the dynamic, multi-layered assessment approach.

Thomlinson (2003) points out that this concept of educating from where the student is in the life cycle is very powerful.

They [students] also were able to integrate family content knowledge with life experiences to assist their understanding of family dynamics. They were able to examine the process of family–their own–in order to understand the family as a constantly changing system influencing belief systems, behaviors, and relationships. Finally they were able to build on what they bring from family experiences, to personalize their approach to practice and learning, and to understand the diversity of ideas and outcomes when applying the family assessment process to learning (Thomlinson, 2003, p. 17).

The *spiral perspective* gave students a greater understanding that families they serve will have multiple problems, with multiple solutions, inter-related with others in the client system. The social work students also realize that the family unit, complete with multiple generations, has unique strength and resiliency coupled with multiple coping strategies to assist members through lifecycle development.

REFERENCES

Ashman, K., & Hull, G. (1993). *Understanding generalist practice.* Chicago, IL: Nelson-Hall.

Ashman, K., & Zastrow, C. (2001). *Understanding human behavior and the social environment.* Pacific Grove, CA: Brooks/Cole Thomson Learning.

Damron-Rodriguez, J. & Lubben, J. (1997). The 1995 WHCoA: An Agenda for Social Work Education and Training. *Journal of Gerontological Social Work, 27* (3), 65-78.

Framo, J. (1992). *Family-of-origin therapy: An intergenerational approach.* New York, NY: Taylor & Francis.

Freedman, M. (2000). New possibilities for the longevity revolution. *Exchange: A Newsletter of Intergenerational Issues, Programs, and Research, 15* (2), pp. 221-227.

Gehart, D., & Tuttle, A. (2003). *Theory-based treatment planning for marriage and family therapists: Integrating theory and practice.* Pacific Grove, CA: Wadsworth.

Peterson, D. A., & Wendt, P. F. (1990). Employment in the field of aging: A survey of professionals in four fields. *The Gerontologist, 35,* 489-497.

Reid, W. J. (1992). *Task strategies: An empirical approach to social work practice.* New York, NY: Columbia University Press.

Scharlach, A., Damron-Rodriguez, J., Robinson, B., & Feldman, R. (2000). Educating social workers for an aging society: A vision for the 21st century. *Journal of Social Work Education, 35* (3), 83-95.

Shulman, L. (1999). *The Skills of helping individuals, families, groups, and communities.* Chicago, IL: F.E. Peacock.

Thomlison, B.(2003). *Family assessment handbook.* Pacific Grove, CA: Brooks/Cole.

U.S. Bureau of the Census. (2000). *The 65 year old population: Census 2000 Brief.* Washington, D.C.: U.S. Government Printing Office.

doi: 10.1300/J083v48n01_09

Developing Geriatric Social Work Competencies for Field Education

JoAnn Damron-Rodriguez, LCSW, PhD
Frances P. Lawrance, PhD, MSW
Diane Barnett, MSW
June Simmons, LCSW

SUMMARY. Preparing social workers to effectively practice with the growing older population requires the identification of geriatric competencies for the profession. The John A. Hartford Geriatric Social Work Initiative provided the impetus and direction for a national strategy to improve the quality of preparation of geriatric social workers. The Geriatric Social Work Practicum Partnership Program (PPP) is the project with the Hartford Initiative that emphasizes field education. The Geriatric Social Work Education Consortium (GSWEC), one of the PPP programs,

---

The authors which to acknowledge Patricia J. Volland, Principal Investigator of the Practicum Partnership Program and Principle Investigators of the PPP demonstration sites: Hunter College/Brookdale Center on Aging: Joann Ivry, PhD, and Rose Dobrof, DSW; UC Berkley: Andrew Scharlach, PhD, and Barrie Robinson, MSSW; University at Albany, SUNY: Anne E. Fortune, PhD; University of Houston: Virginia Cooke Robbins, MSW; University of Michigan: Ruth Dunkle, PhD, and Lily Jarman-Rohde, MSW.

This study was funded by grants from the John A. Hartford Foundation and the Archstone Foundation.

[Haworth co-indexing entry note]: "Developing Geriatric Social Work Competencies for Field Education" Damron-Rodriguez, JoAnn et al. Co-published simultaneously in *Journal of Gerontological Social Work* (The Haworth Press, Inc.) Vol. 48, No. 1/2, 2006, pp. 139-160; and: *Fostering Social Work Gerontology Competence: A Collection of Papers from the First National Gerontological Social Work Conference* (ed: Catherine J. Tompkins, and Anita L. Rosen) The Haworth Press, Inc., 2007, pp. 139-160. Single or multiple copies of this article are available for a fee from The Haworth Document Delivery Service [1-800-HAWORTH, 9:00 a.m. - 5:00 p.m. (EST). E-mail address: docdelivery@haworthpress.com].

initiated the development of competencies for work with older adults. GSWEC utilized Geriatric Social Work White Papers and the pioneering work of the Council on Social Work Education's (CSWE) Strengthening Aging and Gerontology Education for Social Work's (SAGE-SW) comprehensive competency list as well as conducted focus groups locally to delineate key competencies for field education. The Coordinating Center for the PPP, located at the New York Academy of Medicine, led in collaboratively developing knowledge based skill competencies for geriatric social work across all 6 demonstration sites (11 universities). The competencies adopted across sites include skills in the following five major domains: values and ethics; assessment (individuals and families, aging services, programs and policies); practice and interventions (theory and knowledge in practice, individual and family, aging services, programs and practice) interdisciplinary collaboration; and evaluation and research. The identified competencies have proven effective in evaluating students (n = 190) pre- and post PPP field education. The implications for further development of competency driven education for geriatric social work are discussed. doi: 10.1300/J083v48n01_10 *[Article copies available for a fee from The Haworth Document Delivery Service: 1-800-HAWORTH. E-mail address: <docdelivery@haworthpress.com> Website: <http://www.HaworthPress.com> © 2006 by The Haworth Press, Inc. All rights reserved.]*

KEYWORDS. Geriatric social work competencies, geriatric/gerontological education, geriatric training, social work competence, social work education

CONTEXT OF COMPETENCY DEVELOPMENT

The demand for social workers with the specialized knowledge and skills necessary to meet the needs of a rapidly growing aging population is well documented (Berkman, Dobrof, Harry, & Damron-Rodriguez, 1997; Hudson, Gonyea, & Curley, 2003; Scharlach, Damron-Rodriguez, Robinson, & Feldman, 2000). However, the identification of the specific practice skills required for social work with older adults is a work in progress for the profession. The development of geriatric social work competencies must be framed within an understanding of the differences and relationships of values, knowledge, and skill in social work practice generally. Additionally, the content of competencies for practice with older adults must be specifically delineated.

Values, knowledge and skill are all fundamental to social work practice (Brown, 1996). Vass (1996), however, asserts that social work values and knowledge are important primarily in their application in practice. Vass states that social work competence is the achievement and demonstration of core knowledge, values and skills. Qualified social work practitioners, therefore, demonstrate "competence in working with individuals, families and groups over a sustained period in an area of particular practice within the relevant legal and organizational framework" (Vass, 1996, p. 3).

Over the last two decades the social work profession has made efforts to identify skills related to competent practice at both micro and macro levels (Dore, Epstein, & Herrerias, 1992; Garcia & Floyd, 1992; Gitterman & Gitterman, 1979; O'Hare & Collins, 1997). Studies have investigated valid assessment of research competencies utilizing self efficacy theory (Holden, Barker, Meenaghan, & Rosenberg, 1999), of student field performance (Bogo et al., 1992), and whether or not the delineation of social work specific knowledge is possible (Thyer, 2002). Specialty-specific competency tools have also been developed to assess, for example, social work students' interviewing skills (Koroloff & Rhyne, 1989). The Council on Social Work Education (CSWE) developed a competency-based generalist curriculum for professional baccalaureate social work (Gardella, 1997). From structured interviews with leaders and employers in health and human services, Dalton and Wright (1999) identified knowledge, skills, and attitudes most desired in social work graduates.

Bogo and colleagues (2002) have further examined the reliability and validity of a measure to evaluate social work student performance. Competency standard development has been conducted in other professions to better evaluate practitioner competence. According to Multon, Brown and Lent (1991), there exists a positive and significant relationship between self-efficacy beliefs, academic performance, and persistence outcomes across subjects and designs in their meta-analysis. In the health field, however, the focus on measuring student competencies tends to focus on professional competencies, a focus primarily motivated by professional associations and licensure requirements and standards. A variety of assessment tools have been developed to measure student competency in the areas of nursing and medicine (Ballantyne, Cheek, O'Brien, & Pincombe, 1998; Levenson, Thornby, & Tollett, 1980; McKinley, Fraser & Baker, 2000; Smith, Marcy, Mast, & Ham, 1984; Zweifler & Gonzalez, 1998).

Multiple professions have identified specific competencies for work with older adults and their families. The American Geriatrics Society (AGS) and the American Association of Colleges of Nursing (AACN) have defined basic competencies for attitudes, knowledge and skills of medical students and nurses, and 30 core geriatric competencies for baccalaureate nursing education (AGS, 2000; AACN, 2000). The Joint Commission on Accreditation of

Healthcare Organizations (JCAHO) include age specific assessment and intervention as an element in their evaluation of health care systems (JCAHO, 2001). Molinari, Kier and Kunik (2002), from surveys of 334 mental health professionals with the Department of Veterans Affairs, proposed age-related competencies in mental health. Bennett and Sneed (1999) surveyed a sample of 70 advanced-level practitioners employed in aging to have them identify the competencies needed for entry-level professionals in aging.

Though the importance of the identification of competencies in social work was recognized and there was movement in some professions to identify geriatric competencies, none were available for social work at the beginning of the Hartford Geriatric Social Work Initiative. The Geriatric Social Work Practicum Partners Programs (PPP), funded by the John A. Hartford Foundation, is designed to increase the number of well qualified social workers available to serve older persons and their families. The PPP aims to accomplish this goal through the development of more aging-rich field practicum sites. The New York Academy of Medicine (NYAM) is the Co-ordinating Center nationally responsible for the PPPs. After an initial competitive application process, 11 proposals were selected for a planning year and 6 PPP programs were granted funding for implementation. The 6 programs include 11 universities as demonstration sites. Selected universities have developed and implemented the PPP in their master's of social work (MSW) education programs beginning in academic year 2000 to 2003.

In 2000, Rosen, Zlotnik, Curl, and Green embarked on a national survey to identify core competencies in social work practice with older adults. Analyzing results obtained from 945 social work practitioners and educators revealed a number of gerontological competencies important to effective geriatric social work assessment, intervention and evaluation. This survey revealed the need for curriculum change as well as development of a standardized assessment tool that aims to further identify social work student competency related to work with older adults. Currently, there is a nationwide effort by the Hartford Geriatric Enrichment in Social Work Education (GeroRich) program to infuse social work curriculum with gerontological content. There is not, however, an available assessment tool to measure students perceived competence in core geriatric social work skills. According to Gordon (1991), the use of self-evaluative tools to assess personal strengths and weakness in practice is necessary in a profession that values monitoring and improving personal practice technique.

This paper describes the process of defining geriatric social work competencies to be used nationally in the PPP education interventions to evaluate student outcomes. These competencies have proven useful in social work field education and are presented as a step forward in the development of competency driven education for social work practice with older adults.

COMPETENCY DEVELOPMENT METHODOLOGY

Geriatric Social Work White Papers

The first step in the process of geriatric competency development was a literature review and synthesis for the purpose of providing a conceptual framework for competency identification. White Papers focused on geriatric social work had synthesized the gerontological social work literature just prior to the beginning of the Hartford Geriatric Social Work Initiative. The first was written under the auspice of the U.S. Bureau of Health Professions (BHP) of the Health Resources and Services Administration. The BHP funds a national network of Geriatric Education Centers that aim to increase geriatric education nationally in all the health professions. The Geriatric Social Work White Paper (Berkman, Dobrof, Harry, & Damron-Rodriguez, 1997) was a part of a series of papers on several health professions used to establish a National Agenda for Geriatric Education. In addition to assessing the state of the art in geriatric social work education and proposing twelve major recommendations for change, the White Paper proposed major theoretical and practice orientations for geriatric social work education. These were: (1) biopsychosocial perspective with an emphasis on the person-in-socio-cultural-context as they relate to physical change and illness; (2) a family systems context for intervention; (3) a life span developmental approach with a focus on normal or healthy growth, development, and adaptation in late life; and (4) recognition of ethnic and cohort differences and the needs of special populations. These perspectives for practice were adopted as the knowledge domains from which to view geriatric competencies.

The White Paper by Berkman et al. (1997) modified the definition of social work from the National Association of Social Worker's (1981) Standards for Classification of Social Work Practice to focus on older adults. This definition of geriatric social work was adopted for the GSWEC competency project. Geriatric social work is: Professionally responsible intervention to (1) enhance the developmental, problem solving, and coping capacities of *older* people *and their families*; (2) promote the effective and humane operating of systems that provide resources and services to *older* people *and their families*; (3) link *older* people with systems that provide them with resources, services and opportunities; and (4) contribute to the development and improvement of social policies *that support persons throughout the lifespan* (Italics are words added to focus on aging; Berkman et al., 1997, p. 221).

This definition of geriatric social work encompasses both direct practice, community organization and policy levels of social work. The GSWEC competency development aimed to address skills required to work with older adults at both the micro and macro levels of practice, as well as to relate to the major knowledge domains identified in the White Paper.

A second White Paper, written for the John A. Hartford Foundation and later published as "Education Social Workers for an Aging Society: A Vision for the 21st Century" (Scharlach, Damron-Rodriguez, Robinson & Feldman, 2000), informed competency development by pointing to the future of geriatric social work practice. Changes in the structure of the family, multiple institutional changes including transformations in health and social services, and increasing diversity of the older population all direct social work to respond with relevant interventions.

GSWEC utilized the synthesis of major knowledge domains in a biopsychosocial framework that related to the life course and family systems participating the framework to issues of diversity in the older population. Figure 1 presents the model that was used to guide the field learning experience for the GSWEC demonstration site. The definition of geriatric social work and the goals of the PPP necessitated that both micro, individual and family practice, and macro, program and policy level practice, be considered in the development of geriatric social work competencies.

FIGURE 1. Conceptual Framework for Geriatric Social Work Practice with Diverse Populations

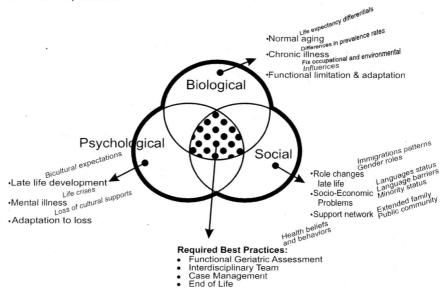

CSWE SAGE-SW

The Council on Social Work Education (CSWE) was a recipient of an award from the John A. Hartford Foundation as the first grantee in the Geriatric Social Work Initiative. The Initiative aims to improve the care of older adults by increasing the capacity of social workers to care for them (Robbins & Reider, 2002). The foci of CSWE's Strengthening Aging and Gerontology Education for Social Work (SAGE-SW) was to assess the current state of gerontological education in social work, to develop competencies for gerontological social work, and to develop aging-related curriculum resources that could be widely disseminated (Rosen, Zlotnik, & Singer, 2002). The Hartford Geriatric Social Work Initiative promoted collaboration between grantees of the various projects in order to create a synergy to enhance the field of geriatric social work. The PPP field education domain of the Initiative integrated the work of SAGE-SW in competency development aimed predominantly for social work curriculum development in the classroom to build competencies for field education.

SAGE-SW conducted a national survey of competencies related to social work with older adults. Phase I of this project included a review of the literature in gerontology to identify gerontological social work competency items, as well as solicitation of gerontology competency items from six national experts. These were refined into 65 competencies organized in three major competency domains: Knowledge about elderly people and their families; professional skills; and professional practice (e.g., respect for cultural diversity, assessing one's own values and biases regarding aging and death) (Rosen, Zlotnik, Curl, & Green, 2000). Phase II sent a survey of the identified items to social work practitioners and faculty, asking them to rate the items as competencies required for generalist practice, those required for advanced practitioners, and those needed by people specializing in working with older people. Thirty-five of the competencies were judged by respondents to be required of all social work practitioners (Rosen, Zlotnik, & Singer, 2002).

This comprehensive SAGE-SW gerontological social work competency development was going on at the same time as PPP efforts to identify geriatric social work competencies for field. Knowledge of and participation in the SAGE-SW process informed the PPP work from the beginning of the effort to foster competence in the field education of graduate students. In addition, at the culminating phase of collaboratively developing competencies to be used nationally for the field education projects, a systematic effort was made to cross reference all SAGE-SW competencies. Core competencies that were essential for all social work practitioners for intervening in the lives of older adults and their families were included as a foundation for field education.

Additionally, since the PPP focus on specialty practice in aging advanced practice competencies identified by SAGE-SW were also included.

The PPP adaptation of SAGE-SW competencies to the field involved operationalizing the items into skill statements as well as conceptualizing the list of competencies into major domains of practice. Further, the competencies were related back to the White Papers to ensure they addressed the frameworks for social work practice, including family systems, diversity, and program and policy development.

GERIATRIC SOCIAL WORK EDUCATION CONSORTIUM (GSWEC): FOCUS GROUPS

In 1998 during the initial planning phase, the lack of commonly accepted competencies for geriatric social work practice was identified by the Geriatric Social Work Consortium of Southern California (GSWEC), one of the six PPP demonstration sites (Partners in Care Foundation, 2000). GSWEC is an inter-organizational alliance comprised of all four social work graduate programs in Los Angeles, four premier regional geriatric social work service agencies designated as Centers of Excellence in field training, and selected other health and social service providers that serve older adults. GSWEC was created and the Partners in Care Foundation, formerly the Visiting Nurse Association Foundation of Los Angeles (VNAF), administered the grant. The goal of GSWEC to formulate "a comprehensive, replicable model for integrated field and academic graduate geriatric social work education" (Partners in Care Foundation, 2002, p. 1). Accordingly, one of the primary objectives of GSWEC was to develop geriatric social work competencies as a foundation for establishing core, integrated field and academic curriculum in aging.

An initial step toward identifying competencies was to ask consumers of geriatric services and social work education what they thought were the important skills needed to serve older adults. Members of GSWEC recruited participants for focus groups, from providers (employers of geriatric social workers), new geriatric social work graduates, older adults and their family care providers. A structured interview schedule was developed, and focus group leaders received a brief training. The groups were audiotaped and transcribed. Analyses were performed using Ethnograph.

Naito-Chan, Damron-Rodriguez and Simmons (2004) report the findings of the focus groups as identifying a number of negative opinions about the current level of skill of social workers in working with older adults. The deficiencies identified in the groups informed the development of the GSWEC competencies. Older adults found it difficult to describe what the social workers provided by way of services and difficulty in knowing how to access social work assistance. These perceptions by older adults further supported the GSWEC aim to identify the skills social workers used in working with older adults.

Both employers and graduates identified conducting geriatric assessments, demonstrating self-awareness, practicing cultural competence, and recognizing the special needs of older adults and their families as among the most important competencies geriatric social workers can possess. Competencies involving knowledge about the impact of ageism and skills in communication, networking, and providing emotional support were also mentioned by both provider groups, albeit less frequently. With respect to the quality of graduate social work education, both employers and graduates expressed varying degrees of dissatisfaction with schools of social work in adequately preparing their students to work with older populations (Naito-Chan et al., in press).

Initially rather than identifying discreet competencies for the field education experience areas of geriatric practice with an evidence based foundation were identified as "best practices." The findings of the GSWEC focus groups suggested the following best practices, which were used to guide the field education model: comprehensive geriatric assessment (CGA), care/case management, and interdisciplinary practice (Figure 1).The focus groups also aided GSWEC in identifying specific competencies related to these best practices. In the first of the three years of implementation of the GSWEC model, the CAL-SWEC framework for child welfare was used as a guide for major areas along which to frame the geriatric competencies. Since CAL-SWEC was familiar to the field instructors across universities, it was decided that adapting the geriatric competencies to the CAL-SWEC format would facilitate acceptance across schools and agencies.

As GSWEC and all the demonstration sites began the first year of implementation evaluation of educational interventions was a priority. GSWEC developed a pre-post evaluation design that included the assessment of these identified competencies. Other demonstration sites also used competencies to guide field experience and in some cases measure student outcomes.

PRACTICUM PARTNERSHIP PROGRAM: COLLABORATIVE EVALUATION OF SKILL COMPETENCIES

The demonstration sites were all required to develop individual evaluation plans. Both process and outcome evaluation was reported to the NYAM at regular intervals. During the first year of implementation a PPP Principal Investigator (PI) meeting was held at the CSWE Annual Program Meeting. At this meeting it was suggested that certain outcomes would be more powerfully measured if the measures were consistent across programs. The goal was to allow for program diversity and at the same time measure certain student outcomes across programs. The NYAM fostered a collaborative approach to evaluation of PPP implementation.

The challenges of this collaborative approach were identified and strategically approached:

- Committee process: how to function as a group, achieve consensus on issues of cross-site evaluation
- Effective communication: how to communicate effectively given the distance, diverse group, busy schedules, people didn't know each other
- Coordination with other evaluation levels: how to avoid duplication, over-evaluating, and conflict

The strengths of a collaborative evaluation model were also identified:

- A larger sample size for measuring student outcomes
- Pooling of knowledge, expertise (design, instrument development and selection, analysis)
- Stronger investment in cross-site evaluation (collaborative vs. to-down) and the potential to compare and contrast elements of success
- More powerful and more relevant dissemination effort by relating PPP models to diverse programs

Through a listserve, conference calls, sharing of all evaluation tools across sites, and meetings at professional and scientific programs consensus, built a common instrument for student assessment. This was accomplished by: respecting the evaluation plans of individual sites, selecting a small core group of instruments for cross-site evaluation, assurance that this was not a comparison of programs, use of secondary data whenever possible and an open forum to share issues and goals. A motivating factor was that the integrated data-base would be shared by all researchers and that a research agenda would be pursued by the PPP.

A major aim of the PPP collaborative evaluation strategy was to develop uniform measures for student competence for working with older adults. Many PPPs had identified several competencies to use in their evaluation. The GSWEC competencies were extensive and therefore used as a foundation for organizing the skill set and addition of other PPP competencies.

The items were based on the CSWE SAGE-SW professional competencies for social work practice in aging. The SAGE-SW project developed these competencies through a literature review and using expert opinions in gerontology (Rosen et al., 2000). These competencies were reviewed for relevance to the educational content of PPP; a majority of the competencies were converted into statements of skills. These and new items with macro, interdisciplinary, and research and evaluation content were then grouped into domains. This was followed by a series of reviews of items for clarity and validity by members of the PPP Evaluation Committee, who are experts in social work and aging. As a result of these reviews and pilot testing, some items were modified, others deleted, and new items developed.

They were then matched against sets of competencies developed by five other PPP sites and additional competencies were identified. All were converted into statement of skills. Members of the Evaluation Committee of the PPP, who are experts in social work and aging, then reviewed these items for clarity and validity. As a result of these reviews and pilot testing, some items were modified, others deleted, and new items developed.

A Tool for Assessing Student Competence in Geriatric Social Work

The following is a description of the tool developed across PPP sites for the assessment of student competence in geriatric social work. The aim was to measure the degree of skill competency of graduate social work students specializing in aging, in working with older adults and their families. The education tool is a 58-item instrument that is divided into 5 domains, some with subsections: Values and Ethics, Assessment (Individual and Family, Aging Services, Programs and Policies); Practice and Intervention (Theory and Knowledge in Practice; Individual and Family; Aging Services, Programs, and Policies); Interdisciplinary Collaboration; and Evaluation and Research. A section for students to comment on their skill in each domain provides them with the opportunity to clarify their ratings, especially as some items are complex. The educational tool was designed as a pre-post test to measure the effect of the PPP's innovative field education programs in aging on the skills of participating graduate social work students who were specializing in aging. This instrument can also be used for educational planning after the pre-test. The scale measures the respondent's perceptions of their level of skill in aging practice as compared to a competent MSW geriatric social worker. Respondents rate each item on a 0-10 scale (0 = not skilled at all; 10 = very skilled). Each domain may be scored by adding the responses to individual items. Table 1 provides examples of the competency items within the major domains.

RESULTS

PPP Students

The student sample (n = 190) reported here consists of social work students with a stated interest in the field of aging and selected to be part of the PPP at

TABLE 1. Examples of Competency Skills by Domain

Competency Domain	Example Skill
I. Values & Ethics	Assess personal bias/values regarding aging Respect diversity among older adult clients
II. Assessment	
Assessment, Individual & Family	Adapt interviewing methods to possible limitations Assess functional needs of family/caregiver
Assessment, Programs & Policies	Identify gaps/barriers in service delivery systems Assess organizational effectiveness to client need
III. Practice and Intervention Theory & Knowledge	Apply biopsychosocial theories in practice with clients Understand/comply with laws/policies related to clients
Individual & Family	Set realistic/mutual goals sensitive to individual capacity Develop clear, timely, appropriate service plans
Programs and Policies	Incorporate a full continuum of services for older client Use strategies that empower older adult, community, etc.
IV. Interdisciplinary Collaboration	Collaborate/communicate with other health professions Advocate on behalf of client with other professionals
V. Evaluation & Research	Evaluate practice/program for effective outcomes Incorporate evaluation outcomes into program/policy

one of the 11 universities implementing the new field models. Table 2 presents the student demographic characteristics. There was a broad age range of students. Over half the students (56%) were in the youngest age category of 20-29. Nine percent of the students were over 50 years of age. Sixteen percent of the students were male. The student body was very diverse, with 48% Caucasian, 18% African-American, 14% Asian-American, 16% Hispanic-American, and 3.5% other groups.

The majority of PPP students are second year graduate students (55%) with most of the remaining students being first year graduate students (27%). Six percent of the students were BSW students and 1% were in advanced standing. Students came from a variety of undergraduate majors: 27% social welfare majors, 16% psychology, and 16% biology, with the rest in other fields. Less than half the students had completed any courses in aging despite their stated interest in the field. The vast majority of the students were full time (82%). PPP students identified as both micro and macro (13%) in their concentrations, with more direct practice students (40%); almost half (47%) of the students did not identify a field of practice (Table 3).

TABLE 2. Student Descriptive Characteristics (N = 190)

Demographic	n	%
Age		
20-29	106	56
30-39	43	23
40-49	23	12
50-59	15	8
60-69	3	1
Gender		
Male	31	16
Female	143	75
Not Specified	16	9
Ethnicity		
Caucasian	92	48
African-American	34	18
Asian-American	26	14
Hispanic/Latino	31	16
Other	6	3.5
Not Specified	1	.5

TABLE 3. Student Educational and Experiential Backgrounds (N = 190)

	n	%
Educational Level During Internship		
BSW	11	6
1st Year MSW	52	27
2nd Year MSW	104	55
Advanced Standing	2	1
Not Specified	21	11
Undergraduate Major		
Psychology	31	16
Social Work/Welfare	52	27
Sociology	20	11
Aging/Gerontology	2	1
Biology	30	16
English/Literature	4	2
History	1	.5
Business	1	.5
Other	15	8
Not Specified	34	18
Completed Courses in Aging		
Yes	88	46
No	89	47
Not Specified	13	7
Enrollment Status		
Full-time	155	82
Part-time	19	10
Not Specified	16	8
Current Concentration		
Micro	75	40
Macro	25	13
Other	21	11
Not Specified	69	36

PPP Student Self-Assessment of Geriatric Social Work Competence

Table 4 presents the mean student competency self-assessments at pre-test and post-test. On a scale of 1 to 10, with lower scores indicating less skill, the mean scores of students at pre-test ranged from 4.29 for Evaluation and Research to 7.9 for Values and Ethics domain. At post-test the mean score range was from 6.79 for Evaluation and Research, to 8.5 in Values and Ethics. Within the Assessment and Practice domains, the mean scores for work with older adults and their families were higher at both pre- and post-test than the assessment and practice means for program and policy level skills. The rank orders of the major domains for geriatric social work competency assessment both at pre and at post students were: Values and Ethics, Interdisciplinary Collaboration, Assessment, Practice and Intervention, and Evaluation and Research. The greatest gain in mean score was in Interdisciplinary Collaboration. The standard deviations for each domain was smaller at post-test than at pre-test.

TABLE 4. Student Competency Scores by Category: 2001-2003 (N = 190)

Category	Pre-test		Post-test	
	Mean	SD	Mean	SD
I. Values & Ethics	7.09	1.96	8.5*	1.17
II. Assessment; Individual & Family	5.47	2.34	7.84*	1.46
Assessment; Programs & Policies	5.12	2.41	7.72*	1.42
III. Practice & Intervention; Theory and Knowledge	5.11	2.44	7.77*	1.42
Practice & Intervention; Individual and Family	5.64	2.32	8.02*	1.36
Practice & Intervention; Programs and Policies	4.48	2.54	7.25*	1.79
IV. Interdisciplinary Collaboration	5.51	2.52	8.09*	2.31
V. Evaluation & Research	4.29	2.62	6.79*	2.25

*p ≤ .0001

Figure 2 presents this information as a bar graph to view the gains in pre-test and post-test scores. This figure provides the results of paired *t* tests to measure the significance of the differences of pre- and post-test self assessments with scores in each domain and sub-area showing statistically significantly higher ratings at post-test (p < .0001).

Figure 3 converts the competency ratings into a percentage of the maximum score in all competency domains. The mean percentage on the overall competency at pre test was 55% and at post test was 76%. This is a score that demonstrates that students when asked to rate themselves as students approaching graduation estimate they have improved substantially in skills in geriatric social work and still have room to grow post graduation. The

FIGURE 2. Student Competency by Category (N = 190)

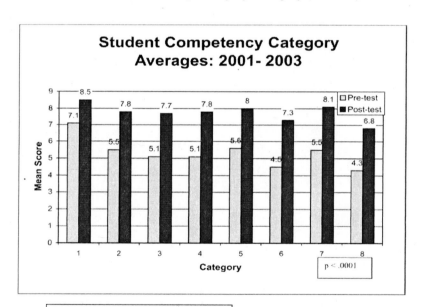

1 **Values/Ethics**
2 **Assessment**: Individual/Family
3 Assessment: Program/Policy
4 **Practice**: Theory
5 Practice: Individual/Family
6 Practice: Program/Policy
7 **Interdiciplinary**
8 **Evaluation/Research**

FIGURE 3. Student Overall Competency Scores (N = 190)
Overall Competency Score 2001-2003

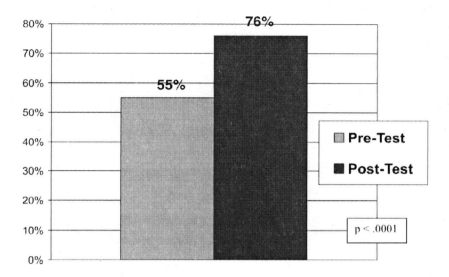

significance of this change in overall score was highly significant as well
(p < .0001).

Limitations

The pooled sample for this pre/post evaluation research is small. Further,
these are a select group of students with an interest in aging. The use of this
tool with a broad group of students with varying levels of interest in aging
could provide a comparison group to the PPP student evaluation. The tool
used only self ratings and field instructors did not uniformly rate students
using the same tool. This instrument has not been subjected to psychometric
testing to determine reliability and validity.

DISCUSSION AND IMPLICATIONS

The incremental and collaborative process of identifying geriatric social
work competencies and using them for evaluation in the field is a promising
step toward quality practicum experiences to prepare social workers for practice with older adults and their families. Relating social work knowledge and

values to skills is essential for effective practice (Brown, 1996; Vass, 1996). The White Papers served as a foundation for the competency development by suggesting knowledge domains of gerontological social work. The bio-psychosocial framework with a family focus and related to diversity was found to encompass the skills for geriatric social work.

Moving past identification of knowledge to skill delineation is increasingly a driving force in the health profession education and practice (AGS, 2000; AACN, 2000; Bennett & Sneed, 1999; McKinley et al., 2000; Stewart et al., 2000). The current context of care requires a new perspectives for social work practice (Reishch & Jarman-Rohde, 2000) and this includes the identification of skills that relate to effective outcomes for the population served (Green & Galambos, 2003; Rosen, Zlotnik, Curl, & Green, 2000). The identification and utilization of specific competencies is a step in this process of training.

The GSWEC focus groups supported the need for social work competencies through statements of both providers and older persons. Older adult participants testified that they were unclear about the role of social workers in assisting the elderly. Providers were clear about the competencies needed by social work practitioners, though, and these included comprehensive geriatric assessment skills.

The SAGE-SW Competencies Project was the foundation for the next step in this development of geriatric competencies for field education. The product of the SAGE-SW project was a comprehensive list of geriatric social work skills that were validated broadly by academics and practitioners in the field of aging. PPP used these to cross-validate the competencies developed by the demonstration projects. SAGE-SW continues to relate the identified geriatric skills to social work curriculum (Green & Galambos, 2002). The SAGE-SW competencies have been related to the CSWE Educational Policy and Accreditation Standards for foundation curriculum to Research (Green & Galambos, 2002). The PPP process described in this article has related the geriatric social work competencies to the field education experience. The field experience is grounded in skill development and, thus, of its nature competency driven (O'Hare & Collins, 1997; Regehr et al., 2002; Spitzer, 2001). Identifying, articulating and providing a conceptual orientation to the skills needed to work with older adults assists in not only evaluating student accomplishment but structuring the teaching and field experiences.

The PPP collaborative was the final stage in the geriatric competency development for field education. It built consensus on the specific competencies, organized and framed the competencies within a conceptual framework, cross referenced each to the SAGE-SW competencies and created action statements that were scaled and used for self assessment. The demonstration sites collaborated to administer the same competency evaluation tool across sites.

Self assessment has been found to be effective in assessing multiple health professional students (Atkins & Wood, 2002; McKinley, Fraser, & Baker, 2000; Gordon, 1991; Stewart et al., 2000). This initial use of the geriatric social work competencies for field has demonstrated the usefulness in assessing student outcomes. The assessment tool positively did not have a ceiling effect and students were able to appreciate their continued need to learn in this area post graduation. The self assessment tool has pointed to areas of strength and challenge in major content areas in geriatric social work. The use of the assessment tool by field instructors to rate students and to compare their own self ratings would add another dimension to the teaching/learning experience. The competencies have also been used by the demonstration sites to structure student contracts, provide integrative seminars, train field instructors, and audit classroom curricular.

Future work requires the 56 item learning tool to be further tested for reliability and validity before it is appropriately used for different populations of social work students. The PPP National Collaborative Evaluation continues working toward the development of a reliable and valid geriatric social work competency instrument. The data presented here on student self rated skill is primarily for illustration of the use of the instrument for evaluation of learning in field education. Further analysis of the content of student skills and its relationship to individual characteristics and institutional variables will be described in future publications.

In addition to competency driven education, the Practicum Partnership Program developed several key components for innovative field education in geriatric social work. Though not described here, these include: university-community collaborative, an expanded role for field instructors, a rotational model of field education across the continuum of care and with diverse populations, and targeted recruitment. The demonstration sites have begun to describe these new field models (Bures, Toseland & Fortune, 2002; Ivry & Hadden, 2002). These innovations in field education, with the focus on competency driven preparation of geriatric social workers, aim to inform the practice of the profession not only for older adults but also for practice across the life span.

REFERENCES

American Association of Colleges of Nursing and the John A. Hartford Foundation Institute for Geriatric Nursing. (2000). *Older adults: Recommended baccalaureate competencies and curricular guidelines for geriatric nursing care.* (Author, New York City, New York).

American Geriatrics Society. (2000). Core competencies for the care of older patients: Recommendations of the American Geriatrics Society. *Academic Medicine, 75*(3), 252-255.

Bennett, J. M., & Sneed, J. (1999). Practice competencies for entry-level professionals in the field of aging. *Educational Gerontology, 25*, 305-315.

Berkman, B., Dobrof, R., Harry, L., & Damron-Rodriguez, J. (1997). Social work. In S. M. Klein (Ed.), *A national agenda for geriatric education: White papers* (pp. 53-85). New York: Springer.

Bogo, M., & Globerman, J. (1999). Interorganizational relationships between schools of social work and field agencies: Testing a framework for analysis. *Journal of Social Work Education, 35*(2), 265-272.

Bogo, M., Regehr, C., Hughes, J., Power, R., & Globerman, J. (2002). Evaluating a measure of student field performance in direct service: Testing reliability and validity of explicit criteria. *Journal of Social Work Education, 38*(3), 385-401.

Brown, H. C. (1996). The knowledge base of social work. In A. A. Vass (Ed.), *Social work competencies: Core knowledge, values and skills* (pp. 8-35). London: Sage.

Bures, R. M., Toseland, R. W., & Fortune, A. E. (2002). Strengthening geriatric social work training: Perspectives from the University at Albany. *Journal of Gerontological Social Work, 39*, 111-128.

Crisp, B. R., & Green-Lister, P. (2002). Assessment methods in social work education: A review of the literature. *Journal of Social Work Education, 21*(2), 259-269.

Dalton, B., & Wright, L. (1999). Using community input for the curriculum review process. *Journal of Social Work Education, 35*(2), 275-288.

Dore, M., Epstein, B., & Herrerias, C. (1992). Evaluating students' micro practice field performance: Do universal learning objectives exist? *Journal of Social Work Education, 28*, 353-362.

Gambrill, E. D. (2001). Evaluating the quality of social work education: Options galore. *Journal of Social Work Education, 37*(3), 418-430.

Gardella, L. G. (1997). Baccalaureate social workers. In R. L. Edwards (Ed.), *Encyclopedia of social work* (19th ed., Supplement; pp. 37-46). Washington, DC: NASW Press.

Gordon, M. (1991). A review of validity and accuracy of self-assessments in health professional training. *Academic Medicine, 66*, 762-769.

Greene, R., & Galambos, C. (2002). Social work's pursuit of a common professional framework: Have we reached a milestone? *Advancing Gerontological Social Work Education.* New York: Haworth Press.

Holden, G., Barker, K., Meenaghan, T., & Rosenberg, G. (1999). Research self-efficacy: A new possibility for educational outcomes assessment. *Journal of Social Work Education, 35*(3), 463-475.

Holden, G., Meenaghan, T., Anastas, J., & Metrey, G. (2002). Outcomes of social work education: The case for social work self-efficacy. *Journal of Social Work Education, 38*(1), 115-133.

Hudson, R. B., Gonyea, J. G., & Curley, A. (2003). The geriatric social work labor force: Challenges and opportunities. *Public Policy and Aging Report, 13*(2), 12-14.

Ivry, J., & Hadden, B. R. (2002). The Hunter experience: Innovations in the field practicum. *Journal of Gerontological Social Work, 39*, 129-144.

Joint Commission on Accreditation in Healthcare Organizations. (2001). *Comprehensive JCAHO accreditation manual for hospitals: The official handbook.* Oakbrook Terrace, IL.

Levenson, A. J., Thronby, J. I., & Tollett, S. M. (1980). Gerontologic and geriatric training in medical school: Curricular preferences shown by medical students, educators, and general practitioners. *Journal of the American Geriatric Society, 28*, 157-163.

McKinley, R. K., Fraser, R. C., & Baker, R. (2000). Model for directly assessing and improving clinical competence and performance in revalidation of clinicians. *British Medical Journal, 322*, 712-715.

Molinari, V., Kier, F. J., & Kunik, M. E. (2002). Obtaining age-related mental health competency: What is needed? *Educational Gerontology, 28*, 73-82.

Multon, K. D., Brown, S. D., & Lent, R. W. (1991). Relation of self-efficacy beliefs to academic outcomes: A meta-analytic investigation. *Journal of Counseling Psychology, 38*, 53-63.

Naito-Chan, E., Damron-Rodriguez, J., & Simmons, W. J. (2004). Identifying competencies for geriatric social work practice. *Journal of Gerontological Social Work, 43*, 59-78.

O'Hare, T., & Collins, P. (1997). Development and validation of a scale for measuring social work practice skills. *Research on Social Work Practice, 7*, 228-238.

Partners in Care Foundation. (2000). *The Southern California Geriatric Social Work Education Consortium: Executive summary.* Burbank, CA: Author.

Reed, C. C., Beall, S. C., & Baumhover, L. A. (1992). Gerontological education for students in nursing and social work: Knowledge, attitudes, and perceived barriers. *Educational Gerontology, 18*, 625-636.

Regehr, C., Regehr, G., Leeson, J., & Fusco, L. (2002). Setting priorities for learning in the field practicum: A comparative study of students and field instructors. *Journal of Social Work Education, 38*(1), 55-65.

Reishch, M., & Jarman-Rohde, L. (2000). The future of social work in the United States: Implications for field education. *Journal of Social Work Education, 36*(2), 201-215.

Robbins, L. A., & Rieder, C. H. (2002). The John A. Hartford Foundation Geriatric Social Work Initiative. *Journal of Gerontological Social Work, 39*, 71-90.

Rosen, A. L., Zlotnik, J. L., Curl, A. L., & Green, R. G. (2000). *The CSWE/SAGE-SW national aging competencies survey report.* Alexandria, VA: Council on Social Work Education.

Rosen, A. L., Zlotnik, J. L., & Singer, T. (2002). Basic gerontological competence for all social workers: The need to "gerontologize" social work education. *Journal of Gerontological Social Work, 39*, 25-36.

Scharlach, A., Damron-Rodriguez, J., Robinson, B., & Feldman, R. (2000). Educating social workers for an aging society: A vision for the 21st century. *Journal of Social Work Education, 36*(3), 521-538.

Smith, M. R., Marcey, M. L., & Ham, R. J. (1984). Implementation and evaluation of a model geriatric curriculum. *Journal of Medical Education, 59*, 416-424.

Thyer, B. A. (2002). Developing discipline-specific knowledge for social work: Is it possible? *Journal of Social Work Education, 38*(1), 101-114.

Vass, A. A. (Ed.). (1996). *Social work competencies, knowledge, values and skills.* London: Sage.

Zweifler, J., & Gonzalez, A. M. (1998). Teaching residents to care for culturally diverse populations. *Academy of Medicine, 73*(10), 1057-1061.

doi:10.1300/J083v48n01_10

Intergenerational Service-Learning: An Innovative Teaching Strategy to Infuse Gerontology Content into Foundation Courses

Harriet L. Cohen, PhD, LCSW
Bonnie Hatchett, PhD
Darlene Eastridge, MSSW, PhD

SUMMARY. This article provides an overview of intergenerational service-learning, an experiential pedagogy that involves students in learning outside the traditional classroom while providing a needed service in the community. Examples of intergenerational service-learning projects are presented that have been successfully utilized by the authors. These projects demonstrate the importance of using reflective practice assignments to help students deconstruct and reconstruct images, beliefs and paradigms about older adults. In addition, problems and opportunities in developing service-learning projects in urban and rural settings and with the Hispanic community are described, as well as some of the types of learning that may result from implementing service-learning experiences in various social work foundation courses. doi: 10.1300/J083v48n01_11 *[Article copies available for a fee from The Haworth Document Delivery Service: 1-800-HAWORTH. E-mail address: <docdelivery@haworthpress.com> Website: <http://www.HaworthPress.com> © 2006 by The Haworth Press, Inc. All rights reserved.]*

[Haworth co-indexing entry note]: "Intergenerational Service-Learning: An Innovative Teaching Strategy to Infuse Gerontology Content into Foundation Courses." Cohen, Harriet L., Bonnie Hatchett, and Darlene Eastridge. Co-published simultaneously in *Journal of Gerontological Social Work* (The Haworth Press, Inc.) Vol. 48, No. 1/2, 2006, pp. 161-178; and: *Fostering Social Work Gerontology Competence: A Collection of Papers from the First National Gerontological Social Work Conference* (ed: Catherine J. Tompkins, and Anita L. Rosen) The Haworth Press, Inc., 2007, pp. 161-178. Single or multiple copies of this article are available for a fee from The Haworth Document Delivery Service [1-800-HAWORTH, 9:00 a.m. - 5:00 p.m. (EST). E-mail address: docdelivery@haworthpress.com].

KEYWORDS. Intergenerational, service learning, social work, pedagogy, education

WHAT IS INTERGENERATIONAL SERVICE-LEARNING?

Service-learning is an experiential pedagogy that involves students in learning experiences outside the classroom. It is a philosophy, a community development model and a teaching and learning methodology (http:// www.nylc.org/sl_definition.cfm). Intergenerational service-learning provides students the opportunity to apply theoretical concepts to real life situations with older adults, moving learning from the traditional classroom to the community, while focusing on genuine problems and solving real community needs. Intergenerational service-learning brings community service activities and the educational curriculum together while focusing on the interaction of older adults and students. It provides for increased collaboration between the academic community and the aging network, including exposing students to older adults and practitioners serving older adults, as well as the service delivery support system. Service learning in addition to providing service to the community and learning for the students also involves an opportunity for students to reflect on their learning experiences.

Service-learning is a both pedagogy/andragogy or a teaching strategy and a goal. It brings together teaching, research, and service, while connecting the academic institution with the needs of the community and the larger society (Astin & Sax, 1998). The five components of service-learning for faculty, students, service recipients, and the community partner include: (1) Planning the experience and identifying the skills and knowledge that may be learned from this experience, identifying community partners, selecting the reading, assignments and grading criteria; (2) Performing the service, analyzing the experience, and reflecting on the lessons learned through writing, discussion and presentations; (3) Receiving the services; (4) Recognizing the students, service recipients, and agencies with publicity, food, certificates and awards; and (5) Evaluating the experience from students, faculty, agency, and consumer/ service recipients' perspectives.

This teaching strategy is particularly useful for preparing students for a liberal arts education and is an extremely good fit for social work education. Colleges and universities who desire to prepare students as concerned citizens and press forward the "social good," have recently begun their mission to advance knowledge, economic development, and community outreach by including educational activities that incorporate service-learning through direct community involvement (Rhoads, 2000). Institutions utilizing this community-building approach encourage community residents and institution professionals to work together in an effort aimed at solving problems and enriching the lives of all its participants (Maurrasse, 2001). With collaboration, this approach relies on strengthening existing partnerships to bring about change in the community (O'Connor & Netting, 1999).

At the same time, social work education focuses on extensive community involvement of the social work students in order for them to understand the dynamics of a multicultural society and develop their skills as empathetic practitioners (Nagy & Falk, 2001). Accredited social work programs have successfully employed a variety of approaches to nurture both the integration of theory and practice or field placement, and the university's approach of service-learning through university-community partnerships (Maurrasse, 2001). This has been achieved by elaborating "faculty-headed field units in existing agencies, the development of school-community learning centers, and university-based practice opportunities" (Rosenblum & Raphael, 1983, p. 67). Today many of these institutions have achieved national recognition (Maurrasse, 2001).

The service-learning experiences through university-community partnerships, similar to the field practicum, benefit the social work student ideally because "communities provide powerful opportunities that complement social work education" (Lawson, 1998). Through the successful integration of university-community partnerships, the student can acquire experience from both the classroom and community placement alike. This can include, but is not limited to, the promotion of leadership through direct community involvement, a closer identification of self as a caring person through exploration, reflection, and understanding (Rhoads, 2000), and a deeper comprehension of the three levels of social work practice–micro, mezzo, macro (Dhooper, Rompf, & Royse, 1999). Simultaneously, this environment allows practicum students to experience learning from the other foundation areas: social work values and ethics, diversity, promotion of social and economic justice, and populations at risk for the enhancement of a multicultural education (Dhooper, Rompf, & Royse, 1993). All of which, as stated by the literature, are also promoted through service-learning (Rhoads, 2000). However, service-learning differs from practicum as mentioned earlier because service-learning is "a philosophy of education that focuses on service to the community as students increase their understanding of a specific population's needs, issues, problems and solutions" (Newman & Tompkins, 2000).

As mentioned above, reflection is an important component of the service-learning experience. Reflection is a thoughtful look at the meaning of one's experiences, individually or in groups (Lucas, 2000). Using reflection, students can better identify what they have learned about themselves, called "process reflection." They can reflect on what they learned about older adults or the aging service delivery system, called "content reflection." Or they can reflect on how they will apply what they learned, or the "so what? reflection" (Mezirow, 1991; Schon, 1983).

Process reflection questions might include, what took you by surprise? When did you feel most engaged? Why? When did you feel least engaged? Why? How did this experience challenge your beliefs about older adults? Content reflection questions might ask students to identify three concepts learned in class and apply the theory to their experience in the community. Compare and contrast the theories learned in class with your observations and experiences with the aging network. Describe the strengths and gaps in the aging service delivery system. "So what" reflection questions might ask students to determine how they will utilize the information they learned in the field. This occurs through a process that incorporates critical decision-making and evaluation of the effectiveness of service-learning. This teaching/learning strategy provides students with an opportunity to expand their knowledge through experience (Brookfield, 1987; Mezirow, 1991).

Faculty may use a variety of reflective practice assignments depending on the teaching strategies used, the type of students, the objectives of the course, and/or the service-learning setting (Cranton, 1994; Cranton, 2000). One type of reflective assignment is the use of critical incident analysis and includes content, process, and so what reflection. Students are asked to describe an incident that occurred during their service-learning experience. They are then asked to reflect critically on their reactions, thoughts, and feelings about the situation. What took them by surprise? What did they learn? How will they use this experience in the future? Another type of reflective assignment is the dialogue journal in which the student writes reflections on one page and the instructor provides feedback or asks critical questions on the opposite page. Students may be given a list of key concepts or phases that they include in their reflection. In addition, students may be given directed readings and asked to reflect on the readings. They may be asked to make class presentations about what they learned or participate in email or chat discussions (Taylor, Marienau, & Fiddler, 2000). Examples of reflective questions will be presented in the service-learning projects described later in the article.

Service-learning is a valuable instructional tool. "Research supports the contention that service-learning has a positive impact on personal, attitudinal, moral, social, and cognitive outcomes" (Bringle & Hatcher, 1996, p. 223). Astin and Sax (1998) conclude from their 1995 evaluation of service-learning that participation during the undergraduate years substantially enhances the academic development of students. Unlike volunteer work, service-learning is course-based and the purpose is to implant a sense of responsibility as the student integrates theoretical knowledge with experience (Bringle & Hatcher, 1996).

BENEFITS AND BARRIERS

An important component of intergenerational service-learning is developing an association with agencies and organizations serving older adults in the community, as well as with older adults. The involvement of community partners can provide benefits and pose barriers in planning intergenerational service-learning experiences. Some of the benefits of working with community partners include:

- Exposing students to older adults, which often results in a change of attitude for students toward older adults and to their own aging process (Newman & Tompkins, 2000; Schwartz & Simmons, 2001),
- Building bridges between the university and the community,
- Exposing students to practitioners working with older adults which challenges students stereotypes about social workers and gerontologists working with older adults,
- Identifying social work practitioners to serve as guest lecturers on various practice issues related to older adults and their families,
- Discovering areas for applied research in gerontological social work practice,
- Providing an opportunity for students to explore their own aging process, and
- Coupling students with community agencies and professionals that are potential employers.

Some of the barriers to establishing relationships with community partners include:

- A previous history of strained relationships between the community partner and the educational institution,
- An organizational structure within the community partner agency that is in transition or chaos,
- High staff turnover rates that affect the stability of student involvement with designated contact persons,
- Funding issues associated with liability,
- Indemnity release forms,
- Transportation of the student to the service-learning site,
- Lack of flexibility of the community organization,
- Misconceptions about the concept of service,
- Lack of an appropriate orientation to identify expectations of all partners–agency, community members, students, and faculty,

- Lack of student flexibility due to course scheduling and other demands,
- Lack of flexibility of the educational institution in relation to understanding the needs of the community partner,
- Student anxiety related to the initial contact with the older adults who will be involved in the service-learning experience, and
- Anxiety experienced by the service recipients about what is expected of them and how much time this will require.

SERVICE-LEARNING PROJECTS

The following section will identify different models of intergenerational service-learning experiences, the kinds of skills and learning experiences provided by each, and the variety of community based agencies that the authors have utilized. The models can be utilized in policy, practice, Human Behavior and the Social Environment, research and/or aging elective courses, with the assignments and reflective questions geared to the content and goals of the course.

Intergenerational service-learning experiences utilized by these authors have included working with an agency serving older adults to plan and implement a conference geared to the needs and interests of older women, interviewing older adults to help them prepare their spiritual legacies and working with a housing facility to conduct focus groups with older adults about transition issues related to moving from independent to congregate living. In addition, two examples will demonstrate challenges and opportunities of working in rural locations. One project reflects the barriers and benefits that occurred while developing an intergenerational service-learning project with a Hispanic serving institution in a rural setting. The final project describes individual service projects that occurred between students and older adults in rural communities.

PLANNING AN OLDER WOMEN'S CONFERENCE

Students in an aging and social work elective class were asked to help plan a conference geared to the interests of older women. Students participated by serving on the Planning and Marketing Committees at an agency that provides an array of services to older adults. Students reviewed the literature about older women and identified program ideas for the workshop session. They contacted distribution sites for the brochures and fliers to attract the attention of the target population. Students also participated during the event by assisting with on-site logistics, registration and breakout sessions. This intergenerational service-learning experience assisted students in meeting the course objectives, which included helping students:

- To gain knowledge of physical, emotional, and spiritual aspects of aging
- To gain knowledge of existing programs, both government and voluntary serving the older adult population
- To gain knowledge about the diversity of older adults and the specific factors affecting women, people of color, lesbians, gay men, etc.
- To identify career opportunities and roles for professionals in the field of gerontology
- To identify one's own attitudes and beliefs about aging and older adults in order to work more effectively with this population

The participation of the students was so successful that at the de-briefing meeting the older volunteers, agency staff, and students overwhelmingly decided that the conference should evolve from that geared specifically to older women to an intergenerational women's conference. The students made suggestions to the planning committee about how to attract younger women, including where to advertise, seminar topics to generate interest, etc. As a result of student suggestions the agency has redesigned their intergenerational women's conference into an annual event that includes daughters and mothers, mothers and grandmothers, granddaughters and grandmothers, sisters and aunts, great aunts and nieces who share a day exploring issues relating to health, social situations, legal concerns, financial and economic planning, and spirituality that affect them as women across the lifespan.

From this experience students developed confidence in their planning skills and they learned about issues affecting older women, that their voices count, and about how lifespan issues affect women across age and racial/ethnic boundaries. They developed confidence in their planning skills. As a result of the students' involvement, the agency learned that the community was open and hungry for multigenerational women's programming. The instructor learned about thinking outside of the box, as the agency staff and volunteers decided to transform the Older Women's Conference into a Multigenerational Women's Conference.

It was important for the students to have an opportunity for class and individual reflections to examine their previous assumptions about older adults and to reflect on their recent experiences with older adults. Students responded to reflective questions in both oral and written forms. Some of the questions included: At what moment during the day did you feel most engaged with what was happening? Why? At what moment during the day did you feel most distanced from what was happening? Why? What action taken by anyone (participant or facilitator) during the day did you find most affirming or helpful? Explain. What action taken by anyone (facilitator or participant) during the day did you find most puzzling or confusing? Explain. What about this experience surprised you the most? This could be your own reaction to what went on, or something that someone did, or anything else that occurs to you. Why? How will you integrate or apply what you learned at the conference with your social work knowledge, skills, values, and/or conscious use of self (Brookfield, 1987)? In addition to the experience gained from the students involved in planning and implementing this conference as a service-learning project, a MSW student working on her gerontology certificate became interested in the conference as a research project. She developed a program evaluation for the Older Women's conference and interviewed students, older women, and the agency staff about the impact of the conference. Thus, students in the class also learned about applied research through this intergenerational service-learning experience. Exposure to older women helped these students to deconstruct negative stereotypes about older adults and replace them with positive and affirming ones.

PREPARING A SPIRITUAL LEGACY PROJECT

This service learning experience was designed to assist students to deconstruct their attitudes, stereotypes and biases about older adults by engaging the students with older adults in exploring how the older adults have made meaning of their lives. Although this service-learning project began as a partnership with a community based agency, because of changes within the administration of the agency at the beginning of the semester for this project, the agency social worker felt she could not participate in the project. Several other agencies were contacted but nothing could be worked out for the class as a whole. As was mentioned earlier, this is one of the barriers in developing service-learning projects. The students suggested that they interview an older family member, which turned out to be an incredible and meaningful learning experience for the students.

The service component of this project involved developing a spiritual legacy with an older family member that could be shared with the students' families. Another component of this assignment was that the students were required to write their own spiritual legacies, which challenged them to think about their own lives with attention to the lessons they have learned, the impact they have made in the world and to explore the values in which they live and make decisions. This process of engaging the students in interaction with family members helped to meet the objectives of this aging and social work course entitled "Assessing and Intervening with Older Adults." By the end of the course, students were expected to:

- Understand the impact of physical, emotional, cognitive and social aging on older adults when assessing and intervening with older adults.
- Assess one's own attitudes, values and biases regarding aging, death and dying.
- Recognize the similarities and the differences in older adults, including specific factors affecting women, people of color, lesbians, gay men, etc.
- Apply professional social work values and practice principles when assessing and intervening with older adults and their families, recognizing the diversity in this population.
- Critically analyze those social forces that are part of the older person's environment (particularly older women, people of color, differently able, gay/lesbian, etc.) and be able to assess the impact of those forces on the client's level of functioning.
- Develop an understanding and appreciation of how older adults make meaning of their life experiences.

The students scheduled time with their older family members and asked them to discuss their values, lessons learned, regrets, turning points, and significant people in their lives. As they interviewed their older family members, the students discovered the human being behind the role of grandmother or grandfather and they also came to understand better how their own values, beliefs, and perspectives had developed. At a time when young people are still individuating from family, these students found a connection with their heritage and their family. It was a transformative experience as they discussed concerns and topics related to living and dying with their older family member. As a result of these discussions the students developed a greater understanding about how their family members made meaning of their lives. The instructor learned how important is it to be present and attentive to the students when they have been given assignments that challenge their paradigms. Students responded to reflective questions about their experiences. What challenged your beliefs, thoughts, and attitudes? What took you by surprise or what happened that you did not expect to happen? What (readings, class discussion, speakers, exercises, etc.) helped you to prepare for the interview with your family member? What would you do differently the next time you interview an older adult? What would you do the same? What new understanding about yourself and your family did you gain from this experience? Based on the interviews with family members and preparing your own spiritual legacy, what is of real value or importance to you and what to your older family member? How do you find meaning in life? How does your older family member find meaning in life? How are your responses to these questions alike and how are they different?

CONDUCTING A FOCUS GROUP

Students in a course entitled "Social Work Practice with Communities and Organizations" learned to conduct focus groups, which explored transition issues related to the housing continuum with older adults. At the end of the course, students will:

- understand how housing policies and the options on the housing continuum, which provide opportunities for older adults to age in place, affect older adults,
- demonstrate an understanding of how the history of an organization or community informs and shapes its current polices, programs, client systems, and positioning in the community,
- conduct or evaluate research that informs social change efforts and apply findings to generalist social work practice across the lifespan with diverse populations,
- understand ethical issues in conducting research with older adults, and
- demonstrate professional use of self, including ability to articulate and manage ethical and value dilemmas, and to apply principles of reflective practice and critical thinking skills to one's own practice with diverse populations across the lifespan.

The setting was an affordable housing community for older adults, targeted to older adults who could no longer live in an independent setting and were attracted to a communal living facility with services designed to support them as frailty increased. These students were exposed to aging content, which included understanding issues effecting both the physical and psychological adjustment to the housing continuum. Students met with the administrator of a recently built affordable housing facility to learn about housing older adults and the transitions that occur as older adults adjust to the housing continuum.

A "mock" focus group conducted in the classroom gave student the opportunity to discuss their own feelings and experiences with personal moves, either from their family home into a dorm, an apartment, or their first home. This helped them to remember their own experiences with moving so that they could be more empathetic to the experiences of the older adults. Also, the mock focus group helped them to understand the content and process of focus groups and how to analyze and integrate the experiences of the participants, as well as their own.

Based on their knowledge of focus groups, previous exposure to older adults and the moving experience the students developed questions for use in a focus group with older adults. They participated in a focus group with older adults at the facility where they learned about the residents' experiences with moving from their own homes into this communal setting. After the focus group, the students analyzed the shared stories and made recommendations to the administrator. Through this experience, the students learned: (1) how to plan and conduct focus groups, (2) how to gather and analyze stories shared by participants, (3) how to understand issues related to housing and housing policy for older adults, and (4) how to interview and communicate with older adults. Students were asked to reflect on content, process, and the "so what" of the experience. Reflection questions included: What did you learn about older adults? How have your views about older adults changed from the beginning of the class through the end of the class? What surprised you about the focus group with older adults? Compare and contrast focus groups for data gathering with at least one other method of data gathering. Explain which one you would choose in the future if contacted by an older adult housing facility. Defend your answer. It became evident from the students' reflections in class and their written reflective papers that as they deconstructed cultural messages about older adults they were developing a desire and interest for working with and advocating for older adults.

INTERVENING WITH MEXICAN AMERICAN OLDER ADULTS

This experience provides another example of intergenerational service-learning, which occurred in a rural setting. It summarizes some of the barriers and benefits of service-learning, as well as principles and concepts discussed earlier in this article. This title of the course is Aging: Cross Cultural Perspectives, which familiarizes students with the requisite values, knowledge, ethics and methods by which social work practitioners can more ably serve the needs of diverse elderly population in the El Paso/Juarez, urban/rural/border region. By the end of the semester the students will be able to:

- Identify and assess the economic, biological, psychological, social and cultural factors that impact the quality of life of older adults.

- Recognize and gain sensitivity to the diversity within the aging population; emphasis will be on older Hispanic and other diverse populations of the El Paso/Juarez, urban/rural/border region.
- Employ a goal oriented planned change approach to the development of intervention strategies.
- Become knowledgeable regarding the utilization of research methods to describe; explain; and predict human behavior in later years.
- Become familiar with social policy issues relevant to aging in American society.
- Apply critical thinking and writing skills in the development of an intervention strategy with older adults.

This class is a part of a social work program at a Hispanic serving institution located along the Texas/Mexico border. The county is primarily rural with many students coming either from Mexico to attend classes or from rural "colonias," unincorporated communities characterized by poverty, high crime, low educational levels, high levels of unemployment, and the lack of running water (TDH, 1995). The majority of the students at the University are the first in their families to pursue a college degree.

As a result, parents of these students are often unable, due to lack of education, language issues, and non-citizenship status to obtain employment offering a livable wage or sufficient income that would allow them to contribute monetarily to the student's education. Thus many of the students must work to pay for living and as well as educational expenses. As a result of these demands, a barrier often associated with the structuring of the service-learning experience was related to time availability. In addition to the time constraints, the anticipation of this new experience was accompanied by some anxiety. This too is a barrier that must be addressed when beginning a service-learning project.

Another issue to be considered in a rural area is that of the availability of partners to provide opportunities for the students. Limited options resulted in more anxiety regarding fitting requirements into specific time schedules. In addition to the time constraints, for many of the students this would be the first service-learning experience and the anticipation was also accompanied by verbalized anxiety and fear of what they considered the "unknown." Much of the anxiety was countered by class discussions related to concepts of aging, demographic profiles and by having older adults come into the classroom to speak and serve as guest lecturers. In addition, students were provided the opportunity to discuss particular concerns and address those concerns on an individual basis. For example, if the student had only a specific slot of time available then a service partner was located who had activities that could accommodate the student's schedule.

The students were partnered with agencies that provided services to older Hispanic (Mexican American) adults who live in El Paso County, a largely rural area along the Texas/Mexico border. To understand the significance of geography and culture one needs to be aware of the demographics of the older adult population in this portion of the Texas/Mexico border and of their specific service needs. Most of the older adult population in El Paso County migrated from Mexico, with 75% of the overall population identified as Hispanic, and primarily Mexican/American. Many of the older adults moved to this area as young adults, and settled in areas now known as "colonias" due to the opportunity for land ownership. These "colonias" are all within 40 miles of El Paso, a city of over 750,000 people. Many of the residents never applied for citizenship and are considered undocumented, a citizenship status that precludes eligibility for some government benefits and services. The educational level of these older adults is lower than the national average with only a small proportion having finished the equivalent of a high school education. A significant proportion lack English language skills.

The older adult partners selected by the students were recipients of services being provided by the limited number of agencies designed to assist with this population. Those services included transportation, nutrition, diabetes adherence, and group home monitoring. The reflections from the students' journals indicated that prior to the service-learning experiences many had limited contact with older adults outside of their own families. A significant proportion of the students had never been to the "colonias." They were unaware of the needs of the older adults in the area and lacked knowledge about the limited resources available to this population. Feelings of desperation were sometimes reflected in the journal writings of the students regarding the time limited involvement with these older adults and the immense unmet service needs. Those insights inspired discussions pertaining to the need to increase the advocacy and brokering role as social workers to expand culturally relevant service delivery to older adults living along the Texas/Mexico border. In conjunction with this process, students started to research policy issues that would impact service delivery, especially policies that excluded non-resident citizens.

The final phase of the reflection process occurred during an event entitled The Celebration of Aging, which took place during the last scheduled class of the semester. The purpose of the event was to show appreciation to the older adults and service partners who provided learning experiences for the students by recognizing their contribution and by the awarding of a certificate. Each student introduced the older adult with whom they interacted. The students had the opportunity to reflect on the significance of their shared experience.

The verbal reflections by the students indicated feelings of gratitude to the older adults for providing them an opportunity to integrate theory with practice, and to apply concepts and theories learned in the classroom to older adults. Most of the students expressed an appreciation for the experience, proclaiming that it provided an avenue to increase their understanding of aging in a way that could only be gained through direct involvement and observation. Students also expressed an increased respect for older adults who persevered in difficult circumstances, despite limited resources.

The course content, as reflected in the course objectives, was evident in the reflective musings of the students. They took a holistic approach to the study of the older adults looking at all issues that affect well-being and productive aging especially in this particular geographic area. The knowledge gained was channel into a productive means of social action. The objectives were achieved through readings and a course pack that addressed all area of the aging process, involvement of older adults as guest lecturers, interface with aging related organizations and service learning experiences with older adults.

Overall, many misconceptions regarding older adults were dispelled as a result of the service-learning experiences and many of the students expressed interest and intentions for working with older adults after graduation. These statements coincide with findings by Hatchett, Holmes, and Ryan (2002) from a survey administered to Hispanic students indicating that an increased familiarity with older adults has a positive impact on attitudes regarding older adults, especially women, and the intention to work with older adults.

PARTNERING WITH INDIVIDUALS IN COMMUNITY AND RESIDENTIAL SETTINGS

In this intergenerational service-learning project students were paired with older adults in a rural, country setting. Some of the service recipients lived independently and some were in residential service settings. Students were paired, either through personal selection or with the assistance of their instructor, with two older adult service-learning partners per student. One older adult partner was dependent upon social services as a result of their physical or emotional state and the other partner was living independently continuing to function in an active lifestyle. The purpose of having two service-learning partners was to explore the conclusions of Schwartz and Simmons (2001) that favorable experience with a population is more likely to heighten attitudes toward a population than unfavorable experiences. Amir (1969) postulates that favorable conditions tend to reduce prejudice; unfavorable ones may increase prejudice and intergroup tension (p. 338). Thus, contact with an elderly population may not in and of itself increase attitudes about a differing group but the experience must be perceived as positive.

The objectives of this course were to help the student define:

- Who are the elderly? How is aged defined?
- How is Engagement and Disengagement theory exemplified in this population?
- What is successful aging?
- How are the attitudes of older adults similar or different as a result of their living and care conditions?
- What restrictions are associated with older adults and how might the restrictions be addressed through advocacy and policy changes?
- Does religion and spirituality play a role in the daily decisions and activities of this population and if so, how?
- How is sexuality an issue for this population?
- How does the transition from independence to communal support occur and do preparations occur for the end of independence and life?

Reflection exercises occurred by way of class discussions and journal writings. Classroom activities included discussions about required and elective readings, interactive activities with the service recipients and the learning experiences of the student as a result of the activities, service needs identified by the student and their service-recipient, social relationship issues, family issues that impacted the social and living conditions of the service recipient, financial issues experienced by the recipients, and issues related to spiritual and religious involvement. Sexuality was briefly discussed but the majority of the students did not feel comfortable approaching the topic with their service recipients. Therefore, most of the reflections about sexuality were presented in a written format that discussed the observations the students made of the older adults and their significant other.

The assessment instruments used to determine student attitudes and interest for working with older adults indicate improved interest regardless of the dependency attributes of the service-learning recipient. Similar activities were conducted with the service recipients regardless of their physical or emotional state. Some of the activities conducted were video histories, photo journaling, written histories of life stories, travels, and where applicable, military experience journals, internet usage, meal preparation, shopping excursions, gardening, and dining out. Many of the older adult participants lacked transportation and the students, after providing sufficient evidence and documentation to address liability issues, transported their participants to various locations of interest. The culmination of the intergenerational service-learning experience was a banquet coordinated by the service-learners and presentations of mementos of appreciation to the service recipients.

The students identified the various life-transitions that the differing older adults were experience but the interactions with the differing population yielded no significant differences on the increase in attitudes. However, the conclusions of this specific study should not be generalized due to the small size of the respective sample (n = 13). Students' written and oral reflections indicated that learning occurred and numerous students stated that they had developed a greater interest for working with older adults and an increased level of comfort with older populations as a result of this experience. Similar to the findings of other researchers the students learned gerontological concepts, how to communicate and interact with the older adults, the complexity of problems faced by older adults, the limitations and gaps in services needed to address the issues of aging (Pine, 1997; Brown & Roddin, 2001).

CONCLUSION

Intergenerational service-learning is a teaching strategy that combines community service with academic learning, helping to prepare students for social work practice with older adults in micro, mezzo, and macro settings. These practice settings are highly beneficial and mutually rewarding to students and to older adults. Intergenerational service-learning can be used in a variety of settings and requires generalist knowledge about aging, including communication skills, assessment and problem solving skills, diversity among older adults, social issues and policies related to aging. Because intergenerational service-learning challenges cultural stereotypes about aging and exposes students to real people and not case studies, it provides a good vehicle for infusing gerontology content into a range of foundation courses that exist within the social work curriculum.

NOTES

1. Funding for these projects was provided by the Corporation for National and Community Service, Learn & Serve Higher Education through a grant to The Association for Gerontology in Higher Education in partnership with Generations Together/ University of Pittsburgh and from the Geriatric Enrichment in Social Work Education (GeroRich) grant funded by the John A. Hartford Foundation through the Council on Social Work Education.

2. At the time of the service learning project, Bonnie Hatchett was on the faculty of the University of Texas at El Paso.

REFERENCES

Amir, Y. (1969). Contact hypothesis in ethnic relations. *Psychological Bulletin, 71*(5), 319-342.

Astin, A. W., & Sax, L. J. (1998). How undergraduates are affected by service participation. *Journal of College Student Development, 39*, 251-263.

Bringle, R. G., & Hatcher, J. A. (1996). Implementing service-learning in higher education. *Journal of Higher Education, 67*(2), 221-239.

Brookfield, S. D. (1987). *Developing critical thinkers: Challenging adults to explore alternative ways of thinking and acting.* San Francisco: Jossey-Bass.

Brown, L., & Roodin, P. (2001). Service-learning in gerontology: An out-of-classroom experience. *Educational Gerontology, 27*, 89-103.

Cranton, P. (1994). *Understanding and promoting transformative learning: A guide for educators of adults.* San Francisco: Jossey-Bass.

Cranton, P. (2000). Individual differences and transformative learning. In J. Mezirow (Ed). *Learning as transformation: Critical perspective in theory in progress.* San Francisco: Jossey-Bass.

Dhooper, S. S., Rompf, E. L., & Royse, D. (1993). *Field instruction: A guide for social work students (1st ed).* Longman Publishing Group. White Plains, NY.

Dhooper, S. S., Rompf, E. L., & Royse, D. (1999). *Field instruction: A guide for social work students (3rd ed).* Longman Publishing Group. White Plains, NY.

Educational Policy and Accreditation Standards, Part 1. Council on Social Work Education.

Hatchett, B., Holmes, K., & Ryan, E. (2002) Attitudes of a predominantly hispanic college sample towards older adults. *Journal of Gerontological Social Work. 37*(2), 45-60.

Lawson, H. (ed.). (1998). *Practice teaching–Changing social work.* Jessica Kingsley Publishers. United Kingdom.

Lucas, E. T. (2000). Journal writing: Enhancing the service-learning experience. In J. M. McCrea, A. Nichols, and S. Newman (Eds). *Intergenerational service-learning in gerontology: A compendium Volume II.* University of Pittsburgh: Pittsburgh, PA.

Marullo, S. & Edwards, B. (2000) From charity to justice. *American Behavioral Scientist, 43* (5), 895-912.

Maurrasse, D. J. (2001). *Beyond the campus: How colleges and universities form partnerships with their communities.* New York: Routledge.

Mezirow, J. (1991). *Transformative dimensions of adult learning.* San Francisco: Jossey-Bass.

Nagy, G. & Falk, D. (2001). Dilemmas in international and cross-cultural social work education. *International Social Work Journal, 43*(1), 49-60.

Newman, S. & Tompkins, C. J. (2000). Building an intergenerational service-learning infrastructure in gerontology. In J. M. McCrea, A. Nichols, and S. Newman (Eds). *Intergenerational service-learning in gerontology: A compendium Volume II.* University of Pittsburgh: Pittsburgh, PA.

O'Connor, M. K. & Netting, E. F. (1999). Teaching students about collaborative approaches to organizational change. *Affilia, 14*(3).

Pine, P. (1997). Learning by sharing: An intergenerational college course. *Journal of Gerontological Social Work, 28*(1/2), 93-102.

Rhoads, R. (2000). Democratic citizenship and service-learning: Advancing the caring self. *New Directions for Teaching and Learning (82),* 37-45.

Schon, D. (1983). *The reflective practitioner: How professionals think in action.* New York: BasicBooks.

Schwartz, L. K. & Simmons, J. P. (2001). Contact quality and attitudes toward the elderly. *Educational Gerontology, 27*(2), 127-137.

Smith, E. D. (2001). The assessment of civic leadership. Retrieved from the Jossey-Bass Higher Education Series Website www.uca.edu/divisions/academic/idc/resources.htm_27k

Taylor, K., Marienau, C., & Fiddler, M. (2000). *Developing adult learners: Strategies for teachers and trainers.* San Francisco: Jossey-Bass.

Texas Department of Health (1995). Associateship for Disease Control and Prevention. Austin, Texas.

Wlodkowski, R. J. & Ginsberg, M. B. (1995). *Diversity and motivation: Culturally responsive teaching.* San Francisco: Jossey-Bass.

doi:10.1300/J083v48n01_11

Increasing Aging
and Advocacy Competency:
The Intergenerational Advocacy
Pilot Project

Joyce Hermoso, MSW
Anita L. Rosen, PhD
Libby Overly, MSW
Catherine J. Tompkins, MSW, PhD

SUMMARY. The Council on Social Work Education's (CSWE) Strengthening Aging and Gerontology Education for Social Work (SAGE-SW) project, funded by the John A. Hartford Foundation partnered with the National Committee to Preserve Social Security and Medicare (NCPSSM) to develop an Intergenerational Policy and Advocacy Project (IAP). This curriculum pilot project, based on a community organization model, was conducted with 13 baccalaureate social work (BSW) and master's social work (MSW) programs across the country and 122 students. The project was one method to pursue CSWE SAGE-SW's efforts to infuse aging content into social work foundation curricula, to support intergenerational teaching, to strengthen social work advocacy skills, and to provide social work students with positive experiences working with older adults.

[Haworth co-indexing entry note]: "Increasing Aging and Advocacy Competency: The Intergenerational Advocacy Pilot Project." Hermoso, Joyce et al. Co-published simultaneously in *Journal of Gerontological Social Work* (The Haworth Press, Inc.) Vol. 48, No. 1/2, 2006, pp. 179-192; and: *Fostering Social Work Gerontology Competence: A Collection of Papers from the First National Gerontological Social Work Conference* (ed: Catherine J. Tompkins, and Anita L. Rosen) The Haworth Press, Inc., 2007, pp. 179-192. Single or multiple copies of this article are available for a fee from The Haworth Document Delivery Service [1-800-HAWORTH, 9:00 a.m. - 5:00 p.m. (EST). E-mail address: docdelivery@haworthpress.com].

Available online at http://jgsw.haworthpress.com
doi:10.1300/J083v48n01_12

Pilot sites were asked to carry out the project as part of an existing course foundation or field practicum course. Project activities included collaboration with a variety of community agencies, holding issues or "town hall" forums in order to educate community members about critical policy issues affecting older adults; making contacts and establishing relationships with local, state and/or federal legislators; and conducting assessments of the service needs of older adults in the students' communities.

Questionnaires, feedback, pre-post evaluations as well as brief accounts of each project are presented. Participants considered the IAP to be a successful project in terms of the objectives of increasing awareness and competency among social work students of aging issues and of promoting intergenerational linkages between older people and social work students. doi: 10.1300/J083v48n01_12 *[Article copies available for a fee from The Haworth Document Delivery Service: 1-800-HAWORTH. E-mail address: <docdelivery@haworthpress.com> Website: <http://www.HaworthPress.com> © 2006 by The Haworth Press, Inc. All rights reserved.]*

KEYWORDS. Intergenerational, policy social work, education, community organization

INTRODUCTION

Infusing aging content into the social work foundation curriculum is one important way to help prepare all social work students with basic aging competence that would adequately meet the needs of a growing aging population. This is the philosophy behind the Council on Social Work Education's (CSWE) Strengthening Aging and Gerontology Education for Social Work (SAGE-SW) project, funded by the John A. Hartford Foundation (Rosen, Zlotnik, & Singer, 2002). In an effort to reach this goal, CSWE SAGE-SW partnered with the National Committee to Preserve Social Security and Medicare (NCPSSM) in 2001 to implement the Intergenerational Advocacy and Policy (IAP) Project. The project sought to foster positive intergenerational activities between social work students and the aging community, and to strengthen social work education in the areas of gerontology, policy, community organization, and advocacy.

The IAP, intended as a single semester curricular pilot project, was one means to address an identified need to develop infusion projects for social work education that incorporated aging and advocacy. Prior to the IAP, the CSWE SAGE-SW Project had conducted a national competency survey of 2,400 social work practitioners and academics both with and without interest in aging (CSWE SAGE-SW, November 2000). Feedback from the competency survey indicated that the sixty-five identified gerontology competencies had limited inclusion of advocacy skills. In addition, data-gathering work by SAGE-SW staff (such as focus groups) suggested that student's first exposure to older adults should not focus on end-of-life or people with severe limitations, but rather on non-institutionalized older persons who were more active and with whom students could communicate (CSWE SAGE-SW, 2000; Rosen, Zlotnik, & Singer, 2002).

The IAP followed the community organization model of practice. Both social work students and older people organized and advocated for major issues affecting seniors. Some examples of these issues include Medicare drug coverage, Social Security reform, transportation needs of older people, issues affecting grandparents raising grandchildren, and older minorities and immigrants. Seniors and social work students were to collaborate on such activities as town hall meetings, legislative analyses, conducting needs assessments, writing to and meeting with legislators, and engaging policy specialists and key community members on these issues.

THE INTERGENERATIONAL APPROACH

In recent years, the intergenerational approach has been advocated by some social work programs to increase awareness, competency, and sensitivity among practitioners, scholars and policy analysts for aging issues (Henkin, Santiago, Sonkowsky, & Tunick, 1997). The concerns and problems of older people are seen, not in isolation, but in relation to issues that are intergenerational. The intergenerational approach is predicated on the belief that the problems that older persons face also affect other generations and vice-versa. It is anticipated that working on aging issues is inextricably linked to working on issues of younger generations, thus making it pointless to compartmentalize the interests of older and younger generations or to pit them against one another (Henkin et al., 1997).

One of the trends resulting from the rapid modernization and industrialization of most societies is the increasing segregation of communities along class, racial, gender, and generational lines (Freedman, 1997). The globalization of economies all over the world have led to greater migration of people to different places thus causing shifts in the demographics and structures of societies. The resulting mélange in some cases led to greater segregation rather than integration. In an effort to assert their own interests, communities come into conflict with groups of other interests. Such communities tended towards allowing conflict to unfold rather than attempt to search for ways to see where their interests may unite (Henkin et al., 1997). Similar types of tension may also ensue between younger and older people. As each age group or generation advocates for its own unique set of interests exclusive of the other, the potential for conflict between generations may arise (Gelfand, 1982 as quoted in Henkin et al., 1997).

The concept of social capital has often been invoked in recent times by social scientists as a notion that may generate solutions to present-day problems of segregation and the demise of healthy community life (Homan, 2004). The idea of social capital surfaced as early as the 19th century when Alexis de Tocqueville wrote an account of the vibrant civic life in America during that period (Freedman, 1997; Putnam, 1995). In the early 1990s, there was a revival of interest among social scientists in the concept of social capital, particularly in studies linking democracy with the vibrancy of civic and community life.

The concept of social capital can, in part, be defined as the existence of social relations that facilitate trust and reciprocity and that enable people to collectively solve shared problems and concerns (Homan, 2004). As a form of capital, social capital has an intrinsic value that could be social as well as economic. However, unlike physical or financial capital, it increases with its use. When people are connected with one another and foster trust and reciprocity, they are better able to facilitate collective resolution of problems (Schmid, 2000; Wilson, 1997).

One way of diffusing the potential for conflict in communities resulting from greater fragmentation and segregation is by helping to build social capital within communities. Generating social capital in a community aids in building relationships between segregated groups. Working towards creating more social relations across generations can help in building relationships between older and younger persons which foster greater understanding and help in bridging their varying interests. An intergenerational approach can help bridge linkages across generations (Freedman, 1997). Intergenerational approaches also provide a way for communities to tap resources of people of all ages (Henkin, Santiago, Sonkowsky, & Tunick, 1997, as quoted in Kaplan, 1997). For example, by virtue of their experience and age, older people are usually looked upon as sources of wisdom and counsel. Younger generations can learn more about life lessons through regular interactions with older adults. Equally, younger people can offer their vitality and knowledge of modern technology in aiding older people to go about their day-to-day activities with better ease amidst a society that is becoming increasingly complex.

Another contribution of an intergenerational approach to building social capital is through the way that it promotes cultural identity and continuity (Henkin, Santiago, Sonkowsky, & Tunick, 1997; Kaplan, 1997). Intergenerational approaches may help in preserving cultural identities in communities.

Through cross-generational relationships, younger people can broaden their knowledge of the past and can thus have better appreciation for their history. Older people can aid younger generations in keeping their cultural identities alive amidst constant and rapid societal changes. Similarly, such relationships also enable older people to understand the youth and assist them in facing the challenges that the future brings. Intergenerational approaches can help weave these traditions and cultural identities and ensure their continuity through time and across generations.

Finally, intergenerational approaches promote the "ideals of common citizenship" (Moody & Disch, 1989, as quoted in Kaplan, 1997). The ideals of true citizenship entail active involvement in the community in ways that build relationships and foster linkages between varying groups. Intergenerational approaches can foster this idea of citizenship between both older and younger people. It encourages its adherents to develop relationships beyond their own age group and to have an appreciation and understanding of the interests of other groups. Moreover, intergenerational approaches foster a consciousness and appreciation towards building relationships and coalitions with groups that are different from one's own. These ideals are essential in maintaining and preserving communities, especially in a world that is transforming expeditiously.

METHODOLOGY

Selecting Pilot Sites

With the intergenerational framework in mind, the IAP project began with assistance sought from an IAP advisory committee, which was composed of expert social work faculty, some members of the SAGE-SW Executive Committee, and staff from the National Committee to Preserve Social Security and Medicare (NCPSSM), the National Association of Area Agencies on Aging, and SPRY. In selecting pilot areas for the IAP, a project development committee laid out a number of criteria and guidelines. The committee did not wish to be too proscriptive to allow for a variety of methods and activities. All participants were promised materials, resource lists, linking sites with community groups, and consultation from the NCPSSM and members of the project development advisory committee. No funding was promised, though the NCPSSM did eventually provide small stipends ($200 or less) to several programs for expenses for community events.

The first guideline was that pilot program faculty should be willing to incorporate the IAP into their foundation curriculum as part of the effort to infuse aging content. By infusing the IAP into a course or courses, social work programs would be better able to sustain the gains achieved through the project as well as its goals of supporting intergenerational approaches, providing an opportunity to link social work students with communities of older people, and giving students positive experiences with the elderly.

Another guideline for participating programs was that pilots must be open to developing and maintaining relationships with various aging stakeholders. These include public and private local organizations, Areas Agencies on Aging (AAA), other seniors' groups such as AARP, Silver Haired Legislatures, Grey Panthers, and state and federal legislators and policy makers. Also, it was strongly suggested that there be a least one contact with congressional representatives during the pilots projects. Nurturing relationships with aging stakeholders could help engender a stronger constituency for aging issues at the local and national levels. Developing and maintaining these relationships was also one strategy for sustaining the project's gains.

Participating programs were also expected to provide feedback and evaluation on the efficacy of the IAP. Assessments were based on the individual project's goals and objectives, chosen in relation to the broader CSWE Educational Policy and Assessment Statement's (EPAS) learning objectives (CSWE, 2001). Pilot faculty must have been willing to administer a CSWE SAGE-SW pre- and post-assessment forms to students which sought to evaluate the students' knowledge and attitudes about aging issues and the implications of these on their career choices. The faculty of each pilot project was also expected to assist in facilitating brief project evaluations to older adults and social work students.

The final guideline for social work programs that were involved with the IAP was that they were to be willing to share their experiences of implementing the project and the lessons drawn from these. The project development committee outlined various modes by which pilots could share and disseminate information about the IAP which included, but were not limited to, developing content for a website to be created for the project, writing articles for publication, and presenting at conferences particularly the Baccalaureate Program Directors (BPD) meeting, the CSWE Annual Program Meeting (APM) and the National Gerontological Social Work Conference (NGSWC).

The committee decided that, based on these criteria, they would invite social work programs to participate in this project primarily through exhibit booths and outreach at conferences such as the Association of Baccalaureate Social Work Program Directors (BPD) and through notification through the CSWE aging-interest Listserve. It was hoped that there would be diversity among pilot sites in terms of program size, geography (East Coast/West Coast), degree programs, and whether or not they were urban and rural social work programs. Choosing faculty who were already undertaking policy or advocacy activities related to aging issues also was seen as a possible way of building on existing initiatives of social work programs and organizations of older people. Social work programs and community organizations with pre-existing relationships with their local area agency on aging (AAA's) was also a useful criterion for selection.

Thirteen (13) sites across the country were involved in this project with 121 students. The sites generally met all of the criteria and the diversity desired. The pilot sites selected for the IAP included the University of North Alabama, St. Mary's College (Indiana), Texas A & M International University, Long Island University (Brooklyn Campus), James Madison University, and Lincoln Memorial University all of which have a baccalaureate program (N = 6); the University of Missouri-Kansas City and California State University-Bakersfield both of which have an MSW program (N = 2); and West Chester University, University of Nevada-Las Vegas, San Jose State University, Southern University at New Orleans, and George Mason University which have combined baccalaureate and master's programs (N = 5).

The IAP Approach

While the IAP was developed as an educational experience for social work students, on a secondary level, it also addressed the various needs of other stakeholders. For one, the IAP sought to meet some of the grassroots needs of the elder community. Issues affecting older persons abound; yet, there is limited grassroots advocacy on these issues and rarely enough intergenerational activities to address them. Though a high proportion of today's cohort of elders votes they are frequently reluctant to engage in political advocacy. At the same time, the population of older persons in America has grown at staggering rates (AoA, 2002) making seniors a significant political constituency. The pilot projects sought to optimize this potential and to act as catalysts to increase grassroots activities, organizing around senior issues in local communities.

There were a number of social work education needs that the IAP also hoped to address. One was the need for more exposure of students to aging issues (Rosen & Zlotnik, 2001; Scharlach et al., 2000). Generally, in social work programs, there has been more enthusiasm or attention given to other age groups and issues that on issues or problems affecting older people. The IAP provided opportunities for social work students to become familiar with issues facing older people. Moreover, working closely with active and interested older persons and advocating for their concerns may include positive perceptions about working with older adults.

The IAP attempted to bring together the needs of both the grassroots older persons and social work students by linking social work programs with the aging community. Through this partnership, the social work students aided senior groups in organizing and mobilizing other seniors to be involved in advocating for aging issues. The project also gave social work students the opportunity to work side by side with active and healthy older persons who have the capacity to advocate for policies affecting members of their age cohort. The hope was that this project would make younger students question the stereotypes they might hold about elders and also give them an opportunity to increase their competencies in both aging and community organization and advocacy. It was expected that as a result of participating in the IAP, students would have a greater familiarity and heightened sense of competence with the aging population and would be more likely to consider entering the field of aging.

Description of the Intergenerational Advocacy Projects

Given this theoretical framework for intergenerational approaches and the project criteria the IAP conducted a variety of community level and advocacy projects. The following is a brief descriptor of each pilot site, which only begins to explain either the complexity or the excitement generated by each of the programs:

- University of Missouri-Kansas City students worked with the Silver-Haired Legislature in Missouri and Kansas to advocate on such issues as Social Security, Medicare, and the Older Americans Act. Students investigated these issues from both a historical and contemporary perspective. The pilot was linked to a social welfare policy course and a foundation year master's level policy course. The goals of this pilot were to identify core professional values and ethics represented in formal policy and its service implications for older adults; and to understand how political forces and advocacy movements initiate and transform social policy.
- St. Mary's College (Indiana) students were required to work with the local AAA and meet with individuals impacted by legislation pertaining to Social Security, Medicare, and the American with Disabilities Act. They worked with legislators and community organizations and organized a Legislative Advocacy Day on campus. The students also met with the state Lieutenant Governor. The pilot was undertaken as part of the Human Behavior and the Social Environment (HBSE) II course.
- Long Island University students worked with a coalition of grandparent groups and community service agency participants who identified issues related to Temporary Assistance for Needy Families (TANF) for community education, direct intervention and advocacy. TANF proved to be an issue with clear intergenerational impact.

George Mason University students organized three seminar teams termed "Social Justice Teams." Two of them focused on grandparenting issues such as housing and grandparents as caregivers while the third one addressed the privatization of Social Security. The grandparenting teams hosted a showing of "Legacy," a documentary film about intergenerational issues in low-income housing, and invited legislators and media to the event. The Women and Social Security team hosted a town hall meeting. The three seminar teams had representation in an overall coordinating committee that was overseen by the Director of Field Instruction. GMU's pilot was linked to a Senior Practicum and Seminar at the BSW level which ran for two semesters.

Students at the Texas A & M International University were asked to gather information about the current state of Social Security and various proposals to reform the program. They were challenged to analyze how the various reform proposals could affect citizens of their community, both current and future beneficiaries, and how they should be enacted. Along with this, the students developed a community education program about the various proposals for Social Security reform. To carry out a community education project that involved holding a town meeting, the students worked with the El Azeteca Economic Development Foundation, a local organization. The pilot was undertaken in conjunction with a Social Welfare Programs and Services course.

San Jose State University students initiated efforts to reach out to Asian-American older adults as well as to a diverse group of seniors. They formed work teams of four to eight members along with older adults in the community to identify local issues of relevance and information needs related to Social Security, Medicare, and Older Americans Act programs. Each class met with representatives of two senior centers for planning purposes. The teams also sponsored community forums for disseminating information and held meetings with legislators and political leaders. In addition, the teams sponsored a mini-conference where they presented results of their research to the campus and the general public. The pilot was related to their course on Generalist Practice.

Students from the University of Nevada-Las Vegas formed an advisory board made up of AARP and Gray Panthers members, the Adult Protective Services staff, and other community representatives. They also collaborated with an advocate for the prescription drug industry and Senator Harry Reid. The students also wrote a position paper to disseminate information to seniors during election year both for U.S. Congress and their state legislature. Moreover, they conducted a town hall meeting and an aging day. The pilot was linked to their John A. Hartford Foundation, CSWE Geriatric Enrichment grant.

University of North Alabama students formed an active steering committee consisting of students, Alabama Silver-Haired Legislators, the local Department of Aging Services, the Northwest Alabama Council on Local Government, and other community organizations. The students were assigned to committees related to various aspects of their pilot (e.g., public relations, event coordination, etc.). The focal point of their project was a town hall meeting at the city's conference center. The pilot was implemented as part of the HBSE II course. Plans were made to maintain the steering committee and to involve succeeding cohorts of HBSE students.

James Madison University students hosted several town hall meetings and focus groups and organized a steering committee on aging issues. The project was carried on to a macro course which students were required to take in their senior year. The pilot was linked to a social policy class for BSW students.

The pilot project of University of California-Bakersfield focused on developing materials that were incorporated into class readings. The program held in-class debates about Social Security privatization. As a result of the readings and discussions, a number of students joined the National Committee to Preserve Social Security and Medicare while other students wrote position papers about privatization of Social Security. The pilot was undertaken as part of an Advanced Social Work Policy course at the MSW level.

The students of the Southern University at New Orleans met in pairs with older adults in the community to assess their knowledge and concerns about Social Security, Medicare, and the Olmstead Act. They wrote up the results of their findings and provided thoughts about steps to be taken to advocate for and with older adults in their community. The students participated in an aging needs assessment telephone survey sponsored by their local Council on Aging. The pilot was related to a course on Social Work Practice with Organizations and Communities.

The Lincoln Memorial University students worked with two senior centers and created tri-fold brochures about Social Security and Medicare. One senior center director worked with students to conduct a survey on the information needs of older people in this rural isolated area of Tennessee. The pilot initiative was linked to a policy class at the BSW level.

West Chester University students, in conjunction with the local AAA, did a community needs assessment of seniors living in their own homes through field visits and other initiatives of reaching out to seniors in their homes. They hosted a town meeting to focus on home and community-based issues. The students also organized a stakeholders meeting involving the state Department of Human Resources, the Social Security Administration, and the Center for Medicaid and Medicare Services. There also was a scheduled visit to

Washington, DC. West Chester's initiatives were linked to their Introduction to Social Work, Practice, and Advanced Policy courses.

RESULTS

Assessing Project Impact

In order to evaluate the impact that the pilot projects had in terms of achieving the learning objectives, student pre- and post-test surveys were administered among the participating social work programs. The survey included questions about the students' area of interests, their experience of working with older persons, their interest in social work with older people, and their career options after graduation. The Facts on Aging Quiz (1977) by Erdman Palmore was added to the last section of the questionnaire to assess the students' knowledge and attitudes about aging. The pre-test was given prior to participating in the IAP pilot project and the post-test was administered before the end of the semester when the pilot projects were implemented.

About fifty percent (50%) of the one hundred twenty-two students surveyed indicated previous experiences with older people came largely from personal relationships with grandparents, great uncles or aunts, or other older family members. Nineteen percent (19%) of students also encountered older people through their volunteer work particularly through their churches. The other experiences of working with older adults were in field placements, employment and volunteer work. A little more than seventy percent (70%) of the students had field placements in non-aging field settings such as child welfare, youth, and families, mental health centers, community organizations, women's shelters, and substance abuse centers. The few that had a placement in an aging field setting were in health or long-term care.

When comparing the students' responses before and after their involvement with the IAP pilot site, there were significant differences in responses on whether they were interested in social work, social policy, or advocacy work with older adults, and whether basic competence in working with older adults was important. The student responses indicated an increase in interest in social work, social policy, and advocacy on aging issues. In addition, the difference in scores between the pre and post tests revealed that the student respondents valued having basic competence in working with older populations.

There was no significant difference in responses between pre and post tests when student were asked whether they would accept a job working with older adults after graduation. These results notwithstanding a little less than half of the students surveyed stated an interest in working in aging after graduation. Those who indicated this interest maintained that they wanted to be more involved in advocacy for aging issues or to work in federal government such as the Commission on Aging pursuing the interests of older people. This suggests that the pilot projects may have positively influenced students' career preferences toward work with older adults after graduation.

DISCUSSION

Upon completion of their projects and reporting on their accomplishments, the participating pilot sites gave general feedback on the strengths of the projects and the other areas for improvement. Generally, the participants considered the IAP to be a successful project in terms of its objectives of increasing awareness and competency among social work students of aging issues and of promoting intergenerational linkages between older people and social work students. One of the major gains of the project was that it provided the initial venue for older people, social work students, and other stakeholders in the community to collaborate on important community issues. The participants recommended that the social work programs should establish and maintain on-going relationships with senior groups in their communities and build new ones as well.

Pilot site faculty with projects that entailed a major community event indicated that event planning was often time consuming but provided valuable learning lessons. Among identified skills were planning, collaboration, and community outreach. In presentations at national conferences and from feedback, these faculty leaders from pilot sites indicated that the IAP project had an unintended benefit for their social work education program through positive, visible, interaction with the community and with the college or university. In a number of cases, there was local media coverage of their IAP program which benefited both the college and the social work program. Some faculty were able to leverage the project into gaining outside funding for their educational activities. Students were given tangible and positive reinforcement for their advocacy activity. In some cases new field practica sites were opened and the IAP also served as an impetus for present and future community organizing and policy advocacy efforts with multi-stakeholder participation.

Another benefit was a substantive example of the IAP as a university-community collaboration model, in which macro social work can be infused in curricula and field education programs. This model can also be used for teaching macro social works regardless of the area of interest.

The pilot sites and other participants of the IAP provided some suggestions for next steps to be taken after completing the project. The first is that social work programs should maintain their presence in the senior advocacy community. One way of maintaining the gains achieved at the community level is by nurturing and building on the relationships already established by the social work programs, their students and faculty, the seniors in their communities and community stakeholders.

Second, social work programs should continue encouraging students to collaborate and advocate with older adults on aging-related issues. Whether they are undertaking this on their own or as part of a program within their curriculum, students should be persuaded to continue being involved in intergenerational efforts.

Finally, the individual pilot project faculty were enthusiastic about documenting their work through publications and presentations. This was suggested so that the IAP model can be incorporated into social work programs as one of many learning activities to infuse aging content and so that other social work programs can easily replicate it. The model can be used in numerous foundation courses and at various levels of social work education so that students' work on these issues will be continued throughout their social work education, as it will be in their careers. The IAP model of infusion of aging and advocacy content into foundation social work curriculum has the benefit of helping social work students experience the value of working with various community stakeholders and older people in a positive intergenerational approach in building and nurturing communities.

REFERENCES

Administration on Aging – AoA. (2002) Profile of Older Americans (2002). Retrieved on-line October, 12, 2003 from the World Wide Web: http://www.aoa.gov.

Council on Social Work Education-CSWE. (2001). *Educational Policy and Accreditation Standards*. Alexandria, VA. Retrieved on-line October, 10, 2003 from the World Wide Web: http://www.cswe.org.

CSWE SAGE-SW (2000) *News From SAGE-SW: Spring Summer, 2000*. Retrieved on-line October 10, 2003 from the World Wide web: http://www.cswe.org/ sage-sw/ resrep/newsletter8.htm.

CSWE SAGE-SW (Nov. 2000). CSWE SAGE-SW National Competencies Survey and Report. Retrieved on-line October 10, 2000 from htttp://depts.washington.edu/ geroctr/Curriculum3/Competencies/CSWESAGE_SWNationalCompetenciesSurv eyandReport.doc.

Freedman, M. (1997). Towards civic renewal: How senior citizens could save civil society. *Journal of Gerontological Social Work, 28*(3), 243-263.

Gelfand (1982). In Henkin, N.Z., Santiago, N., Sonkowsky, M., & Tunick, S. (1997). Intergenerational programming: A vehicle for promoting intra and cross-cultural understanding. *Journal of Gerontological Social Work, 28*(3), 197-209.

Henkin, N. Z., Santiago, N., Sonkowsky, M., & Tunick, S. (1997). Intergenerational programming: A vehicle for promoting intra and cross-cultural understanding. *Journal of Gerontological Social Work, 28*(3), 197-209.

Homan, M.S. (2004). *Promoting Community Change: Making It Happen in the Real World.* CA: Thomson Brooks/Cole.

Kaplan, M. (1997). The benefits of intergenerational community service projects: Implications for promoting intergenerational unity, community activism, and cultural continuity. *Journal of Gerontological Social Work, 28*(3), 211-228.

Palmore, E. (1988). *The Facts on Aging Quiz: A handbook of uses and results.* New York: Springer.

Putnam, R. (1995). Bowling alone: America's declining social capital. *Journal of Democracy, 6*(1), 65-78.

Rosen, A. & Zlotnik, J.L. (2001). Social work's response to a growing older population. *Generations, 25*(1), 69-71.

Rosen, A., Zlotnik, J.L., & Singer, T. (2002). Basic gerontological competence for all social workers: The need to "gerontologize" social work education. *Journal of Gerontological Social Work, 39*(1/2), 25-36.

Scharlach, A., Damron-Rodriguez, J., Robinson, B., & Feldman, R. (2000). Educating social workers for an aging society: A vision for the 21st century. *Journal of Social Work Education, 36*(3), 521-538.

Schmid, A. A. (2000). Affinity as social capital: Its role in development. *Journal of Socio-Economics, 29*, 159-171.

Wilson, P. A. (1997). Building social capital: A learning agenda for the twenty-first century. *Urban Studies, 34*(5/6), 745-760.

doi: 10.1300/J083v48n01_12

Developing an Aging Prepared Community: Collaboration Among Counties, Consumers, Professionals and Organizations

Laura Bronstein, PhD
Phillip McCallion, PhD
Edward Kramer, MA

SUMMARY. This paper reports on a collaborative process to create an "aging prepared community" in a four county region. The process benefited from a generous grant from the John A. Hartford Foundation that supported an 18 month planning period which included input from service providers and a vast array of aging persons and their families, including particular efforts to reach underserved populations from multicultural, inner-city and rural communities. Under the umbrella of the Elder Network of the Capital Region, the process is now beginning its implementation period with foci on the following: linking health, social service and faith communities; developing accessible health education and wellness programs; creating and implementing a regional system of information and assistance; and mounting a media campaign. doi: 10.1300/J083v48n01_13

Development of this article was supported by an Aging Prepared Community Grant from the John A. Hartford Foundation, awarded to the University at Albany and to the New York State Office for the Aging. However, any opinions expressed here are those of the authors.

[Haworth co-indexing entry note]: "Developing an Aging Prepared Community: Collaboration Among Counties, Consumers, Professionals and Organizations." Bronstein, Laura, Phillip McCallion, and Edward Kramer. Co-published simultaneously in *Journal of Gerontological Social Work* (The Haworth Press, Inc.) Vol. 48, No. 1/2, 2006, pp. 193-202; and: *Fostering Social Work Gerontology Competence: A Collection of Papers from the First National Gerontological Social Work Conference* (ed: Catherine J. Tompkins, and Anita L. Rosen) The Haworth Press, Inc., 2007, pp. 193-202. Single or multiple copies of this article are available for a fee from The Haworth Document Delivery Service [1-800-HAWORTH, 9:00 a.m. - 5:00 p.m. (EST). E-mail address: docdelivery@haworthpress.com].

KEYWORDS. Aging prepared, service delivery and access, aging persons, collaboration, planning

THE NEED FOR "AGING PREPAREDNESS"

There is an increasing population of people ages 65 and older due to longer life expectancies, lower fertility rates, and the influx of the Baby Boom Generation into this age category (Riche, 2000). Despite some common characteristics, this and future older populations are more diverse than any preceding one in terms of ethnicity, income level, education, family configurations, living arrangements and health status (Dobrof, Mellor, Pine, & Saul, 2000). For example, while many of today's elderly are in better health, better educated and more affluent than earlier cohorts, this is juxtaposed by the existence of poverty and an increasing gap between the haves and have-nots (Center on Budget and Policy Priorities, 2000; Dobrof, Mellor, Pine, & Saul, 2000).

In addition, it is projected that between the years of 1995 and 2025, minority populations of people 60 years and older will increase dramatically (Sutton, 1999) creating a need to be increasingly attentive to the impact of culture on service delivery. Some related concerns are that ethnic minority groups in the U.S. continue to lag in level of health care coverage as well as on most other health indicators including life expectancy and disease rates (Keigher, 1999). While many minority elders are reported to have a greater need for health and social services than white elders, they have far lower rates of service utilization, health coverage and access (Keigher, 1999; Scharlach, Damron-Rodriguez, Robinson, & Feldman, 2000).

The support of elderly people, particularly those with chronic conditions, has traditionally fallen upon family caregivers. Elderly spouses are the first line, but increasing numbers and age among the cohort of elderly are placing greater demands upon the children of the elderly (Toseland, Smith, & McCallion, 2001). Middle-aged caregivers in these sandwich generations often experience concurrent financial, emotional and physical costs. One study "found that women who spent time helping their parents, either with basic personal activities or with errands and chores, cut back their work hours by 550 hours per year, or 58 percent. This loss in work hours translates into about $10,300 in forgone wages per caregiver per year in 1998 dollars" (Lo Sasso & Johnson, 2002, p. 4). There are many other potential employment complications that are experienced as a result of caregiving, including having to take less demanding jobs, retiring early, turning down promotions and career advancements, losing job benefits, taking leaves of absence, and taking time off from work (Briar & Kaplan, 1990; Ory et al., 1999). These findings support growing recognition that the aging of the nation is a concern for *all* generations in society.

There is also increasing awareness that needs are differentially felt by those living in urban, suburban and rural areas, where there is a high degree of variation in services and access to these services. All of these trends support the need for a different approach to community support of aging citizens. The growing numbers make it an imperative.

AGING PREPAREDNESS AND NEW YORK STATE

According to the U.S. Census, New York State's older population continues to grow faster than its overall population, with the largest growth occurring among the oldest age group, older women, and minority elderly (Sutton, 1995). The current over 65 population in New York State is 2,423,797 (970,512 are men; 1,453,285 are women). New York State has the third largest number of elderly (65+) following only California (3,614,632) and Florida (2,734,145). The elderly in New York State who are over 65 equal 13.3% of the total population and consistent with national trends are increasingly diverse (Sutton, 1995). Trends also show an increasing gap in incomes between downstate metropolitan counties and upstate rural counties, with poverty rates among the elderly highest in the most rural counties in New York (Krout & Maiden, 2000). These population projections and corresponding needs are causing aging providers and policymakers to consider their impact upon services and service delivery, including those of public social service agencies.

In New York State this growing aging awareness has prompted the Governor to launch Project 2015 requiring *all* state agencies to develop plans to better address the needs of the aging population. Project 2015 brings aging demographics to the forefront of every state agency including those not usually charged with paying primary attention to the needs of the aging. There is recognition that aging trends have an impact on all age cohorts. For example, increasing numbers of grandparents are becoming guardians for their grandchildren and over half of these grandparents in New York State are racial/ethnic minorities (Burnette, 2000). Therefore child and family oriented service providers must also be assisted to have an aging sensitivity and focus if they are to successfully serve their core population.

With an increased aging cohort and their increasing diversity and needs, comes an expanding need for high quality long-term care alternatives in New York State. For one, most people are reported to want to remain and age at home whenever possible. Presently, community based resources to support people aging in place are extremely limited especially for those living alone and those with complex medical and/or cognitive impairments such as dementia. Secondly, states are under increasing pressure to respond to the Supreme Court's Olmstead decision, a mandate to care for persons who are elderly and/or who have disabilities, in the least restrictive environment. Aging preparedness in New York State is therefore also seen in the context of expanding long-term care alternatives.

In responding to these national and statewide demographic projections and corresponding needs for community-based care, the John A. Hartford Foundation has targeted initiatives to support proactive planning as opposed to reactive responses to the aging of society. As one of its initiatives, the Foundation awarded a planning grant to the University at Albany and New York State Office for Aging to support the development of an "aging prepared" community in the Capital Region of New York State. The project has conducted an in-depth needs assessment of the four counties of the Capital Region, targeted the prevention of unnecessary hospitalization and institutionalization and developed an implementation plan with initiatives that make the Capital Region a good place to grow old.

The Capital Region, while it has unique features, appeared an ideal location to pilot aging prepared processes that might be both successful and replicable elsewhere. The four county region has three major urban areas, rural communities and suburban developments. Services and resources tend to be concentrated in the urban areas, particularly the city of Albany. There are over 80 elected governmental bodies in the region, something that speaks to high interest in governance and management of critical community issues but also presents potential barriers to collaboration and regional approaches.

BUILDING COLLABORATION IN THE PLANNING PERIOD

Over 600 representatives of state and local government, foundations, health networks, insurers, caregivers, employers, aging services providers, faith communities, and aging persons themselves participated in the planning activities and approximately 80 agencies and faith communities committed to participating in the implementation plans that resulted. Together they implemented a planning process using a mixed methodology: (1) interviews with aging consumers, (2) interviews with key decision-makers and opinion shapers including political leaders, aging advocates, faith community leaders and health system administrators, (3) targeted focus groups and interviews around transportation, discharge planning, underserved communities, information and referral, and faith community linkage, (4) community forums, (5) review of existing health and aging related databases, (6) examination of current service delivery, (7) identification of barriers to continued community living, (8) identification of barriers to effective service delivery, (9) meetings with national experts who had developed innovative solutions in other communities, and (10) development of an implementation plan. Particular efforts targeted outreach to those whose voices are not easily heard, e.g., the frail elderly, seniors living in poverty and those living in remote, rural areas. Also, to "do business differently" became a primary focus of the activities and the planning process involved relationship-building among a wide constituent and provider base.

A regional approach to care seemed ideal. For example, there were many cases identified where a resident of County A may be going for tests at a hospital at County B, relying upon transportation from their local Area Agency on Aging which will take the person only as far as the county line; not much help for the individual in keeping medical appointments but also presenting concerns for county and local offices for aging, and other service providers bound by funding and regulatory restraints.

The planning process did find needed services that were not available, but more often services existed, but were inadequately utilized due to difficulties in access, including limited and/or inflexible transportation options and the lack of a simple system of information and referral/assistance. In meetings, providers themselves frequently talked about difficulties they experienced accessing services for their family members, usually ending their stories with, "and if *I* can't locate services, what does this say about the general public's ability to find services!"

Seniors and providers also noted difficulties in sorting through information that is available. For example, the region was found to support many health education and disease prevention efforts for seniors but there was limited success in getting this information communicated to those needing it. Often seniors described being bombarded by so many and sometimes conflicting messages about changing their diet, exercise, sleep patterns, medications, etc. that it seemed easier to ignore them all. A similar difficulty was found in getting information out to caregivers so that they can plan for their loved one's needs as opposed to reacting in the face of a crisis. A further gap was adequate links between health care and supportive services providers. There were stories of seniors being discharged to home from hospitals only to find that service plans weren't solid enough to maintain the person at home, and so days later they were back in the hospital. One discharge planner told of a

90-year-old woman who claimed to have someone at home to take care of her upon discharge. It was only when she was re-admitted days later, that the discharge planner learned that the person she referred to as her caretaker was her son who lived 500 miles away. Finally, while many service gaps applied to all seniors, it emerged from the data collection process those in the inner city, those in rural communities and members of multicultural communities were particularly limited in their ability to access services.

Despite these challenges, a number of Capital Region strengths came to light through the planning process. For one, there is high interest in improved effectiveness of senior services at all levels of the community. Secondly, despite frustration at how to make change, there is interest in doing things differently. Third, there is a desire by local seniors to be part of the solution. The Capital Region already has a number of very active and successful consumer-led organizations including the Capital District Senior Issues Forum and ROUSE: Rensselaer Organizations United for Senior Endeavors. As the State Capital, the Albany area has many seniors who retire from state work and who are bright, informed and interested in finding meaningful ways to be involved and contribute to their community. This leads into the fourth strength, an already existent network of volunteers. While many of these volunteers are retired state workers, many others have retired from an array of other (often less well-paying) jobs and participate in one of the senior groups noted above or through their religious community. And fifth, key agencies in the community committed to supporting the planning initiative through coordinating with one another to develop services to meet newly identified needs to the extent possible, to reduce duplication and redundancy in service delivery and to intensify shared learning opportunities.

Needs, strengths and commitment molded a four-pronged plan to make the Capital Region more aging prepared and the project was renamed: The Elder Network of the Capital Region (ENCR) to highlight the move from planning to implementation.

ENTERING THE IMPLEMENTATION PHASE

The Elder Network of the Capital Region is committed to enhancing the well-being and sustaining older adults' independence by connecting currently available health and related services and creating new capacity to fill major gaps, as these are identified.

This work will be accomplished by:

CREATING a consortium of health and human services agencies, state & local government, faith communities, and the university with the active participation of older persons themselves to prepare communities and individuals for aging.

CONSTRUCTING a sustainable web-based information and assistance capacity to enable older persons and their families to access services available throughout the Capital Region, in person, by telephone, or over the Internet.

INCREASING awareness, education and training to promote wellness, illness prevention, and safety practices among older persons.

PARTNERING among health care providers, local faith based organizations and volunteers to improve post-hospital discharge care for older persons.

Seven high priority issues were identified in the planning process in order to improve capacity and build upon the region's strengths:

- Address the information deficit
- Improve hospital discharge coordination by engaging seniors and faith community staff as community-based liaisons
- Plan for volunteer and formal transportation supplements to target medical and other appointments, as well as needs for medications and groceries
- Partner formal and informal caregivers to sustain maximum independence of older adults as long as possible
- Redesign senior centers to be central sites for health education, supplemental transportation, and information and assistance
- Improve levels of good health practices by targeting increased immunizations, exercise and falls prevention programs.
- To address these issues, the relevant stakeholders including participating governmental, health, aging services and advocacy programs and representatives, have endorsed the following initial four-pronged work plan for ENCR.

INFORMATION AND ASSISTANCE (I&A)

ENCR is working with local software companies to create and maintain a web-based information resource with mapping capabilities. Related training on its use for discharge liaisons, volunteer care teams and caregivers are being developed. One agency in each county will be designated as the key I&A Resource Center. Each will access the web based information resource and offer telephone and in-person assistance on service, eligibility and supplemental transportation requests. Agencies in the region, older adults and their care-givers will also be able to access and utilize the resource themselves. Over the four years of our implementation phase we estimate that information and assistance (I&A) will be provided to 5,000 seniors and caregivers, and I&A duplication and overlap will be reduced.

Health Education and Wellness

ENCR is developing, publicizing and implementing a region wide health prevention education program, in collaboration with NYSOFA, the Depart-ment of Health, health networks, insurers and pharmaceutical companies. Proven strategies are being used to increase levels of immunizations, healthy lifestyles and falls prevention. Education and volunteer support efforts also address disease management and palliative care concerns. These areas have been chosen because they have the potential to have the largest impact on rea-sons for hospitalizations and premature institutionalization. Faith communi-ties and a broad range of providers are supporting this component of the implementation plan.

Health and Faith Program

To reduce avoidable hospital re-admissions and institutionalization in long-term care facilities, five health networks in the region have agreed to work with faith communities and the county-based I&A resource centers to improve post-discharge care. Faith communities representing different denominations will be linked to each health provider. Congregations have been identified which include a large number of at-risk seniors, and which have leadership committed to working with seniors and health providers. A key member of the congrega-tion will receive a stipend and will lead volunteer efforts within each faith com-munity. The health providers and the faith communities will work together to develop, implement and monitor discharge plans, and will learn from one another under the ENCR umbrella. Faith communities will serve their surround-ing neighborhood as well as their own congregants. Over a four-year period, we estimate that 600 older adults will be helped by this component of ENCR.

Raising Awareness Through a Media Campaign

ENCR will address communication problems in aging services and care including: programs doing good work that the public knows little about; seniors knowing what they need to do in terms of good health practices but needing encouragement to do so; and caregivers not knowing where to turn despite the availability of supports. Good programs and practices not known and not used will not lead to good outcomes. A print/TV/radio and public service announcement campaign over four years will be an integral part of ENCR's efforts. The University's Advancement Office will provide a staff member to coordinate media efforts with assistance from an advisory committee drawn from the various media outlets in the Capital Region.

Governance and Evaluation

An overall governing board for ENCR is drawn from community leaders representing the whole region. Similarly, each of the four prongs of the implementation project will be guided by a working committee of relevant stakeholders, responsible to work with ENCR staff to implement the work plan. Committee members will be drawn from the agencies, faith communities and the region's seniors. An evaluation effort will document ENCR development and outcomes and prepare for and support replication efforts within New York State and beyond. The evaluation will tap existing databases on hospital, nursing home and emergency room use, gather data on health indicators, measure consumer knowledge and satisfaction and assess related costs. Data on the process of implementing ENCR will also be gathered to support development of replication materials. Initial evaluation efforts are beginning and are comprised of qualitative methods including content analysis of daily process notes; minutes of meetings; focus groups; and individual interviews with providers and clients. These data will be analyzed and used to develop quantitative methods of measuring progress towards ENCR's goals.

CONCLUSIONS

The coming and present increase in the aging population of the United States has been much heralded with predictions of dire consequences for Medicare, Social Security, and other programs, greater self-advocacy by Baby Boomers as they age and realignments of work and family to accommodate both increased caregiving and a smaller, young workforce. At times, however, it appears that the response by society to these predictions is in inverse proportion to its concerned reaction to these realities–very concerned but not doing anything too different. It appears that such inertia is related to a lack of vision of how things could and should be different, beliefs that there will not be the needed resources, concerns to "protect" resources for current service populations and providers and the need to address what are seen as more pressing or solvable concerns for other populations. There are efforts to redress this inattention, particularly by the Administration on Aging, by individual states (for example, New York and Florida) and by philanthropic foundations (for example, John A. Hartford Foundation and Robert Wood Johnson Foundation). The planning process that resulted in ENCR recognizes that aging is a cross-generational concern; solutions here will address multiple social problems, makes better use of resources, includes those currently and those yet to be served and offers a vision for living successfully in the community into old, old age.

REFERENCES

Briar, K.H. & Kaplan, C. (1990). *The U.S. caregiving crisis.* Silver Springs, MD: The National Association of Social Workers, Commission on Family and Primary Associations.

Burnette, D. (2000). Grandparents as family caregivers. In R. Kriss & M.J. Mellor (Eds.). *Project 2015: The Future of Aging in New York State.* (pp. 77-85). Albany, NY: New York State Office for the Aging.

Center on Budget and Policy Priorities (2000). *Poverty rate hits lowest level since 1979 as unemployment reaches a 30 year low.* Author: Washington, DC.

Dobrof, R., Mellor, M.J., Pine, P.P., & Saul, S. (2000). Introduction. In R. Kriss & M.J. Mellor (Eds.). *Project 2015: The future of aging in New York State.* (pp. v-vii) Albany, NY: New York State Office for the Aging.

Keigher, S.M. (1999). Reflecting on progress, health and racism: 1900-2000. *Health & Social Work, 24*(4), 243-248.

Krout, J.A. & Maiden, R.J. (2000). Living in the community: A rural and nonrural comparison. In R. Kriss & M.J. Mellor (Eds.). *Project 2015: The future of aging in New York State.* (pp. 43-48). Albany, NY: New York State Office for the Aging.

Lo Sasso, A.T. & Johnson, R.W. (2002). Does informal care from adult children reduce nursing home admissions for the elderly? *Institute for Health Services Research and Policy Studies at Northwestern University:* 1-38.

Ory, M.G., Hoffman, R.R., Yee, J.L., Tennstedt, S., & Shulz, R. (1999). Prevalence and impact of caregiving: A detailed comparison between dementia and non-dementia caregivers. *The Gerontologist, 39*(2), 177-185.

Riche, M.F. (2000). America's diversity and growth: Signposts for the 21st century. *Population Bulletin, 55*(2), 1-54.

Scharlach, A., Damron-Rodriguez, J., Robinson, B., & Feldman, R. (2000). Educating social workers for an aging society: A vision for the 21st century. *Journal of Social Work Education, 36*(3), 521-538.

Sutton, D.L. (1995). *Demographic Projections to 2025.* Albany, NY: New York State Office for the Aging.

Toseland, R., Smith, G., & McCallion, P. (2001). Helping family caregivers. In A. Gitterman (Ed.), *Handbook of social work practice with vulnerable and resilient populations* (2nd ed.) (pp. 548-581). NY: Columbia University Press.

doi: 10.1300/J083v48n01_13

Social Work and Aging
in the Emerging Health Care World

Barbara Berkman, DSW
Daniel Gardner, PhD
Bradley Zodikoff, PhD
Linda Harootyan, MSW

SUMMARY. Social work practice with older adults and their families is increasingly recognized by the profession as a major field of practice in a wide range of health care and community-based settings. This article reviews emerging trends and issues in the fields of aging and health care, drawing on gerontological health care research which bridges these areas. Given the growing number and diversity of older adults in our society, and dramatic changes in the organization and delivery of health care, the authors suggest skills and competencies essential to enhancing the well-being of older adults and their families in the 21st Century. doi: 10.1300/J083v48n01_14 *[Article copies available for a fee from The Haworth Document Delivery Service: 1-800-HAWORTH. E-mail address: <docdelivery @haworthpress.com> Website: <http://www.HaworthPress.com> © 2006 by The Haworth Press, Inc. All rights reserved.]*

KEYWORDS. Health care, geriatric social work practice, intergenerational families

---

[Haworth co-indexing entry note]: "Social Work and Aging in the Emerging Health Care World." Berkman, Barbara et al. Co-published simultaneously in *Journal of Gerontological Social Work* (The Haworth Press, Inc.) Vol. 48, No. 1/2, 2006, pp. 203-217; and: *Fostering Social Work Gerontology Competence: A Collection of Papers from the First National Gerontological Social Work Conference* (ed: Catherine J. Tompkins, and Anita L. Rosen) The Haworth Press, Inc., 2007, pp. 203-217. Single or multiple copies of this article are available for a fee from The Haworth Document Delivery Service [1-800-HAWORTH, 9:00 a.m. - 5:00 p.m. (EST). E-mail address: docdelivery@haworthpress.com].

INTRODUCTION

Historically, the social work profession has separated the issues of aging from the field of health and mental health. This has been most evident in social work education programs in the development of specializations and concentrations in aging as distinct from those in health, mental health and disability. A growing body of research has shown that social work practice with older adults and their families–once virtually the exclusive concern of geriatric social work, but increasingly recognized by the profession as a major focus of services in a range of health care and community-based settings–entails engagement with intersecting biological, psychological, socio-environmental, cultural, political and economic contexts that are entwined with aging in American society (Berkman & Harootyan, 2003). Health care social work in the 21st Century requires the development and application of evidence-based knowledge that reflects the interrelatedness of traditionally circumscribed fields of practice. Given the dramatic growth in the numbers and proportion of older adults in our society and in the financing, delivery and technological advances of biomedical health care, it is time to bring the concepts of aging and health care together in social work educational programs, practice, policy and research.

This article presents an overview of emerging trends and interrelated issues in the fields of aging and health care, drawing from current gerontological health care research which bridges these two areas. The authors use a multidimensional approach to address critical problems facing older adults and their families that exemplify the intersect between biopsychosocial and socio-cultural domains. We then identify the specific social work knowledge and skills needed to address these emerging trends effectively, and suggests promising future directions for research, policy and practice in the interrelated fields of aging and health.

Over the past 10 years, Americans have witnessed dramatic changes in health care delivery stimulated by advances in technology and new approaches to the financing of health care. Health care is increasingly delivered in community-based ambulatory settings where care is provided by a vast array of medical specialists. Patients with chronic conditions move in and out of health care systems more rapidly than in the past and their interaction with all health care professionals is likely to be time-limited and episodic (Shortell, Gilles, & Devers, 1995; Volland, 1996).

There have been equally significant changes in the demographics of aging. People are living longer because of advances in public health, health care technology and service delivery. The statistics that highlight the increasing proportion of the population older than 65 years and the increasing diversity of this population are now familiar to us all. At the end of this decade, the baby boom generation will begin to turn 65, and by 2050, 20% of the total U.S. population will be 65 years and older (U. S. Bureau of the Census, 2000a). The fastest growing segment of the older population is the group aged 85 years and older, which is expected to grow from 4 million in 2000 to 19 million by 2050 (U.S. Bureau of the Census, 2000b). By 2050, about one third of the elderly population will be composed of Blacks, Hispanics, Asians and other minority groups (U.S. Bureau of the Census, 2000c; U.S. Special Committee on Aging, 1996).

These radical transformations in health care delivery and in the older population create new roles and challenges for social workers in health care. In the emerging health care environment, most social workers will find themselves working with larger numbers of older adults and their families than in the past, especially with the growth of aging multigenerational families. Among their patients, health care social workers will see larger proportions of older adults who present in multiple roles, as family members, as caregivers, as care recipients, and as sophisticated consumers of health and social services. Regardless of their specialty, health care social workers will require a deeper understanding of the rapidly changing political, economic, social and cultural contexts that affect health care delivery to older persons. Knowledge of these trends, as well as of the growing body of evidence-based knowledge on the biopsychosocial factors associated with practice with older persons, will strengthen health care social workers' competencies in meeting current needs and in designing the innovative interventions of the future.

MAJOR TRENDS AFFECTING THE HEALTH AND WELL-BEING OF OLDER ADULTS AND THEIR FAMILIES

Chronic Illness

Aging itself is associated with increased vulnerability to a variety of chronic physical and mental health conditions. Chronic illnesses and conditions such as diabetes, heart disease and cancer are enduring and episodic in nature, and often require monitoring and management for extended periods (Burnette & Kang, 2003). In older adults, chronic illnesses contribute to declines in functioning and quality of life, and are related to increases in mortality and health care costs. Chronically ill older patients, the majority of whom are living in the community, present complex interacting medical and psychosocial problems. Along with their families, they require special interventions from community-based social workers to access and utilize social and health care services effectively.

Chronic physical and mental conditions that diminish an older adult's capacity to function independently often lead to the need for long-term care in community or residential settings. However, there are still significant gaps in knowledge about geriatric mental health among both formal and informal caregivers. For example, despite our recognition that mental and physical health are inextricably linked, the emphasis on medical intervention in long-term nursing home care continues to overshadow attention to psychological and social needs (Adamek, 2003). Unfortunately, America's current reimbursement policies in institutional long-term care promote a limited unilateral approach focused on medical interventions.

Diversity of the Aging Population

The older adult population is increasingly diverse in terms of age, race, ethnicity, gender and socioeconomic status. For example, in the next 50 years the proportion of Hispanic individuals aged 65 or older is expected to triple, representing an estimated 16% of the population (Federal Interagency Forum on Aging Statistics, 2000). Health care professionals must be especially cognizant of the cultural diversity among elders who confront serious physical and mental health problems as there are greater disparities in health care delivery and access to care in later life among diverse groups (Maramaldi & Guevara, 2003).

Intergenerational Families and Caregiving

Aging occurs primarily within a familial context. An individual's experience of physical and mental illness profoundly influences and is influenced by his or her reciprocal relationships (or lack of relationships) with family members and other caregivers. Today, there are significant changes in outcomes of patient care stimulated by technological advances in biomedicine and pharmacology. People are living longer with complex chronic physical and mental health conditions (Berkman, Silverstone, Simmons, Howe, & Volland, 2000). The leading causes of morbidity and mortality are almost all related to chronic diseases, resulting in episodes of illness over a lifetime of chronic complex processes (Paulson, 1994). These elderly people often have significant activity impairments and quality-of-life issues. They will represent an increasing percentage of persons served by social workers. Social workers who will be valued in health care will be those who have the necessary knowledge and skills needed to work effectively with older people and their families.

Changes in longevity and in health care have led to changes in the expectations for family involvement in care of older adults (Hooyman & Kiyak, 2002; Scharlach et al., 2000). Families are increasingly expected to be responsible for home care needs. With the number of beneficiaries of the Medicare Home Health Program rising significantly, there has been a simultaneous increase in the pressure placed on families. Recent national surveys suggest that one in four households was involved in helping to care for a family member aged 50 years or older (NAC/AARP, 1997). More than 9 million people in the United States are informal caregivers. At the same time, there is a reduction in the numbers of family members available to provide care because of geographic distances and increased workforce participation.

One risk associated with the increased burden of family caregiving is elder mistreatment. As with other types of family violence, elder abuse is believed to be under-reported and under-diagnosed, due to a lack of thorough assessment and knowledge of the problem among health care professionals. Although most social workers are aware of the individual and societal costs of elder mistreatment, there is little known about the incidence, the precipitating factors, the consequences, and treatments that are effective. There remains a serious need for empirical research, comprehensive planning and policy to address this multifaceted public health concern (Paveza & VandeWeerd, 2003).

Older persons are not only receiving care, they also are providing it. Half of all people caring for elderly family members are themselves older than 60 years of age (NAC/AARP, 1997), and there are 2.5 million families in the United States that are maintained by a grandparent. A growing number of older women have assumed the role of custodial grandparents, due most often to the biological parent's substance abuse, incarceration, physical disability or death. Poindexter and Boyer (2003), who study older relatives caring for grandchildren whose parents are living with HIV/AIDS, note that although custodial grandmothers can derive emotional rewards (e.g., companionship, pride and a sense of mastery) from their caregiving roles, assuming parenting responsibilities in later life is developmentally dissonant, and can negatively affect their psychosocial and physical health. Innovative responses to the needs of caregivers are required if persons with disabilities are to remain in the community with quality of life (McCallion & Kolomer, 2003).

Cost-Containment, Decentralization and Fragmentation in Health Care

Americans live in a changing political, economic, and social world that is aging. The rising cost of health care in the second half of the last century has led to radical changes in the public and private financing of health care. Efforts to contain the costs of care have resulted in the implementation of a variety of managed care and prospective payment systems in physical and mental health care (Berkman, 1996; Naleppa, 2003; Robert, 2003).

Americans are witnessing dramatic changes in the financing of health care delivery. The increasing corporatization of health care delivery systems in the United States is having a profound impact on health care professionals who work with older adults. Currently, health care is skillful in its ability to provide high quality, technologically advanced acute care, but the ability to meet chronic care needs is limited because the service and financing systems are complex and fragmented into many mini-systems. There is an overlapping, confusing array of service providers–ranging from the federal government to state and local governments, the proprietary sector, the voluntary sector, and the family. Under managed care particularly, there is movement toward more community-based services. There is the decentralization of expensive diagnostic services to out-of-hospital sites and increasing use of ambulatory procedures and services that were once done on an inpatient basis (Shortell et al., 1995; Berkman, 1996).

These changes increasingly complicate the ability of elderly patients and their families to access and use the often multiple systems of care effectively. It is not surprising that with this increasing fragmentation of service delivery even the most competent elders and their families have difficulty deciphering the eligibility requirements of different programs. They and their families require special knowledgeable interventions from social workers in order to access and use social and health care systems effectively. Health care is beginning to respond to the increasing need for continuity of care through the creation of community-based networks linking service providers to a continuum of health care that includes long-term care, rehabilitation, home care, and community social services. Thus, there is new opportunity for social workers to serve the aging population through the continuum of care based on predetermined vulnerable points in a chronic illness (Berkman, 1996).

Community-based options have also emerged for long-term care (Lee & Gutheil, 2003; Robert, 2003). Alternatives to nursing home care, such as community residential care and home health care, have grown in use during the past 15 years. Valuing the philosophy of "aging in place," such services offer more individualized care in less institutional settings (Semke, 2003; Lee & Gutheil, 2003). Despite individual and family preference for alternatives to nursing homes, community residential care is still in its infancy. The move away from institutional care toward community residential care may have preceded the development of more socially oriented models of care that are needed to maximize the health and well-being of older persons (Semke, 2003). And there are both threats and challenges to the provision of psychosocial services posed by the new Prospective Payment System (PPS) in Home Health Care (Lee & Gutheil, 2003).

Consumer-Centered/Consumer-Directed Care

The view that illness is a chronic process raises the question of whether an acute episode can be prevented, placing much more importance on consumers in determining their health care needs and outcomes. The focus of care becomes primary care, with an emphasis on disease prevention and health promotion. The growing empowerment of older adults who wish to participate in decision-making regarding their own health care and treatment, is shifting the decision-making role away from the physician to the patient. Patients and their families are increasingly seeking more active participation in health care decision making as they are faced with more complex clinical choices.

Accordingly, the philosophies of consumer-centered care and consumer-direction have grown increasingly popular in health and long-term care services. Representing a continuum of approaches based on levels of consumer involvement in designing and implementing their own care, "'consumer-direction' has become part of the lexicon among state and some federal policy makers" (Stone, 2000, p. 8). Consumer-centered services specifically prioritize the needs of clients over the needs of professionals. Consumer-directed supports empower older adults and their families with increased choice and control over their own care. An example is the development of better standardized measures to assess consumer satisfaction with home care services (Geron & Little, 2003), and the call for improved quality of life outcome measures representing the consumer's perspective (Robert, 2003).

SOCIAL WORK KNOWLEDGE AND SKILLS NEEDED TO MEET THE CHALLENGE OF THESE TRENDS

These major trends affecting the health and well-being of older adults and their families present a significant challenge to social work education to ensure that the necessary knowledge and skills are addressed in the curriculum. There are several key knowledge areas that are essential to effective social work practice with an aging population in a rapidly changing social, political and health care environment.

Knowledge About Health and the Emerging Health Care World

Social workers must continuously build upon their knowledge of basic mechanisms of health promotion, illness prevention and the impact of illnesses and treatment on older individuals and families. As diagnosis and treatment become more specialized and older adults cope with a greater variety of medical disciplines, social workers are faced with the challenge of knowing about disease-specific medical and psychosocial issues across the range of medical specialty areas (e.g., cardiology, oncology, neurology, psychiatry, endocrinology, and rheumatology). Now more than ever, it is increasingly essential to apply a holistic bio-psychosocial approach to understanding physical and mental health, one that takes into account an individual's complete medical and psychiatric presentation in addition to their coping capacities and social support resources (Berkman, 1996; Netting & Williams, 1998).

Knowledge of mental health and illness, specifically regarding manifestations of psychopathology and symptomatology in later life, is an essential piece of understanding that has been clearly missing in some health care settings. Raising awareness among social workers and other health professionals of the indicators of geriatric mental health concerns (including depression, dementia and developmental disabilities) and their treatment can make significant contributions in clinical settings.

In addition, it is essential to understand the workings of health care systems, financial structures, and processes (including prospective payment and managed care systems), as well the availability of public and private resources that support health maintenance and rehabilitation (Berkman, 1996). Social workers must be familiar with eligibility requirements for these resources, and know how to disseminate the information effectively among older individuals and their caregivers.

Practice Skills in Health and Aging

Social work practitioners in health care and aging must strengthen their foundation skills and develop new skills in order to keep pace with the velocity of societal change. Many of these skills are familiar to gerontological social work practitioners, in that they have and will continue to form the core skill-base of the field. Biopsychosocial assessment, counseling and case management over the continuum of care, family practice and advocacy for the needs of individuals and their families will remain the essential practice skills of social workers in health care and aging. In some areas, social work practitioners will find new ways to accomplish familiar tasks. We will adapt to new modes of information technology and integrate our knowledge of rapidly developing scientific advances in the treatment of disease. This will enhance our abilities to address the psychosocial implications of these discoveries for older patients and their families. Additionally, as evidence-based knowledge on psychosocial interventions is disseminated more rapidly in our information-intensive environment, we will be expected to modify and to adapt our practice skills and intervention techniques at a rate of change much faster than we have experienced in the past.

Cultural Competency Skills

Social workers must remain sensitive to the interactions among health and age, race, ethnicity, gender, and socioeconomic status, and must practice competently and creatively with older individuals and families from a variety of cultural backgrounds. Social workers, by virtue of their bio-psychosocial perspective and training, are strategically well positioned on interdisciplinary teams to assess the impact of both health care recipients' and health care providers' cultures on the effective delivery of health services. It is also essential to facilitate communication among patients, families, and health care providers about culturally related perceptions of wellness, illness and treatment. Self-awareness, cultural competence and sensitivity to the influences of culture are essential for promoting health and preventing illness among older adults of all cultural backgrounds. Cultural competency and the use of social brokerage and advocacy skills to meet the needs of vulnerable older populations will grow in importance.

Standardized Assessment

Comprehensive, bio-psychosocial geriatric assessment has long been the principal tool with which a social worker develops an appropriate response to the needs of older individuals and families (Geron & Little, 2003). Standardized measures that cover physical, psychological and social functioning are used for preventive screening and early identification of individual and family needs, to demonstrate the need for social work involvement, to monitor the effectiveness of intervention and to ensure accountability (Berkman, 1996; Robert, 2003). The assessment tools that best support clinical and policy practice aims of social work practitioners are comprehensive in scope; functional in design; uniform across users; incorporate established measures; balance psychometric precision with practicality; support objective and multiple sources of information; are easy to read and administer; and are culturally sensitive (Geron & Little, 2003).

Social relations are an essential component of physical and mental functioning in later life, and assessment of the extent and strength of social supports is therefore an important element of an older person's health and well-being (Lubben & Gironda, 2003; Lubben, 1988). Older adults often lack the social ties and related resources that promote emotional and psychological adaptation to illness (Lubben & Gironda, 2003; Takamura, 1999). Research is needed in further developing measurement tools, identifying risk factors for social isolation and developing interventions that integrate the importance of supportive social ties to quality of life in older adults and their families.

CASE MANAGEMENT SKILLS

In the midst of dramatic changes in health care, it is a challenge for health care social workers to define their roles and their unique contributions to multidisciplinary health care teams (Netting & Williams, 1998). Berkman (1996) has suggested that social workers are uniquely qualified to perform two basic, overlapping roles in health care settings. *Clinical specialists* teach older adults about health and health promotion, counsel and advocate for individuals and families to help them better manage health conditions and treatment, and collaborate with multidisciplinary health care teams around psychosocial issues, patient and family management, treatment adherence, and ethical issues. *Clinical case managers* engage in education, counseling and social brokerage designed to guide older individuals and their families through the health care system and gain access to essential resources. Naleppa (2003) has emphasized the value of task-centered brief treatment as an intervention modality for case management within the continuum of care. Geriatric social work case management can ensure integration and promote "seamless service" across the continuum of care.

Intergenerational Family Practice

The family has long been a core concern of social work assessment and intervention (Germain & Gitterman, 1996; Woods & Hollis, 2000). It is essential, however, to broaden our understandings of health promotion, illness prevention and treatment in order to incorporate an intergenerational and family systems context. Kropf and Wilks (2003) suggest, for example, that practice with family caregivers and with custodial grandparents is enhanced by the use of family therapy to help clarify boundaries, roles and functions. In their work they highlight intervention approaches to help grandparents with their health care needs and social functioning and present an innovative intervention for custodian grandparents who may typically be outside of existing service networks. Social workers must also promote "family practice" in health settings, by communicating familial concerns and advocating that the health care team view and treat families as the primary unit of care (Berkman, 1996; Volland, 1996).

Social workers, trained in a bio-psychosocial perspective that views an individual in the context of person-in-environment, know the importance of intergenerational social relationships in later life. In a health care system that views the older individual as the unit of care, social workers must identify and address the psychosocial needs of family members and other caregivers, as well as communicate their concerns to other health care professionals. We must also support and advocate for families' efforts to care adequately for the health and long-term care needs of their elder kin, and for those older adults who provide care for family members.

Research and Evidence-Based Practice

Social workers can demonstrate the benefits of assessment, case management and clinical intervention by focusing on research outcomes in their case planning and by using evidence-based interventions (Vourlekis, Ell, & Padgett, 2001). The application of "best practices" and developing "critical path models" are preferred methods to monitor and improve practice with older adults, and to demonstrate the effectiveness of social work interventions (Berkman & Harootyan, 2003). Empirical evaluations of practice modalities and approaches are also increasingly important in this outcomes-oriented health care environment. Research is also an essential component of advocacy for increased funding and policy-making that enhances the lives of older adults and their families. Social workers will need to be flexible, knowledgeable and independent in their practice. Research will become an increasingly vital part of developing, evaluating, and implementing effective and efficient services. There are critical gaps in our knowledge of health concerns and conditions that necessitate empirical study. For example, research is needed on the incidence and prevalence, and the detection and etiology of elder mistreatment (Paveza & VandeWeerd, 2003).

Advocacy and Empowerment Skills

Social workers must intervene actively on multiple levels to ensure the development and delivery of "a just and quality" system of care for older adults and their families (Lee & Gutheil, 2003). Practitioners are ideally positioned to advocate within health care systems to balance the desire for cost-efficiency and successful outcomes with services that best meet the needs of older adults and their families. In today's constantly changing health care environment, practitioners must feel comfortable shifting among and integrating their roles and skills in micro-level, meso-level and macro-level intervention. Chadiha and Adams (2003), for example, suggest that empowerment strategies that build upon the strengths and problem-solving capacities of older Black women are best implemented through collaboration and teamwork with a variety of health care providers, across various levels of practice.

Skills for Ethical Practice

Given current trends, it is probable that geriatric social workers will increasingly be called upon to serve as family therapists, mediators, consultants and advocates in addressing complex ethical dimensions of medical decision-making, particularly in the arena of end-of-life care. Ethical issues involving the decision to continue or withhold life-sustaining interventions at the end of life are particularly prominent in the current health care environment, especially in hospitals where the majority of deaths of older persons occur. Outcomes of medical treatments, in many cases, affect not only the health, longevity and quality of life of older patients but also, increasingly, of their caregivers as well. Mediating among the individual needs, perspectives, values, responsibilities and quality of life of all members of an intergenerational family system demands the highest skill level of ethical practice.

FUTURE DIRECTIONS AND IMPLICATIONS FOR SOCIAL WORK

Many of the demographic, social, economic and political trends described in this article are expected to continue well into the 21st century, as will evolutions in health care and in the practice of health care social work. The expansion and diversification of the older adult population will most likely generate increasing demand for health care services such as home health and community-based long-term care (Cornman & Kingson, 1996). As society grows older and a greater proportion of adults experience chronic illnesses and conditions, our expectations of later life will change dramatically with respect to employment, housing, social relationships, independent functioning and quality of life. In fact, the notion of what constitutes "productive" aging is an evolving construct in the research literature as reflected by these changes in society at large (Morrow-Howell, Hinterlong, & Sherraden, 2001).

Given the present characteristics of the baby boomer cohort, older adults of tomorrow will be more confident, will remain in the workforce longer and will be more active in advocating for themselves in terms of health resources and health care policies (Silverstone, 1996). There will be continued growth of consumer-directed care in physical, mental and long-term care. The ability of older adults to take control over their care will need to be balanced, however, with the cost-effectiveness of services and the needs of the larger population.

Diminishing economic resources and competing needs among an increasingly diverse population might lead to a decline of public financing of health care (including social security) for older adults (Cornman & Kingson, 1996).

Finally, aging families will continue to absorb a growing share of the care and support of older adults, and a larger proportion of families will include multiple intergenerational care arrangements.

In summary, social work practice in health care is inextricably linked with social work practice with an aging population. Moreover, it is increasingly clear that it is no longer possible to view aging as solely the purview of social workers that specialize in gerontology. Given current and future demographic shifts, the profession as a whole will be at a costly disadvantage if it ignores the needs of older adults and their families. Social work practitioners, educators, researchers and policy-makers must "fully embrace gerontological practice" (Scharlach et al., 2000, p. 525) and develop, implement and evaluate intergenerational approaches to meet the evolving needs of this population.

It is time to bring the concepts of aging and health care in social work together in social work educational programs, policy considerations, practice, and research. We need to address the shortage of trained, competent practitioners and educators in aging, and infuse gerontological content throughout social work curricula in bachelors and masters-level programs (Scharlach et al., 2000; Volland, 1996). Moreover, we must address the negative attitudes and myths about work in aging that may prevent social workers from participating in this emerging and rewarding field of practice.

Finally, the future of social work in aging relies on our ability to generate meaningful research into the epidemiology and theoretical bases of health-related psychosocial problems, and to develop and evaluate effective interventions for addressing these concerns. As social workers in health and aging, we are fortunate to work in a field of practice that provides abundant challenges and opportunities to have a positive impact on people's lives.

REFERENCES

Adamek, M. (2003). Late-life depression in long term care: Social work opportunities to prevent, educate and alleviate. In B. Berkman and L. Harootyan (Eds.). *Social Work and Health Care in an Aging Society*. New York: Springer Publications.

Berkman, B. (1996). The emerging health care world: Implications for social work practice and education. *Social Work*, 541-553.

Berkman, B. & Harootyan, L. (Eds.). (2003). *Social Work and Health Care in an Aging Society*. New York: Springer Publications.

Burnette, D. & Kang, S. (2003). Self-care by urban, African American elders. In B. Berkman and L. Harootyan (Eds.). *Social Work and Health Care in an Aging Society*. New York: Springer Publications.

Chaditha, L. & Adams, P. (2003). Physical health and economic well-being of older African American women: Toward strategies of empowerment. In B. Berkman and L. Harootyan (Eds.). *Social Work and Health Care in an Aging Society.* New York: Springer Publications.

Cornman, J. & Kingson, E. (1996). Trends, issues, perspectives and values for the aging of baby boom cohorts. *The Gerontologist, 36*(1), 15-26.

Federal Interagency Forum on Aging-Related Statistics. (2000). *Older Americans 2000: Key Indicators of Well-Being.* FIFAS. Washington, DC: U.S. Government Printing Office.

Germain, C. & Gitterman, A. (1996). *The Life Model of Social Work Practice, 2nd Edition.* New York: Columbia University Press.

Geron, S., & Little, F. (2003). Standardized geriatric assessment in social work practice with older adults. In B. Berkman and L. Harootyan (Eds.). *Social Work and Health Care in an Aging Society.* New York: Springer Publications.

Hooyman, N. & Kiyak, H. (2002). *Social Gerontology: A Multidisciplinary Perspective, 6th Edition.* Boston: Allyn and Bacon.

Kropf, N. & Wilks, S. (2003). Grandparents raising grandchildren. In B. Berkman and L. Harootyan (Eds.). *Social Work and Health Care in an Aging Society.* New York: Springer Publications.

Lee, J. & Gutheil, I. (2003). The older patient at home: Social work services and home health care. In B. Berkman and L. Harootyan (Eds.). *Social Work and Health Care in an Aging Society.* New York: Springer Publications.

Lubben, J. (1988). Assessing social networks among elderly populations. *Family Community Health, 11,* 42-52.

Lubben, J., & Gironda, M. (2003). Centrality of social ties to the health and well-being of older adults. In B. Berkman and L. Harootyan (Eds.). *Social Work and Health Care in an Aging Society.* New York: Springer Publications.

Maramaldi, P. & Guevara, M. (2003). Cultural considerations in maintaining health related quality of life in older adults. In B. Berkman and L. Harootyan (Eds.). *Social Work and Health Care in an Aging Society.* New York: Springer Publications.

McCallion, P. & Kolomer, S. (2003). Aging persons with developmental disabilities and their aging caregivers. In B. Berkman and L. Harootyan (Eds.). *Social Work and Health Care in an Aging Society.* New York: Springer Publications.

Morrow-Howell, N., Hinterlong, J., & Sherraden, M. (2001). *Productive aging: Concepts and challenges.* Baltimore: Johns Hopkins University Press.

Naleppa, M. (2003). Gerontological social work and case management. In B. Berkman, and L. Harootyan (Eds.). *Social Work and Health Care in an Aging Society.* New York: Springer Publications.

National Alliance for Caregiving/American Association of Retired Persons. (1997). Family Caregiving in the U.S.: Findings from a National Study. Washington, DC.

Netting, F. E. & Williams, F. (1998). Can we prepare geriatric social workers to collaborate in primary care practices? *Journal of Social Work Education, 34*(2), 195-210.

Paveza, G. & VandeWeerd, C. (2003). Elder mistreatment and the role of social work. In B. Berkman and L. Harootyan (Eds.). *Social Work and Health Care in an Aging Society.* New York: Springer Publications.

Poindexter, C. & Boyer, N. (2003). Strains and gains of grandmothers raising children in the HIV pandemic. In B. Berkman and L. Harootyan (Eds.). *Social Work and Health Care in an Aging Society*. New York: Springer Publications.

Robert, S. (2003). Home and community-based long term care policies and programs: The crucial role for social work practitioners and researchers in evaluation. In B. Berkman and L. Harootyan (Eds.). *Social Work and Health Care in an Aging Society*. New York: Springer Publications.

Scharlach, A., Damron-Rodriguez, J., Robinson, B. & Feldman, R. (2000). Educating social workers for an aging society: A vision for the 21st century. *Journal of Social Work Education, 36*(3), 521-538.

Semke, J. (2003). Older adults with dementia: Community-based long-term care alternatives. In B. Berkman and L. Harootyan (Eds.). *Social Work and Health Care in an Aging Society*. New York: Springer Publications.

Shortell, S., Gilles, R. & Devers, K. (1995). Reinventing the American hospital. *Milbank Quarterly, 73* (2), 131-159.

Silverstone, B. (1996). Older people of tomorrow: A psychosocial profile. *The Gerontologist, 36*(1), 27-32.

Stone, R. (2000). Consumer direction in long-term care. *Generations, 24*(3), 4-9.

Takamura, J. (1999). Getting ready for the 21st century: The aging of America and the Older Americans Act. *Health and Social Work, 24*(3), 232-238.

U.S. Bureau of the Census. (2000a). Census 2000 summary file 1 (SF 1). Washington, DC: Author.

U.S. Bureau of the Census. (2000b). Population projections of the United States by age, sex, race, Hispanic origin, and nativity: 1999-2000. Washington, DC: Author.

U.S. Bureau of the Census. (2000c). Projections of the total resident population by 5-year age groups, race, and Hispanic origin with special age categories: Middle series, 2050 to 2070 (NP-T4-G). Washington, DC: Author.

U.S. Special Committee on Aging. (1996). GAO report to the Chairman. Washington, DC: Author.

Volland, P. (1996). Social work practice in health care: Looking into the future with a different lens. *Social Work in Health Care, 24*(1/2), 35-51.

Vourlekis, B., Ell, K. & Padgett, D. (2001). Educating social workers for health care's brave new world. *Journal of Social Work Education, 37*(1).

Woods, M. & Hollis, F. (2000). *Casework: A Psychosocial Therapy, 5th Edition*. New York: McGraw-Hill.

doi: 10.1300/J083v48n01_14

End-of-Life Care
and Social Work Education:
What Do Students Need to Know?

Marlene Belew Huff, LCSW, PhD
Sherri Weisenfluh, LCSW
Mindy Murphy, MSW
Pamela J. Black, MSW

SUMMARY. Social workers are major service providers to people who are facing end-of-life issues including the terminally ill and their families. Yet, exemplary models for social work education and intervention methods are limited in rural states. A statewide survey conducted in Kentucky found only two social work courses dedicated to end-of-life care currently being offered by accredited undergraduate and graduate institutions. Another statewide survey found that many hospice social workers are relatively inexperienced and have a need and desire for more education on death, dying and loss. Also, unique cultural, economic and

Special thanks to Ms. Amy Little and Ms. Pamela Handshoe, without whose help this article would not have been written.

The Kentucky Project is funded by a Social Work Leadership Development Grant from the Open Society Institute's Project on Death in America as part of an effort to develop leadership on end-of-life issues across the country.

[Haworth co-indexing entry note]: "End-of-Life Care and Social Work Education: What Do Students Need to Know?" Huff, Marlene Belew et al. Co-published simultaneously in *Journal of Gerontological Social Work* (The Haworth Press, Inc.) Vol. 48, No. 1/2, 2006, pp. 219-231; and: *Fostering Social Work Gerontology Competence: A Collection of Papers from the First National Gerontological Social Work Conference* (ed: Catherine J. Tompkins, and Anita L. Rosen) The Haworth Press, Inc., 2007, pp. 219-231. Single or multiple copies of this article are available for a fee from The Haworth Document Delivery Service [1-800-HAWORTH, 9:00 a.m. - 5:00 p.m. (EST). E-mail address: docdelivery@haworthpress.com].

geographic areas, such as Appalachia are enigmas when it comes to the provision of end-of-life care. This partnership provides a varied perspective on delivery of end-of-life care services with an emphasis on social work interventions and education. doi: 10.1300/J083v48n01_15 *[Article copies available for a fee from The Haworth Document Delivery Service: 1-800-HAWORTH. E-mail address: <docdelivery@haworthpress.com> Website: <http:// www.HaworthPress.com> © 2006 by The Haworth Press, Inc. All rights reserved.]*

KEYWORDS. Death education, social work, elderly

INTRODUCTION

Broderick (1988) states that a decade ago, death was a subject less likely than sex to be found in most college curriculum but the commitment to the subject varies from discipline to discipline. Today, thousands of colleges and universities are involved in death education. In 1994, for example, Dickinson, Sumner and Frederick found that of 270 baccalaureate social work programs, 71 included "at least a lecture" on death. Sixty-four of the undergraduate social work programs reported that they "integrated death into another program" with only 36 offering a "complete course" on the subject. The most popular format for death education to be delivered to social workers was a combined lecture and discussion format.

Research conducted by Channon (1984) indicated that death education is needed among various healthcare professionals. Channon surveyed 454 respondents, "Have you known a relative or friend who has died?" Overwhelmingly, 92.7% replied in the affirmative. Most of them identified the dead person as being a relative or a grandparent (58.5%). Two other interesting questions were asked, "Have you ever seen a dead person?"; 52.7% of the respondents reported that they had seen someone who was dead. However, only 8.5% had actually been present when someone had died.

Many death and dying offerings are supplemented with video-tapes and "field trip" often using the dying person as "teacher." Occasionally, social work programs reported asking the students to share their own feelings toward, and experiences with, death and dying. In a few of the complete courses cited by Bordewich (1994) specific articles and textbooks were assigned to students. So, most social work students reported that they graduated having experienced "a lecture or two" on death and dying but rarely reported that they had completed a full course.

According to Dickinson, Sumner and Frederick (1994), the most reported reasons social work and other professional programs do *not* include complete courses on death and dying were: (1) students can take death and dying courses offered through other programs; (2) such an offering has not been discussed/approved by the faculty; (3) time constraints in the curriculum; (4) no need for such an offering in the curriculum, and (5) limited available faculty that can teach the course.

DEATH EDUCATION IN SOCIAL WORK

Social workers have been described as the hub of interdisciplinary efforts to provide comprehensive medical and support services to dying clients (Blackman, 1995). Social workers are the only healthcare professionals that focus solely on the psychosocial aspects of death and dying, working directly with the family and client in adjusting to the life-threatening illness as well as obtaining resources that enhance quality of life for the longest period of time (Sheldon, 1993; Loscalzo & Zabora, 1996). Thus, social workers are one of the primary healthcare professionals that are in need of death education.

In addition to the learning modules integrated into the social work curriculum, field placements can provide students with opportunities to develop skill through working with dying clients and their families. In the past, dying has usually taken place in various institutions but hospice and palliative care agencies have relocated many of the eventual deaths to the home. As early as 1977, Cassidy identified two major teaching objectives that can be achieved in the field: (1) helping students examine their own personal reactions to death and dying, and (2) assisting students to develop sufficient self-awareness in such a practice situation that their feelings can be consciously controlled.

Field placements are one of the most effective ways for students to learn to assess the capacity of the dying individual to handle the crisis, the amount of support needed for acceptance (to a greater or lesser extent) to occur. Learning the ways that a dying individual can maintain satisfying human relationships even in the final stages of life and helping significant others cope with the death can be best learned in the field or "going to the place where the dying client lives."

Dimensions of Death Education

Through the years, health professionals have tried to identify core competencies and devise formal statements of expectations for undergraduate and graduate programs in various disciplines (Blank, 1995). None of the identified competencies are particularly useful for social work curricula and, in fact, have not been comprehensive in setting forth the competencies needed for consistently excellent care of dying individuals for physicians either (Steel, 1996).

Corr (1995) identified a need for death education in four major areas: *cognitive* or the intellectual because it provides factual information about death-related experiences and tries to assist students in understanding and interpreting those events. An *affective* dimension of death education allows social work students (and others) to struggle with feelings, emotions, and attitudes about death and dying.[1] A *behavioral* dimension that explains the reasons that people act as they do in death related situations. Finally, the *valuation* dimension has to do with how death education can help to identify, articulate and affirm the basic human values subscribed to by all social workers (NASW Code of Ethics, 2003). In short, these dimensions relate to what people know, how they feel, how they behave and what they value.

Goals of Death Education

The mission of death education among social work professionals is to ensure that every one of us who deals directly with dying individuals and their families has foundation knowledge in dealing competently and compassionately with seriously ill and dying clients. Because each health professional faces somewhat different tasks and issues in serving dying clients, their professional education should reflect these differences.

There are several goals of death education. Above all, education about death, dying and bereavement seeks to *enrich the personal lives* of those to whom it is directed. Death education is ultimately meant to assist individuals in understanding themselves more fully and to appreciate both their strengths and weaknesses inherent in being human. A second goal of death education is to *inform and guide individuals in their personal transactions with society*. It does this by making them aware of services that are available to them as well as their options in dealing with end-of-life matters such as living wills and funeral practices.

A third goal of death education is to *prepare individuals for their public roles as consumers*. Death is associated with many social issues such as assisted suicide, euthanasia, and organ and tissue donation. Such issues expand well beyond the individual into a realm of public policy that makes us responsible for the outcomes. A fourth goal of death education is to *support individuals in their professional and vocational roles*. Death education can assist social work students, for example, in providing services to dying clients through a high quality educational program.

A fifth goal of death education is *to enhance the ability of individuals to communicate effectively about death-related matters*. Effective communication is essential when one is addressing death-related topics that may be challenging for many people (Strickland & DeSpelder, 1995). The final goal of death education is to *assist clients in appreciating how development across the human life course interacts with death-related issues* (Corr, Germino & Pittman, 1995).

SOCIAL WORKERS AS "CONTEXTUAL INTERPRETERS"

Social workers are educated to become "contextual interpreters." Although the tasks for gerontological social workers who are working with dying individuals vary, being a contextual interpreter for elders may include:

- Helping the family/caregiver put the factual information about the disease into context and dealing with the emotions provoked by that information;
- Helping the family/caregiver understand the biology of the active dying process;
- Helping the family/caregiver recognize that there may not be a time when the healthcare professionals directly say that death is imminent; and,
- Helping the family/caregiver deal with the lack of control over the dying process (Bern-Klug, Gesser, & Forbes, 2001).

Coluzzi et al. (1995) reports that 75% of the supportive counseling provided to individuals with cancer was from social workers as reported from various agencies that provides services to dying individuals. Elders that are dying can expect to receive social work services that include psychosocial screening, assessment, counseling, referral, and practical assistance with financial resources but are not limited to these activities. The needed services provided to a specific elder are individualized. In 1995, for example, Coluzzi et al. report that 75% of supportive counseling provided to individuals with cancer was from social workers.

METHODOLOGY

The goal of this research was to better understand the educational needs of social work students who are working with dying clients.[2] Our outcome measure was a manual that addressed these educational needs *prior* to entering the field placement/internship where direct client contact occurred. In order to reach this goal, nine student focus groups were conducted in this Midwestern state. The majority of the participants were female (94%), from rural areas (100%), engaged in a variety of field placement or internship (e.g., hospitals, nursing homes and hospice) situations. Fifty-three of the focus group participants were undergraduate social work students while 136 of them were graduate students.

The following questions were applied consistently throughout the nine focus groups:

- How many of you have had training in dealing with end-of-life issues? What kind of training?
- How many of you have dealt with end-of-life issues in your field placements/internships and/or life experiences? Did you feel adequately prepared for this?
- What topics do you suggest be included in an end-of-life manual for social work students?
- How can students be better prepared to deal with mortality issues?
- Do students placed in settings that deal with end-of-life care need additional training in self-care? In setting boundaries between the professional self and the client?
- Do you think that death and dying issues are different in rural areas such as Appalachia? Are your perceptions of differences in rural areas based on personal experiences with such populations?
- What are some things that you think you would need to learn in order to be prepared to work in rural areas?
- What other questions should be addressed in an end-of-life manual for social work students?
- What prevents students from choosing a field placement/internship with hospice or any other agency dealing that deals with death and dying?

Analysis

A summary of the answers to each question is outlined below:

1. How many of you have had training in dealing with end-of-life issues? What kind of training?

Only 5% of the social work students reported taking a full course in death education. Among those 5%, none of the students reported feeling "confident" in entering a field placement that required direct social work intervention with dying individuals.

Nearly 12% of the participants reported that they had attended a community grief and bereavement group that proved helpful to them personally. However, the participants doubted that the information presented in the self-help and/or support groups would be particularly useful in successfully completing upcoming/current field placements.

When asked about the most beneficial parts of the formal training received, the students reported that communication tips and a review of the exceptional need to listen to the dying clients were most valuable. Students found the concrete pieces of information to be most helpful. One focus group participant stated, "There was a table of "do's and don'ts" for communicating effectively that never left my side during the first weeks of the field placement at (the hospice agency). We had role played difficult client situations in class but working with a 'real' client was very different. I didn't want to make a mistake."

Almost 98% of the focus group participants that were assigned to field experiences/internships at hospice agencies were required to complete a "volunteer" training program. The students reported that, in the absence of formal classroom instruction, the volunteer training contained invaluable content on various aspects of death and dying. Those students assigned to other facilities and institutions in which death was not expected to routinely occur did not receive such training and were at a particular disadvantage if one of their clients did, indeed, die during the learning experience.

2. How many of you have dealt with end-of-life issues in your field placements/internships and/or life experiences? Did you feel adequately prepared for this?

Only one student had significant experience in working with dying clients. She had completed one undergraduate field practicum/internship and felt very unsure about entering into another one. Unfortunately, the same student's client died prior to completion of her formal training and according to her,

I never fully felt comfortable (in the field practicum) after that (the death). The client died during my first week at the agency! Everyone thought that he was (medically) stable but I learned (the hard way) that death can be unexpected. This client was the first person that I ever knew who had died! Here I was holding their hand! (crying). I didn't know what to do. I felt angry and wanted to yell at my instructor, *"Why didn't you prepare me for this?"*! I deserved more information.

Focus group participants that had experienced multiple losses were at a advantage over those that had not experienced such losses in two distinct ways. First, those students who were "experienced" with death were able to deal with the emotional ramifications of a client's death through the development and use of a self-care plan. One of the ways that respondents had learned to manage stress and anxiety, for example, was through specific cognitive-behavioral techniques. One focus group respondent reported,

> After three of my grandparents died within a two year period, I learned that death was a part of life that couldn't be avoided. I also figured out that I wasn't invincible. When my first grandparent died, I didn't handle it well. I would call it a "complicated grief response." Just two years later, I learned to keep a journal, practice positive self-talk and take time to relax.... This made all the difference.

Second, social work students that had multiple personal death experiences were more aware of the resources and information that the family might need during this time. For example,

> When my first client had died, my great aunt had passed away six months prior. Because of (the nature of) her death, I had learned about living wills, funeral costs, burial plots ... and the like. I was fortunate to be able to help my client with all of this information.

3. Do students placed in settings dealing with end-of-life care need additional training in self-care? In setting boundaries between the professional self and the client?

All of the respondents were very concerned about their lack of ability to care for themselves and the effect that it might have on their dying clients. The participants identified concerns about their knowledge of techniques that would address such issues as stress management, spiritual conflict and personal mortality issues. Many of the students were very unsure about their ability to transform their knowledge into an action plan that would assist them in maintaining their health. One student reports that,

> I found that I had pushed myself beyond my limits. I wasn't sleeping or eating well. I began to have panic attacks. My heart beat faster (than normal) and I begin to sweat. I just lost my ability to have fun (with life). I thought that it was my client's situation (dying) but I found that I simply wasn't handling my life well. Since I began a program of self-care, I have returned to 'normal'. Plus, I love working at (the hospice agency).

Another focus group respondent reports that she too has had difficulty in balancing her field experience/practicum with maintaining a healthy balance in her personal life. She comments,

> I found that the only way that I could deal with the stress of work was to meditate in the mornings, eat right and get plenty of rest. Otherwise, I couldn't deal with the death that I saw in my clients ...

The most troublesome aspect of self-care as perceived by the social work students surrounds the ability to "leave work at work." In all areas of the field experiences, focus group participants were struggling with boundary settings between the situations encountered at the field site with their personal life circumstance. Many students were seeking out death education resources outside the social work classroom. For example, one respondent indicated,

> I found that all of my evenings were filled with thoughts of the individuals that I had worked with throughout the day. My family told me that I had "changed." I knew that I needed to separate work from my personal life but I didn't know how (to do this). I didn't feel comfortable about speaking up in my practicum (field) class. The other students didn't seem to know (or care) about the dying experience. I registered for a self-care course through the community education program. I didn't get what I needed from the social work classes.

4. Do you think that death and dying issues are different in rural areas such as Appalachia? Are your perceptions of differences in rural areas based on personal experiences with such populations? What are some things that you think you would need to learn in order to be prepared to work in rural areas?

Seventy-five percent (75%) of the respondents were working primarily with diverse populations during at least one of their field/internship experiences. Sixty percent (60%) of the student's clients were from the Appalachian mountain region which has a particular cultural belief surrounding death that those outside the region find difficult to understand. One respondent that had just completed a field practicum/internship with a hospice agency reported,

> During the last day of life, (the client's family) began to gather for the death. They came from the mountains and hollows nearby. There seemed to be hundreds of them! The room was filled with people (seemingly) waiting for the death to occur. People prayed, wailed, collapsed on the floor.... I didn't know what to do. When (the client) died, people hugged and touched the body for a very long time. It was all very strange to me.

Twenty percent (20%) of the respondents reported that their clients were of Hispanic descent[3] while 15% of the social work students were engaged in services with African Americans. Needless to say, each cultural group has unique and valuable death practices and the respondents reported feeling undereducated in the culture of each. This feeling of inadequacy was particularly true of students working with Hispanic or African American cultural death practices primarily because the majority of the students originated from Appalachia or had relatives who live there. So, some level of cultural understanding of Appalachian death practices was reported to exist among the majority of the students. A few of the students reported never have encountered *people* that were of Hispanic or African descent much less an actual client. For example, one social work student relates,

> I had always lived in (a very rural area). Then I came to (the university) to study social work. During my field placement at (a local nursing home), I met my first African American person. His mother was dying and although some of the customs were strange to me, I was surprised to find that we were more alike than different. I learned more about death and culture from (the African American male) than I ever did in a class.

5. What topics do you suggest be included in an end-of-life manual for social work students? What other questions should be addressed in an end-of-life manual for social work students?

The social work students that participated in this research were able to identify several areas of information essential for effective learning to occur in the field. The eight most identified issues that the students felt *unprepared* deal with in the field were:

- The process of active dying;
- Cultural variations on the death event;
- The stages of death and grief reactions;
- Professional social work roles associated with serving dying clients;
- Legal, medical and moral issues related to dying;
- Service referrals most commonly requested by dying individuals and their families (e.g., funeral arrangements, estate planning).
- Anticipatory/complicated grief reactions
- Family adjustment to death

Results obtained from the analysis of the student-centered focus groups, the resulting manual contained the following learning objectives:

- To enable the student to recognize death as a normal response to life;
- To help the student understand the dying process;
- To enable the student in recognizing the defense mechanisms used in coping with death by the dying individual, the family and the social work student themselves;

- To help the student recognize the adaptational patterns used in the resolution of stress surrounding the death of clients and in the restitution of adaptive social functions.

6. What prevents students from choosing a field placement/internship with hospice or any other agency dealing that deals with death and dying?

Unanimously focus group participants identified that a lack of knowledge about death was the biggest reason that they did not choose a field placement/internship in which clients were likely to die. Other reasons included (1) fear of the active dying process; (2) personal issues of mortality; (3) negative experiences with death in the past; (4) fear of cultural differences; (5) lack of a peer group with whom to share field experiences; and/or (6) a fear of being emotionally overwhelmed without the resources to deal with such an intense state. The comments of two social work students summarized the reasons that field experiences with dying individuals are not sought as often as one could expect:

> I feel as if my profession has failed me in a way. If I were to choose a field experience working with dying people, I wouldn't be able to handle it and I wouldn't take all of the responsibility for that. None of the social work classes that I have taken (including field-based courses) have given more than one or two days of information about death. How could I be confident about choosing such a field placement?

The second student reports,

> My goal is to work with elders.... I haven't thought about death very much. When I think of my own death, I become very afraid. I'm not sure that I can help others with death yet and I'm not sure how I can go about this.....Education is not enough. I need support and some type of emotional understanding of the dying process. I know that I haven't found what I need in the social work classes that I have taken.

CONCLUSION

Death education in social work undergraduate and graduate programs is essential for developing the knowledge, skills, and values advocated for in this paper. However, experience in the field along with the ability to process client situations in the classroom setting is as important or more so. In addition, as the role of "contextual interpreters" change within the dynamic arena of policies, organizations and medical technologies, death education cannot end upon graduation. Continuing education is necessary to ensure competence among professional social workers.

NOTES

1. This particular aspect of death is especially helpful to students who have not yet encountered death in any personal way.

2. The focus group research was not limited to elders that were dying. The authors conducted a thematic analysis of the focus group responses. This analysis revealed four distinct areas of social work knowledge that students perceived necessary to work with elders that are dying as they answered the focus group questions. These areas are: (1) educational content; (2) conceptual issues of dying; (3) emotional issues; (4) therapeutic social work interventions.

3. Hispanic people are the most recent group of individuals to migrate to the area in which the research was completed. Currently, all healthcare professionals are struggling with cultural competence in regard to Hispanic elders that are dying.

REFERENCES

Bern-Klug, M., Gessert, C., & Forbes, S. (2001). The need to revise assumptions about the end-of-life: Implications for social work practice. *Health and Social Work, 6*: 38-48.

Blackman, R.A. (1995). Helping the terminally ill face death with dignity. *Quality Letter* March: 19-23.

Blank, L. (1995). Defining and evaluating physician competence in end-of-life patient care: A matter of awareness and emphasis. *Western Journal of Medicine, 163*: 297-301.

Bordewich, F.M. (1988). Mortal fears: Courses in "death education" get mixed reviews. *Atlantic Monthly,* 30-34.

Cassidy, H. (1977). Helping the social work student deal with death and dying. In E. Prichard, J. Collard, B. Arcuth, A. Kutscher, I Sutland, & H. Lefkoutz (Eds.). *Social work with the dying patient and the family.* New York: Columbia University Press.

Channon, L.D. (1984). Death and the pre-clinical medical student: Experiences with death. *Death Education, 8*: 231-235.

Coluzzi, P.H., Grant, M., & Doroshow, J.H. (1995). Survey of the provision of supportive care services at the National Cancer Institute-Designated Cancer Centers. *Journal of Clinical Oncology, 13*: 756-764.

Corr, C.A. (1995). Death education for adults. In I.B. Corless, B. B. Germino, & M.A. Pittman (Eds.), *A challenge for living: Dying, death, and bereavement.* Boston: Jones & Bartlett.

Dickinson, G.E., Sumner, E.D., & Frederick, L.M. (1992). Death education in selected health professions. *Death Studies, 16*: 281-289.

Loscalzo, M.J. & Zabora, J.R. (1996). Oncology social work and palliative care in the United States. Unpublished paper.

National Association of Social Workers. (2003). NASW Code of Ethics. Washington, DC.

Sheldon, F. (1993). Education and training for social workers in palliative care. In *Oxford Textbook of Palliative Medicine*, D. Doyle, G.W.C. Hanks, & N. MacDonald (Eds.): Oxford University Press.

Steel, R.K. (1996). Analysis of residency review requirements. Paper presented for conference on the education of physicians about dying: Hackensack University Medical Center, New Jersey.

Strickland, A.L. & DeSpelder, L.A. (1995). Communicating about death and dying. In I.B. Corr, B.B. Germino & M.A. Pittman (Eds), *A challenge for living: Dying, death and bereavement.* Boston: Jones & Bartlett.

doi: 10.1300/J083v48n01_15

Environmental Issues Affecting Elder Abuse Victims in Their Reception of Community Based Services

Nancy N. Barker, CSW, PhD
Maureen V. Himchak, PhD, LCSW

SUMMARY. This study examined the dominant factors that predict the utilization of services by 129 identified elder abuse victims who reside in the community. Utilizing the Andersen Model, services accepted or rejected were analyzed from individual, family and environmental perspectives. Results indicated that service utilization is related to three "need" factors: (1) Victim has cognitive and ADL impairments, (2) Victim has poor health status (self rated), and (3) The abuser is financially dependent on the victim and is also the primary caregiver of the victim. "Enabling" factor (1) Victim lives alone. "Predisposing" factors (1) Abuser is substance abuser and (2) Abuser is female. A great proportion of the elder abuse victims in this study accepted services from an agency that provided a single entry point into the service system and had highly trained personnel utilizing a case management approach. doi:10.1300/J083v48n01_16 *[Article copies available for a fee from The Haworth Document Delivery Service: 1-800-HAWORTH. E-mail address: <docdelivery@haworthpress.com> Website: <http://www.HaworthPress.com> © 2006 by The Haworth Press, Inc. All rights reserved.]*

[Haworth co-indexing entry note]: "Environmental Issues Affecting Elder Abuse Victims in Their Reception of Community Based Services." Barker, Nancy N., and Maureen V. Himchak. Co-published simultaneously in *Journal of Gerontological Social Work* (The Haworth Press, Inc.) Vol. 48, No. 1/2, 2006, pp. 233-255; and: *Fostering Social Work Gerontology Competence: A Collection of Papers from the First National Gerontological Social Work Conference* (ed: Catherine J. Tompkins, and Anita L. Rosen) The Haworth Press, Inc., 2007, pp. 233-255. Single or multiple copies of this article are available for a fee from The Haworth Document Delivery Service [1-800-HAWORTH, 9:00 a.m. - 5:00 p.m. (EST). E-mail address: docdelivery@haworthpress.com].

KEYWORDS. Elder abuse victims, service utilization, Andersen Model, case management

INTRODUCTION

Elder abuse, also known as elder mistreatment, is not a new phenomenon. Elder abuse is another facet of family violence. However, it was the last form of family violence to be brought to the public's awareness resulting in increased concern to the issues of elder mistreatment and the suffering of its victims (Quinn & Tomita, 1997).

While reported rates in the elder population range anywhere from 4% to 10% (U.S. House of Representatives, 1990a), the number of elder abuse reports can be expected to rise because Americans are living longer. The National Elder Abuse Incidence Study (NEAIS, 1998) estimates that there are approximately 44 million people age 60 and over in the United States who have been abused. Increased longevity will impact on society by the growing amount and visibility of the elderly. Today the elderly are one in every eight persons in the United States; by the year 2030 this proportion is expected to rise to one in five (U.S. Census, 1996).

America's elderly are not homogeneous. In fact, gerontologists, social workers and other professionals are becoming more aware of the cultural and ethnic diversity of America's elders. Current projections by the U. S. Bureau of Census (1996) indicate that by the year 2050 ethnic minorities will comprise nearly half (47%) of the United States population.

America's elders are an integral part of families. Families are the traditional caregivers of their impaired elderly, and the elderly generally prefer these informal caregivers in a hierarchical order: spouse, child, relative, friends and neighbors (Cantor & Brennan, 1993). As the "graying" of America continues and informal supports thin out, the well-being of elderly persons will be best served by strong informal supports with effective formal collaborative efforts (Stevenson, 1996).

In order to develop policies and programs to target the vulnerable elder abuse victims, gerontologists, social work practitioners, policymakers and social work educators must understand the complex factors that contribute to an elder's decision to accept or reject services from the formal service delivery system. The results of the current study of identified elder abuse victims (n = 129) highlights three important factors. First, the influence of the elder victim's informal network on the acceptance/rejection of services must be considered with an awareness to ethnic and cultural differences. Practitioners must also be aware of the concurrent responsibilities to the victim and to the victim's abuser who is often a needy family member. Second, in the current fragmented service delivery system it is essential that the concept of case management, along with its variety of knowledge bases and skills, is employed. Lastly, much emphasis is placed on the interconnectedness of the social worker engaging other agencies in partnerships to address all the needs of this vulnerable population.

LITERATURE REVIEW

Elder Abuse as a Subset of Family Violence

Elder abuse is possibly as old as the concept of "family." Violence in the family has ancient roots in mythical, biblical and literary accounts, as exemplified by the stories of Oedipus, Cain and Abel, and King Lear, yet elder abuse has been referred to as one of the most hidden or "invisible" social problem in our society (Kosberg, 1998). A nationally representative sample of American families was studied and the findings were entitled: *Behind Closed Doors: Violence in the American Family.* Strauss, Gelles, and Steinmetz (1980, p. 4) concluded: "The American family and the American home are perhaps as or more violent than any other American institution or setting with the exception of the military, and only then in time of war." In this context family violence relates to spousal abuse, child abuse and elder abuse. While this statement may be dramatic, it clearly reflects the extent of violence in the American family.

Elder Abuse Research

From the initial "discovery" of elder abuse as a social problem, there have been major difficulties and controversies over definitions of elder abuse. At the policy, practice and research levels the lack of consensus over standardization of elder abuse definitions has resulted in inconsistencies in assessment, reporting, prevalence estimates, service delivery, education, and data collection. The four germinal elder abuse studies, basically descriptive and exploratory, reflected various behaviors (including those of commission and omission) considered as elder abuse. One of the first of these studies, completed by O'Malley, Segars, Perez, Mitchell, and Knuepel (1979), defined elder abuse in descriptive terms, rather than categories. Block and Sinnott (1979) defined four types of abuse: physical, psychological, material and medical; while Douglass, Hickey, and Noel (1980) defined four different categories: passive neglect, active neglect, verbal or emotional abuse and physical abuse. The last of the germinal studies was by Lau and Kosberg (1979), who defined four categories of abuse: physical, psychological, material, and violation of rights.

As elder abuse research matured, definitional and categorical variations emerged. In 1987, the Federal response to the definitional issue of elder abuse and mistreatment was included as part of an amendment to the Older American Act (OAA). This amendment applied to all 50 states through the State Offices for Aging and the local Area Agency on Aging. In New York City this local area agency on aging is known as the Department for the Aging or DFTA. Three major categories of mistreatment were identified and defined: abuse, neglect, and exploitation. While the OAA guidelines are used as a framework, each of the fifty states has continued to define elder abuse and mistreatment differently.

The basic difficulty in defining elder abuse can be attributed to the various perspectives that have attempted to define elder mistreatment according to the particular lens of the viewer. Therefore, elder abuse can be defined differently from the parties of abusive situations (such as the victim, the caregiver, and the dependent adult child), agencies that respond, service systems (such as Protective Services for Adults, social service, medical and criminal justice), and legislation and policies (federal, state and local levels).

Tatara (1993) examined the states' diversified definitions in a recent national survey, which revealed a considerable similarity among the descriptions of elder mistreatments. Despite similarities there exists differences in specific terminologies, resulting in little consensus regarding standardized categories and definitions. In addition, each type of mistreatment does not always occur in isolation and a victim may suffer from more than one type of abuse concurrently.

The first wave of elder abuse research also identified impairments that forced an elderly person to become dependent on caregivers, as well as the resulting stress incurred by the primary caregiver, usually an elder abuse victim's daughter. The second wave of research addressed some of the methodological shortcomings of first wave and more importantly, challenged some of the first wave findings. Utilizing more rigid research techniques, this second wave of research moved beyond the impaired elder and the stressed caregiver theories. Findings from this wave indicated other predictors that result in elder abuse, most notably, the characteristics of the alleged abuser.

Currently, many etiological theories and explanations for elder abuse exist as researchers and practitioners examine abusive behaviors to identify predictive factors and high-risk situations that may contribute to elder abuse. An overview of significant risk factors related to elder abuse include: socio-economic level, marital status, substance abuse, personal problems, isolation, gender, cultural heterogeneity, housing and societal violence (Kosberg & Garcia, 1995).

In addition, as we approach the new millennium, demographers have predicted an increasingly "gray" population that is more ethnically diverse.

According to the U.S. Bureau of the Census (1996) demographic projections anticipate that ethnic minorities will comprise nearly half (47%) of America's population by 2050. Elder abuse research and literature has matured, but one significant gap in our knowledge is the impact of culture, ethnicity and life-style differences on elder abuse victims, their families and informal supports, and the formal service system. This gap is primarily due to early research whose subjects were primarily White. It is critical for policy planners and practitioners to understand the unique service needs, barriers to accessing services, and strategies for expanding those barriers, among different ethnic groups in their communities.

Elder Abuse Definitions

For the purpose of this study the definitions selected to describe the various types of elder abuse are taken from the research of Wolf and Pillemer (1984). This set of elder abuse classifications are used by the New York State Governor's Task Force for Elder Abuse and the New York City Elder Abuse Coalition of which the West Side One Stop is a member agency.

Physical Abuse–The infliction of physical pain or injury, or physical coercion (confinement against one's will). Examples include slapping, bruising, sexual molesting, cutting, lacerating, burning, physically restraining, pushing, shoving.

Psychological Abuse–The infliction of mental anguish. Examples include: demeaning, name calling, treating as a child, insulting, ignoring, frightening, humiliating, intimidating, threatening, isolating.

Financial Abuse–The illegal or unethical exploitation and/or use of funds, property, or other assets belonging to the older person.

Neglect–The refusal or failure to fulfill a caretaking obligation. Isolation or lack of attention. Examples include: non-provision of food or health related services, abandonment, the abuser doesn't talk to the victim, the abuser doesn't respond to the victim's questions. (Note: This definition collapses the categories of active and passive neglect.)

Incidence and Prevalence Rates of Elder Abuse

Researchers have suggested that the prevalence rates of elder abuse range anywhere from 4% to 10% of the older population (U.S. House of Representatives, 1990b; Hudson & Johnson, 1986). Actual prevalence rates estimate the total number of elder abuse cases in a given population at a given time. Tartara (1993) collected national data that estimated 1.57 million elderly persons were victims of domestic abuse and mistreatment in 1991. Estimates of elder abuse have consistently increased every year since tracking began in the 1980s.

Recent findings by the National Elder Abuse Incidence Study (NEAIS) estimated the incidence of elder abuse in America. Incidence rates estimate the number of new elder abuse cases over a specified period of time. NEAIS (1998) reported approximately 551,000 elderly persons were mistreated in domestic settings during 1996. The NEAIS research, which utilized their seven elder abuse definitions or categories, is arguably a monumental milestone in the elder abuse field.

The latest incidence and prevalence reports, however, do not negate the continued hidden nature of elder abuse. NEAIS (1998) reported that for every elder abuse incident reported, five are unreported. This last statistic validates the "iceberg" theory of elder abuse, that is, elder abuse response systems receive reports of only the most noticeable types of mistreatment, but a larger number of incidents are undetected and unreported (NEAIS, 1998).

Responses to Elder Abuse

The U. S. Congress has played a key role in the nation's mistreatment of elders as a social problem (Wolf, 1996). Congress amended the Older Americans Act (OAA) in 1987, to address the nation's mistreatment of their elders. In 1990, Congress appropriated funds to the states through OAA for the development of public education, outreach and prevention programs. The specific content of state legislation and the actual implementation of an elder abuse reporting and response system(s) were left to the states. Many states modeled their elder abuse reporting laws on already existing child abuse laws. This was in spite of the fact that adults are legally entitled to make decisions about their lives (unless declared incompetent by a court of law) which is not a right extended to children.

Most states include elder abuse and neglect in their existing statutes dealing with "protective" services for adults unable to protect their own interests. All fifty states have legislation that defines elder abuse and mistreatment, creates mandatory or voluntary reporting systems, and develops response systems. In general, state reporting laws require specific designated professionals to report any case of suspected elder abuse to a specific agency. The New York State Adult Protective Services (APS) has a voluntary reporting system, and is limited to adults, 18 years of age and above, who are a danger to themselves or others, and who are unable to care for themselves. Unless a victim is impaired, APS in New York City will not respond. This has resulted in a service gap for unimpaired elder abuse victims.

Elder Abuse and Service Utilization

This study reviewed the literature relating to community based services for elders to tease out predictors that contribute to service use. Connecting vulnerable elder abuse victims with appropriate services is a much neglected subject. Krout (1983a) in his seminal study of social service utilization by the elderly found: underutilization of services; negative attitudes about services; a general unawareness of services; and correlates of service use that were not clearly understood. In addition, a demographic profile of service users emerged for the elderly: over 70, living alone, female, widowed, with limited informal social support, and reporting below average health. From the initial literature on service utilization by the elderly, knowledge of services has been cited as a critical factor. Knowledge of services refers to the information needed prior to service use, such as knowledge of service, knowledge of procedures and knowledge of need (Yeatts, Crow, & Folts, 1992).

Service utilization literature is replete with risk factors that promote or inhibit service use by elderly persons including gender (Penning & Strain, 1994); age (Penning, 1995); living arrangement (Webber, Fox, & Burnette, 1994); informal supports (Logan & Spitze, 1994); increased disability (Mutschler & Callahan, 1990); ethnicity (Mui & Burnette, 1994; and Miner, 1995); poverty (Meyer & Bartolomei-Hill, 1994, and Yeatts, Crow, & Folts, 1992); marital status (Ozawa, 1995); specific disease, such as Alzheimer's (Webber, Fox & Burnette, 1994); and need (Dill, 1993).

In general, researchers have noted that increased age, race, poverty, functional disability and cognitive impairment were identified as risk factors contributing to elder abuse (Lachs, Williams, O'Brien, Hurst, & Horowitz, 1997). These factors are also correlated with an increased need for services by elder abuse victims. "Need" factors have been identified as the most important predictors of formal service utilization (Andersen-Newman, 1973).

Cantor and Brennan (1993) have identified pathways, or factors that promote service utilization by elderly persons. In their examination of pathways or linkages to service use several indicators emerged: perceived need, having a previous connection to the formal service system, poor health, a small and/or weak informal support system, inadequate income, and lower involvement with neighbors.

Family caregiving has traditionally been synonymous with "informal" social support. Research has examined the concept of social support and its affect on service utilization by elderly persons (Miner, 1995; Penning, 1995; Logan & Spitz, 1994), often with contradictory conclusions. It has become common wisdom that most older persons express a distinct preference for community based health and social services for continued support to remain in their communities. Equally important is the elders' distinct preference for care by their informal supports, presented in hierarchial order according to the compensatory theory: family members, friends and neighbors (Cantor & Brennan, 1993). When an elder requires emotional, social and/or physical support, the elder prefers to appeal to their "informal" supports. While the elderly prefer their informal supports, they do seek out and receive services from the formal support system (Krause, 1990). "Formal" support refers to the use of services from the formal service system. There is evidence that formal supports are used to compensate or substitute for unavailable informal supports (Cantor & Brennan, 1993). Miner (1995) has also found evidence that racial differences impact the "interplay" of informal and formal supports.

There still remains a significant gap in service utilization research of what kinds of services elder abuse victims need and accept. Berman (1994) notes that there are a plethora of service utilization studies for the elderly, but relatively few relate specifically to the victims of elder abuse. Two recent studies on service utilization and elder abuse have contributed to the knowledge of service use by abused elders. Vinton (1988) reported two important predictors of service use: "able" elders rejected more services than disabled elders and elder abuse victims abused by male abusers were more likely to reject services. Berman (1994) reported that elder abuse victims were less likely to initiate services when victims: lived with their abusers, suffered from financial abuse, and suffered from mental health problems.

Case Management

Case management can be described as an intervention strategy focusing on the continuity of care for vulnerable people. Case management emerged as a respond to America's fragmented and complicated service delivery system (Moore, 1992; Rothman, 1992; Roberts-DeGennaro, 1993). In the case of elder abuse, services to mitigate abusive situations include the victim and the abuser, especially if the abuser is a family member. A range of services may be available for the victim and the abuser; however, many services necessitate referrals to other network agencies. Case managers navigate the various offerings appropriate for the client that may include housing, health, mental health, social service, criminal justice, legal and social services. Case management has been used to assist elder abuse victims, as exhibited by the One Stop Agency used for this study's sample.

Theoretical Framework

In the current research the Andersen-Newman Model (1973) provides the framework for examining the utilization of health and social services by elder abuse victims. The most important aspect of utilizing this model is the contribution it can make to theory about behavioral patterns of service usage. Identifying predictors is the first step in establishing a theory about service behavioral patterns of services used. Through this understanding of predictors and subsequent barriers, strategies can be developed to overcoming barriers to service utilization by elder abuse victims.

Andersen (1968) conceptualized health service utilization as behavior patterns influenced by many concurring factors leading to service utilization. Andersen proposed three categories: (1) client must be "predisposed" to receive services; (2) "enabling" factors promoted access and availability to services, and (3) the "need" for services must be perceived. The major questions in this early research were identifying the factors that contributed to the differential utilization of health services by families.

This theoretical model has been modified by Andersen and his colleagues (Aday & Andersen, 1974; Aday, Andersen, & Fleming, 1980; Andersen & Newman,1973.) The Andersen-Newman model (1973) has been widely used to predict the use of health and social services by older people, including service utilization by abused elders (Cantor & Brennan, 1993; Vinton, 1988). Modifications to this model have allowed investigators to examine the acceptance or rejection of services, as well as other contributing factors influencing access, availability and barriers to services. It is expected that need factors will more fully predict service utilization. While need factors are expected to be the primary factors in service utilization, this model hypothesizes that service utilization is a result of the "interaction" of the predisposing, enabling and need factors.

For the purpose of this study, the conceptual model is referred to as the Andersen-Newman Model (1973) as modified (see Figure 1).

In the above model the predisposing factors refer to individual and environmental characteristics that may predispose a person to utilize formal services. The enabling factors refer to the social and economic conditions that may assist an individual to access formal services. The need factors in this model are the most significant indicators of service utilization and reflect the actual cause for service use. The last component in this framework, the outcome, is service utilization as measured by the actual amount of services used.

Service utilization research has observed service outcomes as acceptance or non-acceptance of services (Vinton, 1988) or volume of service use (Penning, 1995). The dependent variable in this study is the amount of services utilized by elder abuse victims. For the purposes of this study, it is hypothesized that this sample, which has been assessed and identified as being

FIGURE 1. Andersen-Newman Model (Modified)

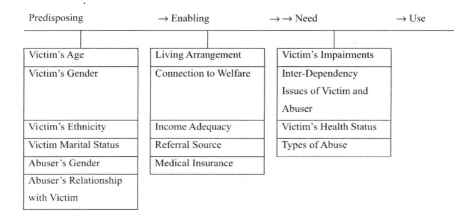

An Operationalized Model of Victims' Anticipated Use of Services

Predisposing	→ Enabling	→ → Need	→ Use
Victim's Age	Living Arrangement	Victim's Impairments	
Victim's Gender	Connection to Welfare	Inter-Dependency Issues of Victim and Abuser	
Victim's Ethnicity	Income Adequacy	Victim's Health Status	
Victim Marital Status	Referral Source	Types of Abuse	
Abuser's Gender	Medical Insurance		
Abuser's Relationship with Victim			

composed of elder abuse victims, will use more services than elderly people will in general.

Based on the literature on service utilization, elder abuse and the Andersen (1968) and the Andersen-Newman (1973) models, this proposed study has focused on the nature of elder abuse, factors contributing to elder abuse, and services utilized. Thus, the modified Andersen-Newman Model (1973) is used to organize a series of independent variables into predisposing, enabling and need categories in order to learn more about the factors which contribute to utilization of services by elder abuse victims. The major hypothesis and the set of sub-hypotheses were based on research findings related to service utilization literature.

Major Hypothesis

The major research question pertains to the factors which affect service utilization by the victims of elder abuse. Thus, the overarching hypothesis of this study is as follows: The most important factor in the utilization of services by elder abuse victims will be the extent of the victim's need factors, followed by enabling factors, and lastly, by predisposing (demographic) factors, which will contribute the least amount of variance.

METHODOLOGY

Sampling Procedure

The specific population studied is a purposive sample of elderly people, 60 years and older, who are identified as having been victims of elder abuse, according to the West Side One Stop for Coordinated Senior Services, Inc. in New York City. The sample is derived from a secondary analysis of case records from this program. The unit of analysis is the abused elder and her or his abuser. To be included in the study sample, the respondent must be at least 60 + years or older, identified by the agency as being a victim of abuse, have a case record of at least two months in duration, and be receiving services from the One Stop Senior Support Project (OSSP) for Abused Elderly Victims during the period of 1993 to 1996. The sample size was 129. This research site was chosen specifically because the case management social workers were educated and trained to identify elder abuse.

Instrument

The data used in this study are based on secondary analysis of case records. Case records consist of demographic data: victim and the abuser, type of abuse, source of referral, and services offered and utilized.

RESULTS

Sample Description

The profile of abused elders that emerges from this sample is overwhelmingly white female, with an average age of 75 years. A significant number of this sample lives with others, reports being widowed or single, has cognitive and/or ADL impairments and reports their health as being "fair." A majority of this sample receives an income below the federal poverty line, and has a previous connection to the welfare system (means-tested entitlement benefits). In addition, a vast majority of this sample had some kind of health insurance (96%), including Medicare, Medicaid, or both (see Table 1).

The profile of the alleged perpetrator that emerges from this sample is a male child, with an average age of 51 years, who lives with the abused elderly victim, is financially dependent upon the elder and has either mental illness or an alcohol and/or substance abuse problem (see Table 2).

Psychological abuse was the most often reported type of abuse (75%), followed by financial abuse (68%), physical abuse (43%) and neglect (33%). The

TABLE 1. Major Demographic Characteristics of Elder Abuse Victims (N = 129)

Victim Characteristics	Number	Percent
Gender	129	
Male	28	22
Female	101	78
Age	129	
Young-old (60-74)	65	50
Old-old (75+)	64	50
Mean Age = 75	Range 60-95	
Ethnicity	129	
White	57	44
African-American	21	16
Hispanic	51	40
Primary Language	129	
English	89	69
Spanish	40	31
Marital Status	129	
Married	23	18
Widowed	59	46
Separated/Divorced	18	14
Single	29	23
Income Adequacy	128	
Poverty Level or Below	71	55
Above Poverty Level	57	45
Health Insurance	128	
Medicare	57	44
Medicare & Medicaid	43	34
Medicaid	23	18
None	5	4
Connection to Welfare	128	
Prior Connection	69	54
No Prior Connection	59	46
Living Arrangements	129	
Alone	33	26
With Spouse	21	16
With Child	50	39
With Other Relative	10	8
With Friend/Boarders	15	11

TABLE 2. Major Demographic Characteristics of Alleged Abusers (N = 114)*

Alleged Abuser Characteristics	Number	Percentage
Age	114	
Mean 51		
Range 16-91		
Gender	114	
Male	72	63
Female	42	37
Ethnicity	114	
White	49	42
African-American	20	18
Hispanic	45	40
Living Arrangements	114	
With Victim	95	83
Not With Victim	19	17
Abuser's Relationship to Victim	114	
Spouse	23	20
Child	56	49
Friend/Boarder	21	18
Other Relative	14	12
Income Adequacy	75	
Below Poverty Line	51	68
Above Poverty Line	24	32
Abuser is Financially Dependent on Victim	113	
No	39	34
Yes	74	66
Abuser is Primary Caregiver of Victim	113	
No	62	55
Yes	51	45
Abuser is Cognitively Impaired	111	
No	75	68
Yes**	36	32
Alcohol/ Substance Abuse	108	
No	68	63
Yes	40	37

*This number reflects identified abusers only. Abusers who could not be specified and those elders who suffered from self neglect were excluded from this descriptive analysis.
**Note: This 32% reflects mental illness (27%) and other (5%).

number of types of abuse reported varied from one to four types; 74% of this sample of elder abuse victims suffered from two or more types of abuse simultaneously. Over three-fourths (77%) of the referrals came from "professionals" and a large proportion of this figure (32%) was referred by One Stop workers who had been trained to identify the signs and symptoms of abuse by an elder abuse specialist. This suggests that educating and training professionals may result in increased appropriate referrals (see Table 3).

With respect to services utilized, the majority of this sample were more likely to use social services (79%), followed by health services (57%), housing services (48%) and finally legal services (41%). The mean number of services utilized by elder abuse victims in this study was 4.2 services (see Table 4).

The top ten services utilized by elder abuse victims in rank order were: (1) Home visits by social worker (62%); (2) Home care (45%); (3) Utilization of police (38%); (4) Visiting Nurse (25%); (5) Reduced transportation fare (23%); (6) Hospital (21%); (7) Elderly Housing Referral (18%); (8) Meals on wheels (17%); (9) Money management (16%); and (10) Order of protection (13%).

Summary of Multiple Regression Analysis

Findings from the regression analysis (see Table 5) indicated that 30% of the variance is explained by the 21 independent variables organized into the Predisposing, Enabling and Need categories according to the Andersen-Newman Model. Among the Predisposing variables only two were significant predictors: (1) Abuser is Female and (2) Abuser (Perpetrator) is Substance Abuser; while only one Enabling variable was significant: (1) Victim Lives Alone. With respect to Need, the two significant need variables underscored the vulnerability of the victim: (1) Victim has Cognitive and ADL Impairments; and (2) Abuser is both Financially Dependent on the Victim and the Primary Caregiver of the Victim. Both the independent Predisposing and Need variables predicted the same amount of variance (12% each, for a total of 24%), followed by the enabling variables at 6%. Ethnicity did not appear to be a significant predictor of the likelihood of using services in this sample.

SUMMATION OF MAJOR FINDINGS

The major hypothesis in this study based on the theoretical Andersen-Newman Model of service utilization was not supported in the multiple regression findings. Predisposing variables, at least in the case of elder abuse victims, were equally as strong as need variables as predictors of the Total Amount of Services Used. The elder abuse victim and abuser characteristics

TABLE 3. Type of Reported Abuse and Referral Source (N = 129)

Variable	Number	Percent
Extent of Abuse		
(# of Types of Abuse Reported)		
2 Types of Abuse	48	37
3 Types of Abuse	36	28
1 Type of Abuse	34	26
4 Types of Abuse	11	9
Type of Abuse		
Psychological	97	75
Financial	88	68
Physical & Sexual	55	43
Neglect	42	33
Referral Source (In Rank Order)		
One Stop Worker	41	32
Home Care Agency	16	12
Friend/ Neighbor	15	12
Housing Agency/	13	10
Social Worker		
Family Member	8	6
Law/ Police	8	6
Referring Social	7	5
Service		
Victim (Self)	7	5
Medical/ Professional	4	3
Clergy/ Church	2	2
Meals-on-Wheels	2	2
Referral (Collapsed)		
Victim (Self)	7	5
Other	122	95

(predisposing variables) contributed as much as need variables in predicting service utilization. Four specific Need variables significantly affect the amount of services used: (1) Victim has Cognitive and ADL Impairments; (2) Victim's "Poor" Health Status; (3) Abuser is Financially Dependent on the Victim and the Primary Caregiver of the Victim; and (4) the type of

TABLE 4. Services Accepted by Elder Abuse Victims—Extent and Type (N = 129)

Variables	Number of Services	No. of Victims	% of Sample
Total Number of Services Used	538	129	100
Mean Services Used	4.2		
White	4.4		
Afro-American	4.2		
Hispanic	3.9		
Extent of Service Use			
High Use (6-12)		36	28.0
Medium Use (3-5)		53	41.1
Low Use (1-2)		29	22.4
No Use (0)		11	8.5
Individual Services Grouped by Type			
Social Services (n = 26)	240	102	79
Health Services (n = 9)	135	73	57
Housing Services (n = 9)	82	62	48
Legal Services (n = 6)	81	53	41

abuse, Neglect. Only Need factors were related to the level of service utilization.

Ethnicity as such did not predict total service use in any of the major categories of the regression analysis. However, in the case of specific services used by ethnic group, there was a trend towards less use of three services by the Hispanic group: Emergency Shelter, Adult Home and Meals-on-Wheels. This does not imply that Hispanics have more or less need for such services, but rather, that cultural factors and the strong emphasis on the family caring for its own may have served as barriers to their use of such services.

Abuser characteristics are important predictors of service use by elder abuse victims. Two Predisposing variables which significantly affect service use were abuser characteristics: (1) Abuser is Female and, (2) Perpetrator (abuser) is a Substance Abuser. This suggests that in the case of elder abuse victims' particular situational factors impact on the victim-abuser relationship in which these situational factors may affect service utilization over and above need factors.

TABLE 5. Hierarchical Multiple Regression Analysis

Factors Involved in the Utilization of Formal Services
Total Amount of Services Utilized (N = 129)

Variables	Beta	Zero order r	% R^2 Change	Cum. R^2
Predisposing				
Victim Characteristics			.04	.04
Victim's Age	.03	.09		
Victim's Gender	.12	.00		
Victim's Ethnicity				
African-American	−.05	.01		
Hispanic	−.09	−.08		
Abuser Characteristics			.08	.12
Abuser's Gender	−.27*	.10		
Abuser is Substance Abuser	.28*	.15		
Abuser is Mentally Ill	−.09	−.08		
Enabling			.06	.18
Living Arrangement				
Victim Lives Alone	.29*	.10		
Connection to Welfare	−.15	−.03		
Referral Source	.05	.07		
Need			.12	.30
Victim's Impairments				
Victim's Cognitive Impairment	.13	.08		
Victim's ADL Impairment	.07	−.04		
Victim's Cog. & ADL	.30*	.20*		
Impairment				
Victim's Health Status	−.11	−.21*		
Type of Dependency				
Abuser is Financially Dependent	.05	−.05		
Abuser is Primary Caregiver	.16	−.02		
Abuser is Financially Dependent on Victim & Primary Caregiver	.31*	.00		
Type of Abuse				
Psychological Abuse	.03	−.04		
Financial Abuse	−.03	.12		
Physical Abuse	−.10	.06		
Neglect	.10	.20*		

*= p < .05
Total Variance Explained: 30%

DISCUSSION

Three of the most common barriers to community service utilization by elder abuse victims according to Wolf and Pillemer (1994) are the fragmented service system, reluctance of victims to accept services, and the shortage of trained personnel. In "Growing Older in New York City in the 1990s" (Cantor & Brennan, 1993) the mean number of services utilized by older New Yorkers as a whole was 1.2 as compared with a mean of 4.2 in the case of the respondents in the current study. Interpretations must be made cautiously, but it appears from the initial examination of these results that the One Stop agency has minimized these structural barriers for their elder abuse clients.

Limitations

All the respondents in this study sample were selected after being identified as elder abuse victims and therefore represent a specific group of elders from the community who are involved with a social service agency based in this respective community. Findings cannot be generalized to all older persons or other elder abuse victims. The very nature of utilizing "secondary" data has automatic limitation, that is, by gathering information from existing case records certain variables were unavailable for analysis. In this study and in the field of elder abuse in general, the most critical factors in comparability are the inconsistent definitions of elder abuse. It is difficult to make comparisons of the current findings with previous research due to these limitations.

Service Systems

Even with adequate knowledge of services, the current service system remains fragmented, and often has a sufficient bureaucratic nature to impede formal service use. One viable intervention to reduce this fragmentation and increase the consistency of services over a continuum for elder abuse victims is case management. Case management allows practitioners to follow elder abuse victims and their perpetrators through the formal service system. Case management can be an effective tool in meeting these varied needs.

Future outreach and education efforts must include computers, especially the Internet. Giffords (1998, p. 243) reports that the world of cyberspace has evolved into a "user-friendly network of exploration." The Internet can provide easy access to relevant empirical and practice knowledge, plus an array of communications, such as e-mail, bulletin boards, on line conversations and chat rooms. While there are concerns about the constraints of data accessibility and additional concerns about confidentiality, coalition building with other service networks for elder abuse victims is critical.

ACCEPTANCE OF SERVICES

Elder abuse is dynamic and involves relationships, especially with family members. A major barrier to service utilization by elder abuse victims has been the reluctance of victims to report abusers who are family members. The findings from this study suggest the importance of understanding the various factors that interplay upon these family relationships. In fact, perhaps the most important finding from this study is that certain abuser characteristics significantly predict increased service utilization of elder abuse victims. Surprisingly, service use by the victim is significantly predicted by gender (female) and substance abuse by the abuser (perpetrator). This might suggest that outreach efforts between formal and informal support system, in this case One Stop and substance abusers, extended normative barriers involving abuser impairments and actually strengthened the adaptive nature of these networks in the best interests of the victim. Thus, this abuser impairment did not interfere with needed service use, and, in fact, promoted service use by elder abuse victims. Practitioners cannot be expected to change the abuser's substance abuse, however, they can understand the dynamics of substance and plan appropriate strategies to meet the elder abuse victim's needs and the needs of the abuser.

Throughout this study, the importance demographic characteristics in predicting service utilization has been emphasized, particularly, the ethnicity of the elder abuse victim. Previous research found that the Hispanic elderly were less likely to use formal services (Cantor & Brennan, 1993). Ethnicity did not emerge as a predictive independent factor in this study. This finding suggests that ethnic minorities in the Upper West Side of Manhattan served by One Stop recognized that the agency was user-friendly and an important resource to mitigate abusive situations. Cultural barriers to service utilization (e.g., language, attitudes about seeking assistance outside the family, and cultural bias toward entitlements) are important. Understanding the sensitive cultural issues that create barriers and developing strategies to overcome them, such as bi-lingual workers, are vital for the acceptance of services by many clients.

Trained Personnel

A reluctance to identify the elder abuse situations by elder abuse victims and their alleged abusers is joined with a lack of problem awareness by aging agencies and staff members. Vinton (1993) found that too often agencies and workers who deal with the elderly do not have appropriate knowledge to identify elder abuse and address elder abuse situations. What is critically needed is a professional shift in attitude among all the agencies and various disciplines that address elder abuse situations. This shift must encompass the understanding of elder abuse as a complex social problem that requires complex strategies and interventions for both the victim and the abuser, especially when they are family members. This shift can only be accomplished through appropriate training and education.

Social Work Research

The Andersen-Newman Model, which was the theoretical underpinning of this study, indicated that need factors will be the most important factors in service utilization, followed by enabling factors, and lastly, by predisposing factors. This was not the case in this study. In using the Andersen-Newman Model in future service utilization studies of elder abuse victims, it will be important to look at abuser characteristics more carefully. The ultimate goal in any elder abuse situation is to stop the abuse. Halting abuse can be accomplished in many different ways, often including a change in living arrangement. The elderly use more services when there is social support (family member(s)) living within the elder's household. There was considerable movement in living arrangements (40%) by victims or abusers during this study that included moving to a nursing home (9%), elder housing referral (9%) and abuser moving out of the victim's household (6%). Research should be conducted on elder abuse intervention outcomes that incorporate these changes in living arrangements. In general, outcome studies can be effective in renewing or reviving political support that is needed for this vulnerable group for aging in place in a safe environment. It is essential that all policy planners, researchers, educators and practitioners work together to integrate and expand the current knowledge about elder abuse in families, so all efforts will dovetail and focus on dealing with this invisible social problem.

REFERENCES

Aday, L. A., & Andersen, R. (1974). A framework for the study of access to medical care. *Health Services Research, 9*, 208-222.

Aday, L. A., Andersen, R., & Fleming, G.V. (1980). *Health care in the U.S.: Equitable for whom?* Beverly Hills, CA: Sage Publications.

Andersen, R. A. (1968). A behavioral model of families' use of health services. Factors that influence use of social services by the elderly. *Research Series 25*, Chicago: University of Chicago.

Andersen, R. A., & Newman, J. F. (1973). Societal and individual determinants of medical care utilization in the United States. *Milbank Memorial Fund Quarterly, 51*, 95-129.

Berman, J. (1994). Maladaptive networks: Elder abuse victims' experience within the service delivery system (Doctoral dissertation, Columbia University, 1994). Dissertation Abstracts International, 6359, 210. (UMI No. 9427032).

Block, M. R. & Sinnott, J. D. (1979). *The battered elder syndrome: An exploratory study.* College Park, MD: University of Maryland.

Cantor, M. H. & Brennan, M. (1993). Growing older in New York City in the 1990's: A study of changing lifestyles, quality of life and quality of care. In *A changing lifestyles, quality of life, and quality study of care*, Vol. 5. New York: The New York Center for Policy on Aging of the New York Community Trust.

Dill, A. (1993). Defining needs, defining systems: A critical analysis. *The Gerontologist, 33*(4), 453-460.

Douglass, R. L., Hickey, T., & Noel, C. (1980). *A study of maltreatment of the elderly and other vulnerable adults.* Ann Arbor, MI: University of Michigan. Institute of Gerontology.

Fulmer, T. & O'Malley, T. (1987). *Inadequate care of the elderly: A health care perspective on abuse and neglect.* New York: Springer Publishing Company.

Giffords, E. D. (1998). Social work on the internet: An introduction. *Social Work, 43*(3), 243-251.

Gonyea, J.G. (1994). The paradox of the advantaged elder and the feminization of poverty. *Social Work, 39*(1), 35-41.

Hudson, M.F. (1986). Elder mistreatment: Current research. In Pillemer, K. A. & Wolf, R. S. (Eds.). *Elder abuse: Conflict in the family.* Dover, MA: Auburn House Publishing Company.

Johnson, I. M. (1995). Family members' perception of and attitudes toward elder abuse. *Families in Society: The Journal of Contemporary Human Services*, 220-229.

Kosberg, J. I. (1986). Victimization of the elderly. Domestic violent public health. Hearing before the subcommittee on children, families, drugs, and alcoholism of the committee on Labor and Human Resources. U.S. Senate. October 30, 1985, Washington DC. U.S. Government Printing Office, 93-94.

Kosberg, J. I. (1988). Preventing elder abuse: Identification of high risk factors prior to placement decisions. *The Gerontologist, 28*, 43-50.

Kosberg, J .I. (1998). The abuse of elderly men. *Journal of Elder Abuse & Neglect, 9*(3), 69-88.

Kosberg, J .I. & Garcia, J .L. (1995). Common and unique themes on elder abuse from a world-wide perspective. *Journal of Elder Abuse & Neglect, 6* (3/4), 183-197.

Krause, N. (1990). Perceived health problems, formal/informal support, and life satisfaction among older adults. *Journal of Gerontology: Social Sciences, 45*, S193-S205.

Krout, J. A. (1983a). Knowledge and use of services by the elderly: A critical review of the literature. *International Journal of Aging and Human Development, 17*(3), 153-167.

Lachs, M. S., Williams, C., O'Brien, S., Hurst, L., & Horowitz, R. (1997). Risk factors for reported elder abuse & neglect: A nine-year observational cohort study. *The Gerontologist, 37*(4), 469-474.

Lau, E., & Kosberg, J. (1979). Abuse of the elderly by informal care providers. *Aging,* Sept.-Oct., 10-15.

Logan, J. R. & Spitze, G. (1994). Informal support and the use of formal services by older Americans. *Journal of Gerontology: Social Sciences, 49*(1), S25-S34.

Meyer, D. R., & Bartolomei-Hill, S. (1994). The adequacy of supplemental security benefits for aged individuals and couples. *The Gerontologist, 34*(2), 161-172.

Miner, S. (1995). Racial differences in family support and formal service utilization among older persons: A nonrecursive model. *Journal of Gerontology: Social Sciences,* 50B(3), S143-S153.

Montoya, V. (1997). Understanding and combating elder abuse in hispanic communities. *Journal of Elder Abuse & Neglect, 9*(2), 5-17.

Moore, S. T. (1992). Case management and the integration of services: How service delivery systems shape case management. *Social Work, 37*(5), 418-423.

Mui, A. C. & Burnette, D. (1994). Long-term care service use by frail elders: Is ethnicity a factor? *The Gerontologist, 34*(2), 190-198.

Mutschler, P. H., & Callahan, Jr. J. J. (1990). Utilizing client experience in developing new service delivery models for care of the aged. *Journal of Gerontological Social Work, 15*(3/4), 49-74.

National Elder Abuse Incidence Study (NEAIS)(1998). National Center on Elder Abuse, U.S. Department of Health and Human Services, Administration on Aging and by the National Center on Elder Abuse at the American Public Human Services Association. Washington, D.C.: U.S. Government Printing Office.

O'Malley, H., Segars, H., Perez, R., Mitchell, V., & Knuepel, G. M. (1979). *Elder abuse in Massachusetts: A survey of professionals and paraprofessionals.* Boston: Legal Research and Services for the Elderly.

Ozawa, M. N. (1995). The economic status of vulnerable older women. *Social Work, 40*(3), 323-331.

Penning, M. J. (1995). Health, social support, and the utilization of health services among older adults. *Journal of Gerontology: Social Sciences,* 50B(3), S330-S339.

Penning, M. J. & Strain, L. A. (1994). Gender differences in disability, assistance and subjective well-being in later life. *Journal of Gerontology: Social Sciences, 49*(4), S202-S208.

Phillipson, C. (1997). Abuse of older people: Sociological perspectives. In Decalmer, P. & Glendenning, F. (Eds.), *The Mistreatment of Elderly People.* London: Sage Publications.

Quinn, M. J., & Tomita, S. K. (1997). *Elder abuse and neglect: Causes, diagnosis, and intervention strategies* (2nd ed.). New York: Springer Publishing Company.

Roberts-De Gennaro, M. (1993). Generalist model of case management. *Journal of Case Management, 2*(3), 106-111.

Rothman, J. (1992). *Guidelines for case management.* Itasca, IL: F. E. Peacock Publishers, Inc.

Stevenson, O. (1996*). Elder protection in the community: What can we learn from child protection?* London: Department of Health Social Services Inspectorate.

Straus, M., Gelles, R. J., & Steinmetz, S. (1980). *Behind closed doors: Violence in the American family.* New York: Doubleday.

Tartara, T. (1993). Finding the nature and scope of domestic elder abuse with the use of state aggregate data: Summaries of the key findings of a national survey of state APS and aging agencies. *Journal of Elder Abuse & Neglect, 5*(4), 35-57.

U.S. Bureau of the Census (1996). *65 + in the America.* Current Population Reports, Special Studies P23-190. Washington DC: Government Printing Office.

U.S. House of Representatives, Select Committee on Aging. (1990a). *Elder abuse: Curbing a national epidemic* (Hearings). Washington, D.C.: Government Printing Office.

Vinton, L. S. (1988). *Correlates of abused elders' anticipated use of services.* (Dissertation). Madison, Wisconsin: University of Wisconsin.

Vinton, L. (1993). Educating case managers about elder abuse and neglect. *Journal of Case Management, 2*(3), 101-105.

Webber, P. A., Fox, P., & Burnette, D. (1994). Living alone with Alzheimer's disease: Effects on health and social service utilization patterns. *The Gerontologist, 34*(1), 8-14.

Wolf, R. S. (1996). Elder abuse and family violence: Testimony presented before the US Senate Special Committee on Aging. *Journal of Elder Abuse & Neglect, 8*(1), 81-96.

Wolf, R. S. & Pillemer, K. A. (1984). *Working with abused elderly: Assessment, advocacy, and intervention.* Worcester, MA: University of Massachusetts Medical Center.

Wolf, R. S. & Pillemer, K. A. (1994). What's new in elder abuse programming? Four bright ideas. *The Gerontologist, 34*(1), 126-129.

Yeatts, D. E., Crow, T., & Folts, E. (1992). Service use among low-income minority elderly: Strategies for overcoming barriers. *The Gerontologist, 32*(1) 24-32.

doi: 10.1300/J083v48n01_16

Research, Macro Practice and Aging
in the Social Work Education Curriculum

Eileen Appleby, PhD
Anne L. Botsford, PhD

SUMMARY. This paper presents a model that used a macro emphasis for teaching research using older adults. Faculty developed the teaching model to address three key areas of concern in the education of Bachelor of Social Work (BSW) students for generalist practice: (1) research, (2) macro-level practice, and (3) aging. The paper explores the nature of these concerns and draws upon previous literature to delineate a teaching model designed to strengthen these areas of generalist practice by integrating content on macro-level concerns and aging into the curriculum of a research course. The development and evaluation of the research course within the context of a community and college project are described, as are the benefits for students, the social work program and the community. Preliminary findings indicate some support for the use of such a model. doi: 10.1300/J083v48n01_17 *[Article copies available for a fee from The Haworth Document Delivery Service: 1-800-HAWORTH. E-mail address: <docdelivery@haworthpress.com> Website: <http://www.HaworthPress.com> © 2006 by The Haworth Press, Inc. All rights reserved.]*

KEYWORDS. Research, aging, macro, generalist, evaluation, curriculum

[Haworth co-indexing entry note]: "Research, Macro Practice and Aging in the Social Work Education Curriculum." Appleby, Eileen, and Anne L. Botsford. Co-published simultaneously in *Journal of Gerontological Social Work* (The Haworth Press, Inc.) Vol. 48, No. 1/2, 2006, pp. 257-279; and: *Fostering Social Work Gerontology Competence: A Collection of Papers from the First National Gerontological Social Work Conference* (ed: Catherine J. Tompkins, and Anita L. Rosen) The Haworth Press, Inc., 2007, pp. 257-279. Single or multiple copies of this article are available for a fee from The Haworth Document Delivery Service [1-800-HAWORTH, 9:00 a.m. - 5:00 p.m. (EST). E-mail address: docdelivery@haworthpress.com].

RESEARCH AND THE BSW CURRICULUM

Integration of theory and practice has been a principal theme historically in social work. However, accommodation between research and practice has been the source of much debate and controversy. More than a decade of discussion passed from the time that Kirk, Osmolov, and Fischer (1976) concluded that practitioners and researchers do not trust each other to Grinnell and Siegal's (1988) proposal of a unified practitioner/researcher role for social workers. Subsequent debates of the practitioner/researcher role, while lively, stimulating, and often perplexing, have failed to resolve this issue within the profession (Kirk, 1996).

For instance, the Task Force on Social Work Research of the National Association of Social Workers (NASW) declared a crisis in social work research in 1991. The Task Force reported that just thirty percent of the NASW members regularly read *Social Work*. Subsequent literature has explored practitioners' reluctance to conduct research (Bradley, 1997; Gerdes, Edmonds, Haslam, & McCartney, 1996; Howard & Jenson, 1999; Weinback & Grinnell, 1995), underscored the importance of research for practitioners (Cournoyer & Klein, 2000; Fortune & Proctor, 2001; Franklin, 1999; Hess & Mullen, 1995; Horner, 2000; Randall, Cowley & Tomlinson, 2000; Williams & Lanigan, 1999) and explicated the role of practitioner as researcher (Beresford & Evans, 1999; Bisman & Hardcastle, 1999; Fook, 2002; Gibbs, 2001).

Just as research has been challenging for the profession, education about research is challenging for social work education. The Task Force observed that despite the emphasis in social work education on integrating research and practice, research methods courses are often taught detached from practice courses (Task Force on Social Work Research, 1991). In addition, the Council on Social Work Education (CSWE) Commission on Accreditation attributed the difficulty satisfying CSWE research requirements to lack of integration of research into the curriculum (Hull & Mokuau, 1994). While some studies have focused on the benefits of integrating technology into the social work curriculum (Finn & Lavitt, 1995; Stone, 1999), there seems to be limited empirical evidence of the benefits of integrating research into the curriculum.

Given the profession's uneasiness with research, it is not surprising that social work students are of a similar mind. Several authors of social work research textbooks have conjectured that the only reason social work students take research is because they are required to do so (Mark, 1996; Rubin & Babbie, 1997). Congress (1993) suggested that required social work research courses are unpopular among students. Other authors have implied that students find research intimidating (Weinbach & Grinnell, 1995; Yegidis & Weinbach, 1996), overwhelming (York, 1997) and "a necessary evil" (Grinnell, 1993).

Royce and Rompf (1992) found that social work students have more math anxiety than non-social work students and Wilson and Rosenthal (1992) found that more than seventy percent of students had moderate or higher levels of anxiety about research and statistics. The uneasy relationship that both the social work profession and social work education have had with research may also contribute to the students' apprehension about research courses.

MACRO PRACTICE AND THE BSW CURRICULUM

Nowhere in the BSW curriculum has the integration of research and practice been more difficult than in the area of macro-level practice. Advocacy on behalf of vulnerable populations with an aim toward rectifying social inequality is an integral part of social work's history. Social work pioneers such as Edith and Grace Abbott, Jane Addams, Dorothea Dix, Florence Kelley, Julia Lathrop, Harry Hopkins and Francis Perkins advocated large-scale social change on behalf of children, the poor and disenfranchised populations.

The more recent history of social work has attested to the profession's greater attention to micro-level practice. This shift has been attributed to the social work curricula's neglecting to teach social work students how to be agents of social change (Wyers, 1991), to the paucity of macro-field placements (Butler & Coleman, 1997; Raber & Richter, 1999) and to the increasing professionalization of social work (Thyer, 1997). In addition, Fisher and Karger (1997) have called for a model of macro practice that includes "the empowerment of citizens, the rebuilding of public life, and the effecting of social change" (p. 132). Responding to a social change agenda is yet another challenge for the BSW generalist curriculum.

AGING AND THE BSW CURRICULUM

A third area of concern for BSW generalist education is preparation of students for practice with special populations such as older adults. With the long-heralded demographic age revolution, dramatic needs for eldercare generalists in a variety of settings are anticipated, with labor force projections suggesting the demand for gerontological social workers could reach 60-70,000 in the next twenty years (Butler, 2001; Rosen & Persky, 1997; Smeeding, Butler & Schaber, 1999). A survey of NASW members (Masters of Social Workers and Bachelors of Social Workers) found that over one-quarter of current NASW members practiced primarily with older people (Peterson & Wendt, 1990) and that the majority of social workers in health care settings served predominately older persons (Damron-Rodriguez & Lubben, 1997). In addition, of all NASW members surveyed, 62% reported the need for knowledge about aging, despite the fact that most practicing social workers receive little or no prior knowledge or skills in gerontology (Peterson, 1990).

In a 1995 survey, 13% of the BSW members of the NASW identified aging as their primary service area (Gibelman & Schervish, 1995, cited in Sharlach, Damron-Rodriguez, Robinson, & Feldman, 2000; Gibelman & Schervish, 1997). Of the BSW graduates surveyed, 16% worked exclusively with older people, yet only 20% of the BSW programs reported offering any aging content (Lubben, Damron-Rodriguez & Beck, 1992), only 9% of the BSW programs offered the opportunity to pursue a concentration in gerontology and only 1% of BSW students took courses in aging. In short, the gap between BSW education and the need for BSWs competent in gerontology is a wide one.

Survey findings have identified major barriers to gerontological education in BSW programs, including a severe shortage of social work educators specializing in aging, cutbacks in federal resources, stigmatizing of social work practice with older adults, inadequate and inequitable salaries and a BSW curriculum already "infused" and "integrated" to near capacity with competing professional interests (Lubben, Damron-Rodriguez, & Beck, 1992; Sharlach et al., 2000).

To address these barriers, several strategies have been introduced by NASW and CSWE. Some of the resources that have been developed for teaching aging in BSW programs are field trips, field placements, guest speakers, videos, interviews with grandparents, life history and eco-map interviews with older people in the community, simulated aging experiences, volunteer work and intergenerational classroom settings (Botsford, 1997; Klein, 1996; Richardson, 1999; Segrist, 1997). In addition, faculty and professional development institutes, workshops and continuing education programs have been developed to upgrade and enrich core content on aging, field practicum and research in aging for social workers and faculty (Association for Gerontology in Higher Education, 1997; Berkman, Silverstone, Simmons, Volland, & Howe, 2000; Damron-Rodriguez et al., 1992; Greene, 1989; Howe, Hyler, Mellor, Lindeman, & Luptak, 2001; Shenk & Sokolovsky, 1999).

Some of the particular challenges for BSW programs seeking to enrich the curriculum with gerontological learning experiences are: (1) defining room and time for gerontological social work content in the BSW curriculum, (2) infusion and integration of content on aging throughout the curriculum, (3) enhancing student perceptions of and experience with diverse older people to encourage practice with this population and (4) developing field placements in innovative aging programs. The model presented here (see Figure 1) illustrates one strategy for BSW programs with the generalist model of

FIGURE 1. Model for Teaching Research that Develops Skill with and Use of Research in Practice

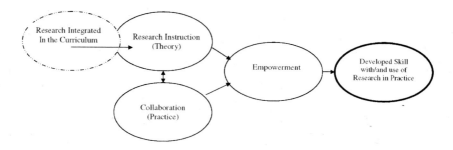

education to address these challenges by increasing content on aging, providing practice experience with older adults and promoting positive perceptions of social work with older adults.

DEVELOPMENT AND IMPLEMENTATION OF THE TEACHING MODEL

Integration of Research

While the literature is rife with a host of issues surrounding the pedagogy of research and macro practice, the literature has also provided a glimpse of possible solutions. Chief among the proposed solutions is the integration of research (Task Force on Social Work Research, 1991; Rubin, Franklin, & Seiber, 1992) and macro assignments (Butler & Colman, 1997; Raber & Richter, 1999) into the curriculum. Other social workers have emphasized the critical role of collaboration in teaching both macro-practice and research (Hess & Mullen, 1995). Larson and Brown (1997), who based their work on the ideas of Freire and Knowles, underscored this message: effective teaching, consistent with the generalist model, is based on collaboration and actual practice. Additional literaure has pointed to the significant role of empowerment of students through knowledge (Congress, 1993; Larson & Brown, 1997). Holden, Barker, Meenaghan, and Rosenberg (1999) consider research self-efficacy a factor in social work empowerment. Once students are empowered, their apprehension about research is reduced. Integrating research content into the curriculum increases students' sense of competence and confidence; they know, and they know that they know. As a result, they develop a sense of their own ability to effect change (Flynn, 1997). Thyer (1997) suggested that research might even have a role in promoting social work's reassertion of its historical emphasis on a just society.

Integration of Macro Practice in the Curriculum

With these three principles in mind–integration, collaboration, and empowerment–the BSW faculty at Marist College developed a teaching model designed to increase students' competencies in the areas of research, macro-level practice and practice with older adults. The goal was to empower students by integrating theory and practice in a classroom research project facilitated by collaboration with the community.

The key to the success of this particular research project was the orderly blend of research in the curriculum. Using Hull and Mokuau's (1994) model for integrating research in the social work curriculum, the authors documented and located the fifteen skills in their curriculum. Readings and assignments related to macro-level practice were similarly identified throughout the curriculum.

The foundation for the students' entering the research course was a rigorous community survey that they completed in their Social Work Methods II course in the semester before the research course. The instrument for the community survey was a comprehensive outline developed by the League of Women Voters (League of Women Voters, Know Your Community, as cited in Zastrow, 1992). The survey included socioeconomic, political, and social welfare demographics of the community. Examples of items were population distribution by sex, age, income, housing patterns, major industries and businesses, recent economic and political trends, and listings of public and private social welfare agencies. Through the process of surveying the community, students learned about needs and gaps in the service delivery systems. This knowledge broadened their thinking about social issues and their experiences with individual clients to the macro-level and increased their awareness of needs and gaps in the service delivery systems. Students integrated this invaluable knowledge and awareness in the Social Work Methods II course, which was designed to introduce students to a macro perspective on practice and research.

Developing the Research Project

The first task was selecting a research project for the semester. Students were in field placements in the community in a variety of agencies. It was suggested to students that they explore the research needs and interests of the agencies in which they were placed and inform agencies that the research class could be a resource for agency projects. In addition, social work faculty were able to assess the potential for research collaboration as community needs were identified. As students informed research faculty of potential research projects, the research faculty used the criteria identified in Figure 2, Criteria for project selection, to make the decision about which project the class would pursue.

Collaboration

The research project was developed by the research and field faculty in conjunction with the community Elder Health Committee (EHC). Although the service providers represented on the EHC had unanimously identified transportation as the number one barrier to older people's accessing health services, data to document the extent of need were lacking. Numerous agencies, including the Alzheimer's Association, the Home Care Association, the Senior Citizens' Association, the Community Action Agency and other groups had each formed committees to address their clients' transportation problems. Despite the agencies, families and clients' perceptions of need, the most recent community needs survey, which had been conducted by a professional consultant, had not identified transportation as a problem for older people, nor had other agencies responsible for service planning in the county.

The BSW field education director, who chaired the EHC, approached the research faculty about the possibility of involving the students in the research

FIGURE 2. Criteria for Project Selection

- The project should provide the opportunity for students to gain research knowledge and skills as defined in the CSWE Curriculum Policy Statement.

- The project should be "hands on" with direct client contact for the students.

- Some aspect of the project should be of interest and challenge to the students.

- The project must have the potential to be completed during one semester (<14 weeks).

- The community group is enthusiastic and knowledgeable, available to the class, committed to the time frame, and accepts potential limitations, such as the development of the questionnaire and the level of statistical analysis.

- Faculty expertise is available to the community group and students.

methods class in assessing older people's transportation needs. After further discussion and using the criteria for project selection, this project was selected. The members of the EHC agreed to attend the second meeting of the Research Methods class to explain their needs.

At the first meeting of the Research Methods class, students were informed of the proposed project and the criteria and rationale used in the selection process. Students were enthusiastic about the transportation aspect of the project, having had personal experience with public transportation in the county, and immediately began empathizing with the older adults. During this discussion, the students in field placements serving older adults provided additional information about how transportation affected the agencies and their clients. With their experiential knowledge about public transportation, the impact on their placement agencies and the effects on clients, the students were engaged and empowered.

Following the faculty's, students' and agencies' acceptance of the EHC project as the class project, the faculty and EHC met to outline the collaborative effort required from EHC. The EHC subsequently agreed to invite over thirty private and public providers of services in the county to a meeting to discuss: (1) the research project and the expected outcomes from agency participation, (2) the research process and one-semester timeframe, (3) development of survey questions, (4) clarification of the role of the agencies in recruiting older people to be surveyed, (5) facilitating students' access to the older people served by the agencies, and (6) planning students' presentation of the findings to the agencies and the community.

The EHC met with the students in the second meeting of the research class to review the agencies' information needs and to develop a "wish list" of questions to be considered for inclusion in the questionnaire. In addition, the EHC members discussed with students some of the special issues in interviewing older people, including cohort characteristics, issues of diverse groups of older people, awareness of functional and sensory limitations and their impact on interviewing, and pacing the interview. They reviewed the demographic predictions for the county; for instance, that the older population in the county would increase from 16.8% to 28.7% in the next twenty years. Since some members of the EHC were themselves older adults, they also spoke to their own concerns about transportation, such as being the spouse of a person with Alzheimer's Disease, having a physical disability, and anticipating loss of driving ability in the next few years. Students who had field placements working with older people in some of the EHC agencies were able to use their experience to serve as consultants on some of the issues in interviewing this population. This class session became an intergenerational one, with students and older professionals engaged in collaboration on a mutual project. Students were impressed with the knowledge, energy and enthusiasm of committee members.

Course Assignments

In addition to the required readings for the course, students were given weekly, albeit minimal but essential homework based mainly on the assigned readings. As an example, an important first assignment was for students to e-mail the instructor to "check-in." This provided the instructor with a beginning assessment of students' technology skills. In turn, the instructor communicated by e-mail with students as a group and as individuals. E-mail was an invaluable tool. Depending upon their schedules, the students then had access to the instructor and the instructor had access to the students according to her schedule. Additionally, the use of e-mail facilitated the asking of questions by the shy, reluctant students about the readings, assignments, or content covered in class. This material was handled in much the way as if it had occurred during class discussion. Frequently e-mail messages from the students began with the disclaimer, "This is a stupid question, but…" This provided the instructor with the additional opportunity to reassure students that it was safe to ask questions and to take risks. Actually, the instructor frequently asked students if their question and the answer could be shared with the class. Additional homework included completing the college's Instructional Review Board Form; using material from the text to construct a table and interpret it; identifying levels of measurement on surveys handed out in class; adapting questions in order to get different levels of measurement; and critiquing a research questionnaire which was handed out.

Early in the course, the assigned readings and lectures focused on the characteristics of the population, the community, and the issue of transportation. In subsequent class discussions, students began to develop questions, based on the EHC's concerns, for the face-to-face interviews with older adults, as well as to consider the realistic limitations of the project given the timeframe and the students' own level of knowledge and skill. Students also addressed the limitations of the specific research approach (i.e., a survey), and the major issues of collecting data on service use. They considered the pros and cons of using various sampling methods and considered the possibility that their findings might or might not confirm the agencies' perceptions of existing need. Within the limits of the timeframe, both agencies and students made genuine efforts to identify diverse subgroups of older people not being served by the agencies and to extend the interviews to them.

Providing the students with choices about the members of their work groups, about the final content and format for the questionnaire, and about how they set up the interviews, and playing to their strengths served to reduce their anxiety about the interviewing process and to increase their interest. Their involvement in these decisions fostered the students' enthusiasm for the project and enhanced cooperation among teams as they divided the assignments.

The strengths-based approach had the effect of empowering the students. For example, gregarious students represented the class by attending constituency group meetings. Less outgoing students volunteered to search the literature either at their agencies, in the college library, or on the Internet. Students whose field placements were directly related to the project in terms of the social problem or the population served as experts to the class. Those with highly developed computer skills were facilitators and teachers for others. The faculty person, as the research project coordinator, located resources and used them to the best advantage for both the students and the project. Two students who were in field placements in agencies serving older adults volunteered to pilot the questionnaire. These experiences support the findings of Lazzari, Banman, and Jackson (1996), who found that joint teaching tasks with faculty empowered students.

Students met with agency representatives to establish a schedule for interviews. The EHC made contacts with their staff to set up the interviews at the agencies. The students were left to their own devices to select the interview sites and schedule the interviews with much discussion of sharing of rides and coordinating schedules. The students' greatest concern about the interviews was that they felt they were too young. They thought the older adults would not take them seriously. In addition, they did not want to hurt anyone's feelings by being condescending. They practiced among themselves. An older, mature student and a shy student with a placement in an adult home demonstrated leadership in this phase of the project. Once the students did go out to conduct interviews and reported to the class on their experiences, their anxieties subsided and the interview process went smoothly. In fact, the faculty had to rein in their enthusiasm to avoid having more questionnaires than students could data enter within the timeframe.

During the semester, a series of small assignments were structured to teach students data entry and analysis. At the first class meeting students completed a five-item questionnaire on physician assisted suicide. The questionnaires were collected and duplicated so that every student had a copy of all of the questionnaires. A class period was devoted to discussing the statistical program and its uses. Students learned about types of data, variables, variable names, variable labels, and values. The first assignment was to name the potential file, number the cases, and name and label the variables. To guarantee the accuracy of the data before moving on to data entry, the instructor checked this assignment. For data entry, the class met in a computer lab and groups entered the data from the assisted suicide questionnaire. Students found the small number of variables and data to be manageable.

Relying on the gerontology content provided throughout the curriculum, as well as by their field placements and contact with the EHC, the students developed and administered a survey to 269 older people who were recruited through EHC. The completed questionnaires were reviewed prior to data entry for purposes of cleaning the data. Every student took a turn at data cleaning and entry. Data gathering, entry, cleaning, and analysis played a critical role in "ownership" of data, which not only increased enthusiasm of the project but also enhanced understanding of the value of research and its contribution to practice. When data entry was completed, each student received a disk copy of the data. Data cleaning, entry and analysis were completed under faculty supervision outside of the classroom.

The students developed and tested their own hypotheses. Two of the hypotheses tested were: (1) There is a relationship between income and transportation needs of older people, and (2) Older people with social and family support perceive themselves as having fewer transportation needs than those without social and family support.

Presentation of the Research Findings

To avoid repetition, since the presentation was made in only one class period, the instructor chose the best problem statement, literature review, methodology, and discussion sections from the groups' papers. Selection was based on the quality of writing and comprehensiveness of material covered. In addition, each presentation was required to include at least one table to illustrate the findings; groups were responsible for making their own transparencies.

The class prior to the presentation was a rehearsal for the presentation. The EHC and their guests were invited to the last class session at which the findings of the project were presented. Programs printed with the names of all the students and their presentations were distributed at the presentation. Each group of students presented their hypotheses, findings and recommendations to the agency representatives for comments and questions.

Findings

Twenty-six different agencies participated in the study. The 265 respondents were predominately white (87%) and female (82%) with an average age of 76. Forty-seven percent were living in their own homes; thirty-two percent, in either senior or adult housing; and twenty-one percent listed their living arrangement as "other," which was probably the home of an adult child or other relative. For the majority of the respondents, someone else, usually an adult offspring, provided transportation to enable them to shop (52%), socialize (47%), and seek medical care (47%).

The qualitative data revealed that older adults felt that they were an imposition on their adult offsprings' time, as many stated that their children had to take time off from work or away from their families to provide transportation. Respondents were most likely to have transportation for medical appointments and least likely to be able to go shopping or socialize where or when they wanted.

Agency representatives were as interested in the students' reflections, experiences and perceptions of older people and of the agencies as they were in their findings about transportation. This exchange provided yet another intergenerational class session and discussion of aging issues. In addition, the survey served the important purpose for the agencies of being able to document the extent and ways in which lack of transportation was a barrier to older people's access to health care services and independent living.

OUTCOMES

From the Students

The effectiveness of the model in addressing the three areas of concern–research, gerontology and macro-level issues–was evaluated using qualitative and quantitative data collected from students, providers and the collaborating committee. Most significant from the viewpoint of promoting the social work students' enthusiasm for and knowledge about gerontology was their experience of interviewing older people in the community and in the process of meeting many diverse older people, families and providers. From their own accounts and discussions in class, it was clear that their stereotypes about older people were shattered. They were exposed to some of the special issues of research with older people, and more than a few students were heard to say, "I never thought I'd be interested in working with older people, but I found I really like talking with them."

From their fellow students in field placements with older people and from the EHC members, they learned many valuable techniques for conducting research with older people (e.g., need for large print type, need to speak clearly in a mid-range voice with mouth visible to the older person, the potential reluctance to discuss financial information, or ask for help, and the potential for having a limited reading level). Their finding that sixty-two percent (101) of the interviewees lived on less than $10,000 a year startled them. They spoke during the presentation about how moved they had been by the loneliness and isolation that many older people expressed. They were surprised by the diversity of older people in terms of family and community roles, health status, mental status, energy levels, and perspectives on life.

Equally important to their understanding of aging was their discovery of the role of family members as the natural support system for older people. In spontaneous class discussions, they began to consider various additional research approaches for studying the families' care-giving roles and to generate questions for getting data on the extent to which access to health, socialization, and shopping depended on the availability of family members.

In addition to learning about older people and their families, they reported that they learned about the broad impact of transportation on older people's lives. They learned about such macro-level issues as the range of community services for older people, the types of services and professionals and the service barriers and gaps. They were also able to make the connections between the macro-level factors that influenced older adults' access to services and the impact on the mental, social and physical well-being of the older individuals they had interviewed.

Having heard first-hand from older people about their transportation problems, students were convinced of the practical and real need for the data they were collecting and were motivated by the fact that their research had social action potential. Their curiosity and concern about the population generally overcame their reservations about the research endeavor. To illustrate to students the importance of disseminating research findings, the faculty submitted the students' final report on the research, which was subsequently accepted for presentation at the annual meeting of the New York State Social Work Education Association, at which four students and two faculty members made the presentation. Students found this a rewarding, affirming experience and their experience served them well in their applications to graduate schools.

From the Agencies

The agencies participating in the survey indicated overwhelmingly positive evaluations of the students' presentations, the usefulness of the findings and the extent to which the survey met their expectations. The EHC made subsequent use of the study to document the priority of transportation for older adults when the United Way conducted a community assessment to determine the agency's funding priorities for the county. The EHC also used the survey in developing a response to a request for proposals from a foundation. The EHC indicated interest in a continuing relationship with the social work program for collaborative research projects in the future. In this regard, the project promoted the visibility of the social work program and the college in the community.

Evaluation of the Course

At the conclusion of the course, students completed course evaluations that were used to assess the impact of this "hands on" community model on their learning about research, macro-practice, gerontology and social action. These evaluations were designed to elicit both quantitative and qualitative responses. Students were asked to respond to five statements about the instructor and five statements about course objectives, grading and instructional materials. For the qualitative evaluation, students were asked three questions: What were the best things about the course; what changes would they suggest; and for additional comments that would be helpful in evaluating the course.

In terms of the qualitative data, students' comments on the best things about the course fell into three general categories: hands on interaction with the community, the value of group work, and exposure to the statistical program. The most frequent comments were about the value of a collaborative community project and the opportunity to develop research skills through practice (e.g., "I liked that the research project was actually being used for a good purpose," "The best thing was going out into the community and doing the research," and "I feel being directly involved in a research study from beginning to end was the best part of this class."). These reports supported the conclusion that the model was successful in empowering students where research was concerned.

In addition to the qualitative responses, students evaluated the workload and rated how much they learned in the course. The vast majority (86%) found the workload heavy and they learned a great deal (83%). That they had learned a great deal was evident in comments on the student evaluations as well as in the findings section of the final papers.

Evaluation of the Effectiveness of the Model

An evaluation of the model in terms of its effectiveness in increasing students' research self-efficacy was conducted using the Research Self-Efficacy (RSE) Scale developed by Holden, Barker, Meenaghan, and Rosenberg (1999). Those authors used the scale with 71 BSW and MSW students. "Because no significant differences between the classes at pre-test or posttest were found ... the classes were combined for the analysis" (p. 469). They found that the differences between the pre-test and post-test mean scores on all of the items and on the total pre and post-test scores were statistically significant ($p = .005$). The alpha reliability of the scale for their sample was .94 at both pre-test and post-test.

The RSE was especially suited for this evaluation since the nine research skills identified in the instrument closely corresponded to those identified by Hull and Mokuau (1994). The RSE tasks also corresponded closely to the tasks identified in the review of the BSW curriculum as either integrated into the curriculum prior to the research course and/or included in the course.

The concept of self-efficacy also corresponded closely to the concept of empowerment, which was the goal of this teaching model. For all of these reasons, the Research Self-Efficacy Scale was selected as a measure of the model's effectiveness. The RSE was administered to the eighteen students in the research class as a pre-test at the beginning of the semester and as a post-test at the end of the semester to evaluate the students' efficacy, defined as their confidence about their ability to perform nine particular research tasks (see Table 2).

Following the procedure of Holden et al. (1999) the Wilcoxon signed ranks test was used to analyze the differences between pre and post-test scores. While the scores on the RSE for the first three items were higher on the posttest, they were not significantly higher. The means of the pre and post-test scores of the remaining six items and the means of the total scores for the pre and post-test were significantly different. The statistical significance ranged from .05 for items C and I, to .01 for items D, E, H, and for the total scores and to .005 for items F, and G. The internal consistency for the RSE for this sample was very good. The Cronbach's alpha was .89 for the pre-test and .97 for the post-test.

These findings supported the hypothesis that students' research self-efficacy increased. They also supported what we had learned earlier, as illustrated in Table 1, about the positive effect on student confidence when content areas are integrated into the curriculum before the research course.

For a variety of reasons, caution should be used in interpreting these results. The RSE is a newly developed instrument with little testing. In addition, the small, nonrandom, convenience sample in this study runs the risk of making a Type I error. However, we believe that it is important to move model development to model testing and the RSE is a step in that direction. In a subsequent study in progress, pre- and post-test RSE scores of students in classes using and not using this teaching model are being compared.

TABLE 1. Research Skills in Professional Foundation Curriculum

Research Skills	Professional Foundation Curriculum					
	Social Work Intro.	Theory & Practice	Methods & II	Social Policy	Social Research	Practicum
Identify independent and dependent variables		X		X	X	X
Conceptualize a research design		X			X	
Conduct a computer search for journal articles		X	X	X	X	
Use abstracts to locate information		X	X	X	X	
Conduct an interview	X	X	X		X	X
Distinguish between descriptive and interpretive behavior					X	X
Write a literature review		X		X	X	
Develop a questionnaire					X	
Set up computer file to enter and analyze data					X	
Identify relevant statistical tests				X	X	
Analyze data					X	
Evaluate own practice						X
Assess validity of an instrument					X	
Critique research	X			X	X	

TABLE 2. Results for Individual Items and the Total Scale on the Research Self-Efficacy Scale (N = 18)

	Pre-Test		Post-Test		
	Mean	SD	Mean	SD	Difference
conduct effective database searching of the scholarly literature?	68.3	18.2	77.8	18.3	9.5
use technological advances effectively in carrying out research (e.g., the Internet)?	73.9	15.8	80	18.2	6.1
review a particular area of social science theory and research; write a balanced and comprehensive review?	60	22.8	73.3[1]	23	13.3
formulate a clear research question or testable hypothesis?	58.3	22.6	80.6[2]	21.6	22.3
choose a research design that will answer a set of research questions and/or test a set of hypotheses about some aspect of practice?	45.6	26.4	76[2]	16.8	31.1
design and implement the best sampling strategy possible for your study of some aspect of practice?	43.9	23.6	71.7[3]	17.6	27.8
design and implement the best measurement approach possible for your study of some aspect of practice?	38.9	25.4	69.4[3]	19.2	30.5
design and implement the best data analysis strategy possible for your study of some aspect of practice?	37.8	26.5	68.3[1]	19.2	30.5
effectively present your study and its implications?	55.6	31	78.9[1]	21.4	23.3
Total Score	53.6	17.7	75.2[3]	17.7	21.6

[1]Difference between pre-test and post-test was statistically significant at p = .05
[2]Difference between pre-test and post-test was statistically significant at p = .01
[3]Difference between pre-test and post-test was statistically significant at p = .005

DISCUSSION AND IMPLICATIONS

This teaching model was designed to meet the challenges of educating BSWs about research, gerontology and macro-level issues–three challenging areas in BSW social work education. While the model was not a guarantee of success, it did provide structure and a process for making decisions about curriculum content and integration of these important areas. Experience with this model demonstrated effectiveness in increasing students' sense of competence about learning to do research, empowering them to connect research with the process of social change and facilitating collaboration between the social work program and the community and gerontology.

There were advantages and disadvantages of this teaching model. The model was time-intensive. Weekly homework assignments and daily attention to e-mail were time consuming. However, the advantages far outweighed these considerations. Since most of the homework was based on some aspect of the readings, the instructor could be reasonably assured that the students were keeping up with the readings. In addition to the homework, one final exam–a comprehensive open-book final exam consisting of multiple choices, true/false, fill in the blank and short essay questions–was given, which all of the students were able to pass.

In addition, experience with this model has prompted suggestions from students, faculty, and agencies for future collaboration between practice and research. As surprising as it was, students suggested that perhaps Research should be a two semester course. Students suggested that their underclassmen colleagues should be made aware of the research project. Students mentioned that when their field supervisor heard about the success of the project, supervisors indicated that their agency would be interested in a research project in the future.

There is a need for practitioners in the field to recognize and apply research to practice and field education. This model facilitated students' orientation to research on two levels. First of all, practitioners were the direct beneficiaries of the research effort. They participated in the formulation of the research initiative, observed the process of the research, and were the recipients of the findings. Perhaps more importantly, the students conducting the collaborative research will be more likely to conduct, understand, and use research findings in their own future practice.

In terms of the future of macro level research with the older population, there is continued need for social workers to be involved in formulating and implementing policy and programs with this growing population. The model described here supports the confluence of the goals of meeting the needs of specific populations and addressing the need for social policy changes at the macro-level.

The next step in developing this model is a rigorous testing of its effectiveness, taking into account the needs of the students, the capacities and capabilities of BSW programs and faculty, and the specific needs of the social work field and the community. As this teaching model continues to be applied, its effectiveness is being empirically evaluated, with measures of students' learning about aging and macro-practice as well as research self-efficacy. Additional research on these educational outcomes of this model is forthcoming.

REFERENCES

Association for Gerontology in Higher Education. (1997). AGHE *collection of syllabi for courses in aging* (Two volumes). Compiled by Program and Publications Committees of the Association for Gerontology in Higher Education, Washington, D.C.

Beresford, P. & Evans, C. (1999). Research note: Research and empowerment. *British Journal of Social Work, 29*(5), 671-677.

Berkman, B. & Harootyan, L. (Eds.) (2003). Social work and health care in our aging society: Education, policy, practice and research. NY, NY: Springer Publishing Co.

Berkman, B., Silverstone, B., Simmons, W., Volland, P., & Howe, J. (2000). Social work gerontological practice: The need for faculty development in the new millennium. *Journal of Gerontological Social Work, 34*(1), 5-23.

Bisman, C.D. & Hardcastle, D.A. (1999). A model for using research methodologies in practice. *Journal of Teaching in Social Work, 19*(1/2), 47-63.

Botsford, A. (1997, October). Educating BSW students for the graying of America. Paper presented at the NYS Social Work Education Association, Colonie, NY.

Bradley, G. (1997). Translating research into practice. *Social Work and Social Sciences Review, 7*, 3-21.

Butler, R. (2001, October). A national crisis: The need for geriatrics faculty training and development. Policy report, International Longevity Center USA, LTD, 60 East 86th Street, NY, NY 10028.

Butler, S.S. & Coleman, P.A. (1997). Raising our voices: A macro practice assignment. *Journal of Teaching in Social Work, 15*, 63-80.

Congress, E.P. (1993). Teaching ethical decision-making to a diverse community of students: Bringing practice into the classroom. *Journal of Teaching in Social Work, 7*, 23-35.

Cournoyer, D.E. & Klein, W.C. (2000). *Research methods for social work*. Boston: Allyn and Bacon.

Damron-Rodriguez, J.A. & Lubben, J.E. (1994). Multidisciplinary factors in gerontological curriculum adoption in schools of social work. *Gerontology & Geriatrics Education, 14*, 39-52.

Damron-Rodriguez, J., Villa, V., Tseng, H., & Lubben, J. (1996). Demographic and organizational influences on the development of gerontological social work curriculum. *Gerontology & Geriatrics Education, 17*(3), 3-18.

Damron-Rodriguez, J., Dorfman, R., & Lubben, J. (1992). A geriatric education center faculty development program dedicated to social work. *Journal of Gerontological Social Work, 18*(3/4), 187-201.

Damron-Rodriguez, J., & Lubben, J. (1997). The 1995 White House Conference on Aging: An agenda for social work education and training. *Journal of Gerontological Social Work, 27*(3), 65-77.

Damron-Rodriguez, J., Villa, V., Tseng, H.F., & Lubben, J.E. (1997). Demographic and organizational influences on the development of gerontological social work curriculum. *Gerontology & Geriatrics Education, 17*(3), 3-18.

Fahey, C. J. (1996). Social work education and the field of aging. *The Gerontologist, 36*, 36-41.

Finn, J. & Lavitt, M. (1995). A survey of information technology-related curriculum in undergraduate social work programs. *The Journal of Baccalaureate Social Work, 1*(1), 39-53.

Fisher, R., & Karger, H.J. (1997). *Social work and community in a private world.* New York: Longman.

Flynn, L. (1977). Social work students confront social justice issues through experiential learning. *Australian Social Work, 50*(4), 21-27.

Fook, J. (2002). Theorizing from practice: Toward an inclusive approach for social work research. *Qualitative Social Work, 1*(1), 79-95.

Fortune, A.E. & Proctor, E.K. (2001). Research on social work interventions. *Social Work Research, 25*(2), 67-69.

Franklin, C.G. (1999). Research or practice: Better than you think? *Social Work in Education, 21*(1), 3-9.

Gerdes, K.E., Edmonds, R.M., Haslam, D.R., & McCartney, T.L. (1996). A statewide survey of licensed clinical social workers' use of practice evaluation procedures. *Research on Social Work Practice, 6*(1), 27-39.

Gibbs, A. (2001). The changing nature and context of social work research. *The British Journal of Social Work, 31*(5), 687-704.

Gibelman, M., & Schervish, P.H. (1995). Pay equity in social work – Not. *Social Work, 40*, 622-629.

Gibelman, M., & Schervish, P. (1997). *Who we are: A second look.* Washington, DC: NASW Press.

Golden, R., & Saltz, C. (1997). The aging family. *Journal of Gerontological Social Work, 27*(3), 55-64.

Greene, R. R. & Knee, R.J. (1996). Shaping the policy agenda of social work in the field of aging. *Social Work, 41*, 553-558.

Greene, R.R. (1989). The growing need for social work services for the aged in 2020. In B.S. Vourlekis and C.G. Leukefeld (Eds.), *Making our case: A resource book of selected materials for social workers in health care* (pp. 11-17). Silverspring, MD: NASW.

Grinnell, R.M., Jr., & Siegel, D.H. (1988). The place of research in social work. In R.M. Grinnell, Jr. (Ed.), *Social Work Research and Evaluation.* (pp. 18-21). Itasca, IL: Peacock.

Grinnell, R.M., Jr. (Ed.) (1993). *Social work research and evaluation* (4th ed.). Itasca, IL: Peacock.

Hess, P.M. & Mullen, E.J. (1995). Bridging the gap: Collaborative considerations in practitioner-researcher knowledge-building partnerships. In P.M. Hess & E.J. Mullen (Eds.), *Practitioner-researcher partnerships* (pp. 1-30). Washington: NASW Press.

Holden, G., Barker, K., Meenaghan, T., & Rosenberg, G. (1999). Research self-efficacy: A new possibility for educational outcomes assessment. *Journal of Social Work Education, 35*, 463-476.

Hooyman, N. & Kiyak, H. A. (2005). *Social gerontology: A multidisciplinary perspective.* (6th edition) Boston: Allyn and Bacon.

Horner, R.D. (2000). A practitioner looks at adoption research. *Family Relations, 49*(4), 473-477.

Howard, M.O. & Jenson, J.M. (1999). Barriers to development, utilization, and evaluation of social work practice guidelines: Toward an action plan for social work. *Research on Social Work Practice, 9*, 347-364.

Howe, J., Hyer, K., Mellor, J., Lindeman, D., & Luptak, M. (2001). Educational approaches for preparing social work students for interdisciplinary teamwork on geriatric health care teams. *Social Work in Health Care, 32*(4), 19-42.

Hull, G.H., & Mokuau, M. (1994). Research in baccalaureate social work programs: A model for integration. *Journal of Teaching in Social Work, 10*, 137-147.

Johnson, Y.M. (1997). Scientist-practitioner: Remaining holes in the debate. *Social Work Research, 21*(3), 196-198.

Kane, M. N. (1999). Factors affecting social work students' willingness to work with elders with Alzheimer's Disease. *Journal of Social Work Education, 35*, 71-85.

Keigher., S., Fortune, A., & Witkin, S. (Eds.) (2000). Aging and social work: The changing landscapes. Washington, DC: NASW Press.

Kirk, S.A. (1996). Practice as science, science as practice [Editorial]. *Social Work Research, 20*, 67.

Kirk, S.A., Osmolov, M., & Fischer, J. (1976). Social workers' involvement in research. *Journal of Education for Social Work, 12*, 63-70.

Klein, S. (Ed.). (1996). *A national agenda for geriatric education: White papers.* Rockville, MD: Health Resources and Services Administration.

Kosberg, J. (1999). Opportunities for social workers in an aging world. *Journal of Sociology and Social Welfare, 26*(1), 7-24.

Langer, N. (1995). Ethnogerontological curriculum: What should we teach and how should we teach it? *Journal of Teaching in Social Work, 11*, 49-66.

Larson, G. & Brown, L. (1997). Teaching research to aboriginal students. *Journal of Teaching in Social Work, 15*, 205-215.

Lazzari, M.M., Banman, N.A., & Jackson, R.A. (1996). Students and faculty as co-teachers: Processes of self-efficacy and educational empowerment. *The Journal of Baccalaureate Social Work, 2*(1), 133-50.

Lubben, J., Damron-Rodriguez, J.A., & Beck, S. (1992). A national survey of aging curriculum. *Journal of Gerontological Social Work, 18*, 157-171.

Mark, R. (1996). *Research made simple: A handbook for social workers.* Thousand Oaks, CA: Sage.

National Institute on Aging. (1987). Personnel for health needs of the elderly through the year 2020. Bethesda, MD: Department of Health and Human Services, Public Health Service.

Peterson, D. (1990). Personnel to serve the aging in the field of social work: Implications for educating professionals. *Social Work, 35,* 412-415.

Peterson, D.A., & Wendt, P.F. (1990). Employment in the field of aging: A survey of professionals in four fields. *The Gerontologist, 30,* 672-684.

Plionis, E.M. (1993). Refocusing undergraduate research teaching: Making conceptualization experiential. *Journal of Teaching in Social Work, 7,* 49-61.

Randall, J., Cowley, P., & Tomlinson, P. (2000). Overcoming barriers to effective practice in child care. *Child and Family Social Work, 5*(4), 343-352.

Richardson, V. (Ed.). (1999). *Teaching gerontological social work: A compendium of model syllabi.* Alexandria, VA: Council on Social Work Education.

Rosen, A. & Persky, T. (1997). Meeting the mental health needs of older adults: Policy and practice issues for social work. In C. Saltz (Ed.), *Social work response to the 1995 White House Conference on Aging: From issues to actions* (pp. 45-54). New York: Haworth Press.

Rosen, A., Zlotnik, J., Curl, A., & Green, R. (2002). *The CSWE/SAGE-SW National Aging Competencies Survey Report.* Alexandria, VA: CSWE.

Rosen, A. (2001). *Strengthening the impact of social work to improve the quality of life for older adults and their families: A blueprint for the new millennium.* Alexandria, VA: Council on Social Work Education/SAGE-SW.

Royse, D., & Rompf, E.L. (1992). Math anxiety: A comparison of social work and non-social work students. *Journal of Social Work Education. 28.* 270-277.

Rubin, A., & Babbie, E. (1997). *Research methods for social work.* (3rd Ed.). Pacific Grove, CA: Brooks/Cole.

Rubin, A., Franklin, C., & Selber, K. (1992). Integrating research and practice into an interviewing skills project: An evaluation. *Journal of Social Work Education, 28,* 141-152.

SAGE-SW (1999, February). News from SAGE-SW: *Strengthening aging and gerontological education for social work.* Alexandria, VA: Council on Social Work Education.

Scharlach, A., Damron-Rodriguez, J., Robinson, B., & Feldman, R. (2000). Educating social workers for an aging society: A vision for the 21st century. *Journal of Social Work Education, 36*(3), 521-538.

Segrist, K. (2000). Statewide gerontology education, training and information technology transfer: Triumphs and tribulations. *Gerontology & Geriatrics Education, 21*(1/2), 81-101.

Sharlach, A., Robinson, B., Damron-Rodriguez, J., & Feldman, R. (1997). *Optimizing gerontological social work education.* A paper prepared for the John A. Hartford Foundation.

Shenk, D. & Sokolovsky, J. (Eds.). (1999). *Teaching about aging: Interdisciplinary and cross-cultural perspectives* (3rd Ed.). Washington, D.C.: Association for Gerontology in Higher Education & Association of Anthropology and Gerontology.

Smeeding, T., Butler, R., & Schaber, G. (July 19, 1999). The consequences of population aging for society. Workshop Report. 60 East 86th Street, NY, NY 10028: International Longevity Center USA, LTD.

Stone, G. (1999). Evaluation of an effort to improve students' attitudes toward technology. *Arête, 23*(3), 46-53.

Task Force on Social Work Research. (1991). *Building social work knowledge for effective services and policies: A plan for research development.* Austin: University of Texas School of Social Work.

Thyer, B.A. (1997). Who stole social work? *Social Work Research, 21,*198-200.

Volland, P. (2000, November). *Geriatric social work practicum development program.* Paper presentation at the 53rd annual scientific meeting of the Gerontological Society of America, Washington, DC.

Weinback, R.W. & Grinnell, R.M. Jr. (1995). *Statistics for social workers.* (3rd Ed.). White Plains, NY: Longman.

Wellons, K. (1996). Aspects of aging in the twenty-first century: Opposing viewpoints. In P.R. Raffoul & C.A. McNeece (Eds.), *Future Issues for Social Work Practice* (pp. 115-124) Boston: Allyn and Bacon.

Williams, J.B.W. & Lanigan, J. (1999). Practice guidelines in social work: A reply, or "our glass is half full." *Research on Social Work Practice, 9*(3), 338-342.

Wilson, W.C., & Rosenthal, B.S. (1992). Anxiety and performance in an MSW research and statistics course. *Journal of Teaching in Social Work, 6,* 75-85.

Wyers, N.L. (1991). Policy-practice in social work: Models and issues. *Journal of Social Work Education, 27*(3), 241-250.

Yegidis, B.L. & Weinbach, R.W. (1996). *Research methods for social workers* (2nd Ed.). Boston: Allyn and Bacon.

York, R.O. (1997). *Building basic competencies in social work research.* Boston: Allyn and Bacon.

Zastrow, C. (1992). *The practice of social work* (4th Ed.). Belmont, CA: Wadsworth.

doi:10.1300/J083v48n01_17

The Impact of Religiousness, Spirituality, and Social Support on Psychological Well-Being Among Older Adults in Rural Areas

Dong Pil Yoon, PhD
Eun-Kyoung Othelia Lee, PhD

SUMMARY. This paper presents the results of a study on the impact of spirituality, religiousness, and social support on the psychological well-being among rural elderly. With a rural community sample of 215 older adults, hierarchical regression analyses found significant associations between dimensions of spirituality/religiousness, social support, and psychological well-being, with spirituality/religiousness inversely related to depression and social support, positively related to life satisfaction. Findings of this study suggest that practitioners need to develop programs or services that are congruent with religious/spiritual beliefs and practices in order to better enhance the psychosocial well-being and improve the quality of life among older persons in rural areas. doi:10.1300/J083v48n03_01 *[Article copies available for a fee from The Haworth Document Delivery Service:*

The authors would like to express their thanks to Dr. Judith Davenport for her continuous assistance and insightful comments on our research. They also would like to thank Yolanda Outlaw, Crystal Massey, and Bernard Rearden who worked as research assistants for data collection.

[Haworth co-indexing entry note]: "The Impact of Religiousness, Spirituality, and Social Support on Psychological Well-Being Among Older Adults in Rural Areas." Yoon, Dong Pil, and Eun-Kyoung Othelia Lee. Co-published simultaneously in *Journal of Gerontological Social Work* (The Haworth Press, Inc.) Vol. 48, No. 3/4, 2007, pp. 281-298; and: *Fostering Social Work Gerontology Competence: A Collection of Papers from the First National Gerontological Social Work Conference* (ed: Catherine J. Tompkins, and Anita L. Rosen) The Haworth Press, Inc., 2007, pp. 281-298. Single or multiple copies of this article are available for a fee from The Haworth Document Delivery Service [1-800-HAWORTH, 9:00 a.m. - 5:00 p.m. (EST). E-mail address: docdelivery@haworthpress.com].

1-800-HAWORTH. E-mail address: <docdelivery@haworthpress.com> Website: <http://www.HaworthPress.com> © 2007 by The Haworth Press, Inc. All rights reserved.]

KEYWORDS. Spirituality/religiousness, social support, life satisfaction, depression, rural elderly, Brief Multidimensional Measures of Religiousness/Spirituality (BMMRS)

INTRODUCTION

Over the past decades, religion has become a topic of great interest to researchers in medicine, nursing, gerontology, and health/mental health disciplines. Especially significant has been an increase in empirical research linking religiosity/spirituality to physical health, emotional and psychological well-being, and quality of life among older adults. Despite methodological limitations and heterogeneity in religious measure, findings of previous empirical studies point consistently, though not unanimously, to a positive effect of religion on health and psychological well-being among elderly individuals (Idler & Kasl, 1997; Koenig et al., 1997; Oman & Reed, 1998; Koenig & Larson, 1998). Some studies have documented a strong positive relationship between religious involvement and coping behaviors in response to negative life events (Koenig, George, & Siegler, 1988; Koenig, Siegler, & George, 1989; Pargament et al., 1990). There are numerous findings linking spirituality with positive well-being among elderly individuals (Levin & Chatters, 1998; Fry, 2000; Fabricatore, Handal, & Fenzel, 2000). In addition, the importance of social support in the treatment of disease and the maintenance of health and well-being also has drawn the attention of researchers and practitioners. The weight of the evidence indicates that perceived support has strong positive main effects on mental health, as well as significant stress-buffering effects (Cohen & Wills, 1985; Wethington & Kessler, 1986). An inverse relationship between the levels of depression and the levels of social support has been shown in a number of studies (Dean, Kolody, & Wood, 1990; Hays et al., 1997; Bothell, Fischer, & Hayashida, 1999; Bosworth et al., 2000).

Although numerous studies document the beneficial impacts of spirituality/religiousness and social support on emotional and psychological well-being, few studies focus on elderly individuals in rural areas where health care and social service are generally limited compared with urban and/or metropolitan areas (Armer & Conn, 2001; Yoon & Lee, 2004). Furthermore, there have been relatively few empirical investigations that have included all three of these variables including spirituality/religiousness, social support, and psychological well-being with the rural elderly. Thus, the researchers examine the relationships of religious involvement, spiritual practice, social support, and psychological well-being among older adults in rural areas.

LITERATURE REVIEW

Characteristics of Life Among Older Adults in Rural Areas

In general, rural communities are often characterized as having low density population, and a paucity of transportation, health care facilities, and social services (Kaufman et al., 2000). Rural elderly individuals are at a greater disadvantage due to these factors and traditional cultural belief systems and they generally have less education, higher poverty rates, poorer health, and higher mortality rates than urban older adults (Bane & Bull, 2001; Buczko, 2001; Rogers, 2002). Although rural older adults were not necessarily in poorer self-reported health, these elderly were significantly poorer in objective health as measured by the number of reported symptoms (Dellasega, 1998). Rural residents rely heavily on social networks to provide social support and other services that more formal agencies often provide in urban areas (Davenport & Davenport, 1982). Although, in most rural and small town communities, older persons often turn to their pastors and religious leaders for help with emotional, mental, and relational problems (Campbell, Gordon, & Chandler, 2002), there are significant groups of older persons who may not have the access or desire to talk with a spiritual care professional.

The Impact of Religiousness and Spirituality on Psychological Well-Being

Religiousness includes personal beliefs (as in transcendent) and organizational practices like church activities and commitment to the belief system of a religion (Zinnbauer et al., 1997). Joseph (1987) defines spirituality as the underlying dimension of consciousness which strives for meaning, union with the universe, and with all things, extending to the experience of the transcendent or a power beyond human-beings. Religiousness and spirituality are often used interchangeably (Kendler et al., 2003; Yoon & Lee, 2004). For a comprehensive and multidimensional examination of these concepts, the measurement of daily spiritual experience, values/beliefs, forgiveness, private religious practice, religious/spiritual coping, and religious support is used in this study.

Religious involvement and spiritual commitment have been positively associated with an array of subjective well-being indicators such as greater life satisfaction, decreased depressive symptoms, optimism, less anxiety, and better emotional adjustment among older adults (McFadden, 1993; Levin, Chatters, & Taylor, 1995; Morris, 1997; Kraaij, Garnefski, & Maes, 2002). Religious involvement may have a positive effect on health perceptions and act as a buffer against the negative impact of physical and emotional problems. Recent research on the relationship between religious faith and depression has generally found that religiosity is associated with lower levels of depression (Hertsgaard & Light, 1984; Catipovic et al., 1995). As a coping mechanism, religious faith and religious/spiritual practices function to ease the grieving or bereavement process for many individuals who may be at risk for depression due to experiencing exceptional circumstances. Among the elderly, religious and spiritual involvement among people experiencing stressful events is significantly associated with lower levels of anxiety (Koenig et al., 1993). In general, some studies investigating religious involvement and well-being have uncovered a strong association between the two constructs (Koenig, 1995; Levin, 1997).

Organizational religious involvement also appears to benefit health through a provision of social supports that buffer stress and enhance coping. Religious people appear to have increased social contact, increased exchanges of assistance, and greater perceptions of support availability and adequacy (Bradley, 1995; Krause, 2002). Indeed, spirituality is typically shaped by a community of individuals who share similar values and experiences and religion has therefore been considered a mechanism of social integration. Mitchell and Weatherly (2000) found that among rural elderly, reduced health status, including functional ability, combined with limited participation in church activities resulted in poorer self-rated mental health and more symptoms of depression.

Yoon and Lee (2004) found that there were significant differences in levels of religiousness/spirituality between White and Non-White elderly in rural areas, with Non-White elderly more likely to practice and participate in religious activities. Religious involvement generally bears a stronger positive relationship with life satisfaction and other aspects of subjective well-being for African Americans than for whites of similar backgrounds (St. George & McNamara, 1984; Thomas & Holmes, 1992). For Native American elderly, religiosity and spirituality were resources that enhanced levels of life satisfaction and lowered levels of depression (Yoon & Lee, 2004).

The Impact of Social Support on Psychological Well-Being

Loneliness, lack of emotional support, and lack of social support may leave elderly individuals vulnerable to physical and emotional problems. Extensive literature documents the salutary effect of social support for various health and well-being outcomes. Elderly individuals who lack social support from both family and friends have decreased physical functioning and lower levels of life satisfaction (Krause, 1987; Aquino et al., 1996; Newsome & Schulz, 1996). According to House and associates (1988), social support among the elderly appeared to have a direct, positive effect in the short-term and to buffer the effect of stress in the long-term. The linkage of social support and depression has been shown in a number of studies, with an inverse relationship between the level of depression and the levels of social support (Dean, Kolody, & Wood, 1990; Bosworth et al., 2000). Bothell and colleagues (1999) found social support to be by far the most powerful predictor of depression among residents living in a low-income senior housing complex. Social support appears to buffer the detrimental effects of depression on the risk of physical decline (Hays et al., 1997). Cohen and Wills (1985) also found evidence that emotional support provided protection against a wide range of different stressful events.

Research Hypotheses

Based on review of previous studies, the literature provides a sound basis for the significance of social support from both family and friends and identifies religiousness/spirituality as a significant contributory factor to psychological well-being. The researchers tested the following hypothesis about the relationship of spirituality/religiousness and social support to psychological well-being among older adults in rural areas: (1) Those who report higher levels of religiousness/spirituality will report higher levels of life satisfaction; (2) Those who report higher levels of religiousness/spirituality will report lower levels of depression; (3) Those who report that they receive higher levels of social support will report higher levels of life satisfaction; and (4) Those who report that they receive higher levels of social support will report lower levels of depression.

METHODS

Sample and Data Collection

The sample for this study came from a rural community survey of 215 elderly individuals, including 85 Caucasians, 75 African Americans, and 55 Native Americans. A convenient sample was used with participants who were actively recruited through senior centers in both West Virginia and North Carolina in 2002. Face-to-face structured interviews were conducted. All participants were interviewed by research assistants who had previous work experiences with older adults, and the interviews lasted about 50 minutes. No participants had difficulty in understanding and answering the questions. At the beginning of each interview, the interviewer explained the purpose and format of the interview, emphasizing the confidentiality of all information collected. All participants signed a detailed informed consent form, and all responses were completely voluntary and anonymous.

Variables and Instruments

Religiousness/Spirituality

To measure various domains of religiousness/spirituality, the Brief Multidimensional Measures of Religiousness/Spirituality (BMMRS) (Fetzer/NIA, 1999) was used. This instrument has been used extensively with multiple populations such as older adults, adolescents, and cancer patients, though it has not been used with this population. Previous studies demonstrated high reliability scores of each sub scale in the BMMRS, ranging .71 to .87 (Kendler, Liu, Gardner, McCullough, Larson, & Prescott, 2003; Yoon & Lee, 2004). For this study, six sub scales were selected that are relevant to the study including daily spiritual experiences, values/beliefs, forgiveness, private religious practice, religious/spiritual coping, and religious support.

Daily spiritual experience measures the individual's experience of a transcendent (God, the divine) in daily life and experience of interaction with God (e.g., "I find strength and comfort in my religion"; "I feel God's love for me, directly or through others."). This sub scale consisted of 6 items with a 5-point response format, which ranged from 1 (never) to 5 (everyday). Higher scores reflect higher daily spiritual experience. Cronbach's alpha was .91 in the current sample.

Values/beliefs measures religious values and beliefs (i.e., "I believe in a God who watches over me"; "I feel a deep sense of responsibility for reducing pain and suffering in the world."). This sub-scale consisted of 2 items with a 4-point response format, which ranged from 1 (strongly disagree) to 4 (strongly agree). Higher scores reflect stronger religious values and beliefs. Cronbach's alpha was .64 in this sample.

Forgiveness measures the degree of forgiveness of self, others, and belief in the forgiveness of the God (e.g., "I have forgiven myself for things that I have done wrong"; "I know that God forgives me."). Most religious traditions attempt to foster beliefs and teach methods that can facilitate forgiveness (Pargament & Rye, 1998). This sub-scale consisted of 3 items rated on a 4-point response format, ranging from 1 (never) to 4 (always). Higher scores reflect greater forgiveness. Cronbach's alpha was .64 for this sample.

Private religious practice measures religious behaviors (e.g., "How often do you pray privately in places other than at church or synagogue?"; "How often do you read the Bible or other religious literature?"). This sub-scale consisted of 5 items with a 5-point response format, which ranged from 1 (never) to 5 (everyday). Higher scores reflect more private religious practice. Cronbach's alpha was .72 in this sample.

Religious/spiritual coping measures additional religious/spiritual practices and beliefs specifically related to coping with life's problems (e.g., "I look to God for strength, support, and guidance."). This sub-scale consisted of 7 items with a 5-point response format, ranging from 1 (not at all) to 5 (a great deal). Higher scores reflect higher religious/spiritual coping skills. Cronbach's alpha was .81 for this sample.

Religious support measures the degree to which local congregations provide help, support, and comfort (e.g., "How much would the people in your congregation help you out if you were ill?"). This sub-scale consisted of 4 items and a 4-point response format was used, which ranged from 1(none) to 4 (very often). Higher scores reflect greater congregational support. Cronbach's alpha was .72 in the current sample.

Social Support

This study also measured the degree of perceived social support participants received outside churches. In general, social support is thought to affect mental and physical health through its influence on emotions, cognitions, and behaviors (Cohen, 1988). To measure perceived social support, the Multidimensional Scale of Perceived Social Support (MSPSS) was used (Zimet, Dahlem, Zimet, & Farley, 1988). This scale measures overall social support scores from family, friends, and significant others. This scale consisted of 12 items and a 4-point response format was used, which ranged from 1 (strongly disagree) to 4 (strongly agree). Higher scores reflect higher perceived support. Cronbach's alpha was .92 in the present sample.

Psychological Well-Being

For this study, life satisfaction and depression were utilized as indicators of psychological well-being, and the Satisfaction with Life Scale (SWLS) (Diener, Emmons, Larsen, & Griffin, 1985) and the Center for Epidemiological Studies-Depression (CES-D) (Radloff, 1977) were used. Cronbach's alpha for these two scales was .84 and .85, respectively, for this sample. The SWLS consisted of 5 items rated on a 4-point response format, ranging from 1 (strongly disagree) to 4 (strongly agree) and the CES-D consisted of 11 items rated on a 4-point response format, ranging from 1 (rare or none of the time: less than a day) to 4 (most of the time: 5-7 days). Higher scores on the SWLS reflect higher life satisfaction and higher scores on the CES-D reflect greater depression.

Data Analyses

Hierarchical multiple regression analyses were performed to determine the relative influence of three sets of variables including demographics, religiousness/spirituality, and social support on dependent variables: life satisfaction and depression. The researchers tested three models for each dependent variable. In Model 1, the independent variable included the demographic variables of age, ethnicity (dichotomously coded as 1 = Non-White and 0 = White), education (dichotomously coded as 1 = > HS diploma, 0 = ≤ HS diploma), annual income (dichotomously coded as 1 = > $10,000, 0 = ≤ $10,000), and living arrangement (dichotomously coded as 1 = living with someone, 0 = living alone). The Model 2 included religiousness/spirituality variables involving daily spiritual experience, values and beliefs, forgiveness, private religious practice, religious/spiritual coping, and religious support. The Model 3 included social support to determine the level of subjective well-being consisting of life satisfaction and depression.

RESULTS

Characteristics of the Participants

As can be seen in Table 1, eighty-five individuals were White (39%), seventy-five African-American (35%), and fifty-five Native Americans (26%). Ninety-two (43%) of the sample had no high school diploma; whereas one hundred twenty-one (57%) of the participants had at least a high school diploma. Forty-one percent were widowed and 33% were married. In terms of annual income, one hundred seventy-seven (83%) reported an income under $20,000, indicating that the majority of the participants were financially below or near the poverty line (DHHS, 2003). Most individuals (97%) were affiliated with a religion: whereas only three percent of respondents had no religion.

Daily spiritual experience scores ranged from 6 to 30 with a mean of 24.6 (SD = 4.2), indicating that respondents reported spiritually experiences most

TABLE 1. Characteristics of the Participants

Variable	Frequency		Percentage
Sex (N = 213)			
Male	82		38.5
Female	131		61.5
Age (N = 209)			
Younger than 71	100		47.8
71-80	78		37.4
Older than 80	31		14.8
M = 72, SD = 7.7, Range = 60-92			
Ethnicity (N = 215)			
African-American	75		34.9
Native American	55		25.6
White	85		39.5
Marital status (N = 214)			
Married	70		32.7
Widowed	88		41.1
Divorced	18		8.4
Single	31		14.5
Other	7		3.3
Education (N = 213)			
Some high school	92		43.2
High school diploma	59		27.7
Some college	38		17.8
College graduate	17		8.0
Above college graduate	7		3.3
Annual income (N = 215)			
Under $10,001	66		30.7
$10,001 to $20,000	111		51.6
$20,001 to $30,000	29		13.5
Over $30,000	9		4.2
Religion (N = 210)			
Protestant	185		88.1
Catholic	8		3.8
Other	10		4.8
No	7		3.3
Living arrangement (N = 208)			
Living alone	107		51.4
Living with someone	101		48.6

days. Elderly respondents reported having strong value and belief in a God (Mean = 6.5; SD = 1.1), ranging from 2 to 8. Forgiveness scores ranged from 4 to 12 with mean of 10.6 (SD = 1.5), indicating that respondents reported often experiencing forgiveness. Most respondents reported practicing religious activities weekly (Mean = 20.1; SD = 4.9), ranging from 5 to 25. Religious and spiritual coping scores ranged from 7 to 28 with a mean of 19.2 (SD = 3.8), indicating that respondents reported using a rather high rate of religious and spiritual coping skills. Most respondents reported receiving religious support (Mean = 10.5; SD = 2.2), ranging from 4 to 16.

By and large, respondents reported that they received social support from family and friends (Mean = 33.8; SD = 8.3), ranging from 12 to 48. Two variables involving life satisfaction and depression were used to measure subjective well-being. Life satisfaction scores ranged from 5 to 20 with a mean of 14.6 (SD = 2.7) and depression scores ranged from 11 to 44 with a mean of 20.3 (SD = 4.3), indicating that respondents were relatively satisfied with their life even though they reported some depressive symptoms.

As shown in Table 2, significant correlations were evident (p < .05) except between values/beliefs and religious/spiritual coping and between values/beliefs and religious support. Social support (.43), religious/spiritual coping (.31), religious values/beliefs (.26), and religious support (.25) positively correlated with life satisfaction. Forgiveness (−.26), social support (−.24), religious values/beliefs (−.21), and religious/spiritual coping (−.20) also moderately and inversely correlated with depression.

Multivariate Analyses

Life Satisfaction. Table 3 indicates that the Model 3 accounts for 31% of the variance in life satisfaction (F = 6.52, p < .001; Adjusted R^2 = .27). In Model 1, no factor relating to a participant's demographic information significantly predicted life satisfaction. In Model 2, as expected, religious/spiritual coping skills and religious values/beliefs significantly predicted life satisfaction, explaining an additional 19% (p < .001) of the variance in life satisfaction. In Model 3, social support was a significant predictor of a subject's life satisfaction, explaining an additional 11% (p < .001) of the variance in life satisfaction. Thus, respondents reporting higher levels of life satisfaction are more likely to: (1) have more religious and spiritual coping skills (beta = .18, p < .05), (2) receive greater religious support (beta = .15, p < .05), and (3) receive more social support (beta = .36, p < .001).

Depression. The results of the regression analyses on depression have been summarized in Table 3. The Model 3 accounted for 21% of the variance in depression (F = 3.89, p < .001; Adjusted R^2 = .16). In Model 1, no factor relating to

TABLE 2. Means, Standard Deviations, and Correlations Among Measured Variables

Variable	1	2	3	4	5	6	7	8	9
1. Daily spiritual experience									
2. Values/beliefs	.42**								
3. Forgiveness	.41**	.21**							
4. Private religious practice	.58**	.40**	.44**						
5. Religious/spiritual coping	.24**	.11	.20**	.40**					
6. Religious support	.20**	.12	.15*	.32**	.42**				
7. Social support	.08	.17*	.10	.04	.18*	.09			
8. Life satisfaction	.24**	.26**	.19**	.18**	.31**	.25**	.43**		
9. Depression	−.14*	−.21**	−.26**	−.07**	−.20**	−.13	−.24**	−.29**	
Mean	24.56	6.49	10.08	20.10	19.20	10.53	33.80	14.56	20.31
Standard Deviation	4.15	1.15	1.46	4.87	3.82	2.21	8.28	2.67	4.30
Range	6-30	2-8	3-12	5-25	7-28	4-16	12-48	5-20	11-44

Note: N = 215, * $p < .05$, ** $p < .01$.

TABLE 3. Summary of Hierarchical Regression Analyses for Variables Predicting Participants' Psychological Well-Being Involving Life Satisfaction and Depression (Standardized Beta Coefficients)

Variable	Life Satisfaction			Depression		
	Model 1	Model 2	Model 3	Model 1	Model 2	Model 3
Demographic Information						
Age	.00	.04	.02	.00	.01	.00
Gender	2.02	2.02	.01	2.08	2.10	2.11
Ethnicity	2.02	.10	.03	2.08	2.18*	2.16
Education	2.05	2.03	2.06	2.05	2.12	2.11
Annual income	.04	.08	.09	.09	.03	.03
Living arrangement	2.03	.01	2.02	2.12	2.13	2.12
Religiousness/Spirituality						
Spiritual experience		.10	.10		.03	.03
Values and beliefs		.16*	.12		2.19*	2.18*
Forgiveness		.07	.04		2.29***	2.28**
Private religious practice		2.08	2.05		.15	.14
Religious/spiritual coping		.30***	.18*		2.28**	2.24**
Religious support		.15	.15*		2.04	2.05
Social support			.36***			2.12
F	.18	3.85***	6.52***	1.02	3.94***	3.89***
ΔR²		.19	.11		.17	.01
R²/Adjusted R²	.01/.00	.20/.15	.31/.27	.03/.00	.20/.15	.21/.16

Note: N = 215, * p < .05, ** p < .01, *** p < .001.

292

a participant's demographic information significantly predicted depression. As expected, in the equation to predict depression, value/belief system, religious and spiritual coping skills, and forgiveness appeared to contribute significantly and explained an additional 17% (p < .001) in Model 2. In Model 3, unexpectedly, social support was not a significant predictor of subject's depression, explaining only an additional 1% of the variance in life satisfaction. Therefore, respondents reporting lower levels of depression are more likely to: (1) have strong religious values and belief system (beta = 2.18, p < .05), (2) possess more religious and spiritual coping skills (beta = 2.24, p < .01), and (3) experience greater forgiveness (beta = 2.28, p < .01).

DISCUSSION

Most of the previous studies investigating the relationship between psychological well-being and religiousness/spirituality have been conducted in urban or metropolitan areas. In general, previously a unidimensional construct has been used to measure religiosity and spiritual well-being. In an attempt to understand the various roles of religiousness and spirituality, this study used the multidimensional scales of religiousness/spirituality and examined its relationship with factors associated with psychological well-being of rural elderly individuals. Simultaneously, the study also investigated how social support played a role in enhancing the levels of psychological well-being among them.

The finding of this study is aligned with previous investigations illuminating the salutary association of religion and spirituality to positive outcomes of general well-being among older adults in urban/suburban areas (Levin, Chatters, & Taylor, 1995; McFadden, 1993; Catipovic et al., 1995; Morris, 1997). The hierarchical regression analyses found positive relationships between religiousness/spirituality and social support with levels of psychological well-being among older adults in rural areas. More specifically, those rural elderly individuals who reported that they were more likely to use religious/spiritual coping behaviors (e.g., looking to God for strength and comfort and working together with God as partner), and who received more religious and social support, reported greater life satisfaction. In addition, those who experienced more forgiveness, had stronger religious belief systems, and were more likely to use religious and spiritual coping skills were less depressed. This rural elderly population drew upon spirituality when they were coping with illness, bereavement, anticipated death, and other adversities. They reported that Bible reading and other religious means set their minds at ease with their problems.

Their faith appeared to operate as a stress buffer, distress deterrent, or stress suppressor.

Inconsistent with previous studies (Dean, Kolody, & Wood, 1990; Bothell, Fischer, & Hayashida, 1999; Bosworth et al., 2000), this study found that perceived social support from family and friends was not associated with depression, but had a strong association with life satisfaction. Perhaps social support can be used as social or external buffering system instead of as an internal coping mechanism for rural elderly individuals. The overall findings support a growing body of literature documenting a positive relationship between social support and life satisfaction and a negative relationship between dimensions of religiousness/spirituality and depression among older adults in rural areas.

The major limitation of this study lies in the generalizability due to the utilization of a non-random and small-size sample. However, the heterogeneity of the sample including diverse geographical regions, ethnic backgrounds, and religious affiliations would increase the generalizability of the current findings. A longitudinal investigation is necessary to examine the effect of religiousness and spirituality over the life span as well as the effects of negative events such as the death of a spouse and the onset of chronic illness. In addition, future research needs to study the oldest-older adults who present serious needs for health care and social support.

In spite of the limitations, this study provides useful information on the impact of religiousness/spirituality and social support on psychological well-being among rural elderly. Results of this study can help service providers to understand and evaluate the roles of religion and spirituality when working with older adults, since a better understanding of this role would facilitate assessment and intervention plans that are strengths-focused. Many elderly clients in mental health settings are powerfully influenced by their sense of spirituality as their thoughts and emotions are rooted in spiritual values and beliefs. Diminishing social resources, death of significant others, and persistent health challenges, common characteristics in later life, provoke elderly to question the meaning and purpose in life. Religiousness and spirituality are so important in the later years that aging has been referring to as a spiritual journey (Bianchi, 1984) and a spiritualizing process (Jones, 1984; Moberg, 1990). By ignoring the spiritual component, mental health professionals fail to focus on the whole person, missing much strength for coping with adversity and loss, as well as a support system important enough to help enhance the quality of life. The clinician can use the assessment to refer the client for the appropriate service, including pastoral care. Rajagopal and colleagues (2002) reported the effectiveness of a spiritually based intervention by using a nondenominational, standardized, replicable, and structured format for praying in the alleviation of subsyndromal anxiety and minor depression among older adults.

Interventions focusing on spiritual perspectives need to be provided and studied to improve general well-being for spiritually-oriented elderly. Thus, social workers should be sensitive to an older person's faith development and cultural values so that the spiritual dimension can be integrated routinely into the assessment and intervention.

It is recommended that practitioners assist in the development of supportive environments that nourish rural life and eventually enhance psychological well-being of rural elderly. In addition, health/mental health professionals should be closely working with faith communities to support the spiritual inclinations of rural elderly. Rural residents rely heavily on social networks to provide social support and other services which more formal agencies often provide in urban areas. Thus, successful rural models that include spiritual care should be based on the context that is germane to rural community life. Such models might include the following: helping rural elderly to develop peer supports and establish a mutual supporting environment, providing mental health professionals with unique training, and expanding linkages with existing health/mental health programs and social services. Health care professionals need to develop programs or services that are congruent with religious/spiritual beliefs and practices in order to better enhance the psychological well-being and improve the quality of life among older adults in rural areas.

REFERENCES

Aquino, J. A., Russel, D. W., Cutrona, C. E., & Altmaier, E. M. (1996). Employment status, social support, and life satisfaction among the elderly. *Journal of Counseling Psychology, 43*(4), 480-489.

Arcury, T. A., Quandt, S. A., McDonald, J., & Bell, R. A. (2000). Faith and health self-management of rural older adults. *Journal of Cross-Cultural Gerontology, 15*(1), 55-74.

Armer, J. M., & Conn, V. S. (2001). Exploration of spirituality & health. *Journal of Gerontological Nursing, 27*(6), 29-37.

Bane, S. D., & Bull, C. N. (2001). Innovative rural mental health service delivery for rural elders. *Journal of Applied Gerontology. 20*(2), 230-240.

Bianchi, E. C. (1984). Aging as a spiritual journey. New York: Crossroad Publishing Co.

Bosworth, H. B., Steffens, D. C., Kuchinbbatla, M. N., Jiang, W. J. Ariasm R. M., O'Connor, C. M., & Krishman, K. R. (2000). Relationship of social support, social networks and negative events with depression in patients with coronary artery disease. *Aging & Mental Health, 4*(3), 253-258.

Bothell, W. L., Fischer, J., & Hayashida, C. (1999). Social support and depression among low income elderly. *Journal of Housing for the Elderly, 13*(1-2), 51-63.

Bradley, D. (1995). Religious involvement and social resources: Evidence from the data set "Americans Changing Lives." *Journal for the Scientific Study of Religion, 34*, 259-273.

Buczko, W. (2001). Rural Medicare beneficiaries' use of rural and urban hospitals. *Journal of Rural Health, 17*(1), 53-58.

Campbell, C. D., Gordon, M. C., & Chandler, A. A. (2002). Wide open spaces: Meeting mental health needs in underserved rural areas. *Journal of Psychology & Christianity, 21*(4), 325-332.

Catipovic, V., Ilakovac, V., Durjancek, J., & Amidzc, V. (1995). Relationship of eight basic emotions with age, sex, education, satisfaction of life needs, and religion. *Psychological Reports, 77,* 115-121.

Cohen, S. (1988). Psychosocial models of the role of social support in the etiology of physical disease. *Health Psychology, 7,* 269-297.

Cohen, S., & Wills, T. A. (1985). Stress, social support, and buffering hypothesis. *Psychological Bulletin, 98,* 310-357.

Davenport, J., & Davenport III, J. (1982). Utilizing the social network in rural communities. *Social Casework, 63,* 106-115.

Dean, A., Kolody, B., & Wood, P. (1990). Effects of social support from various sources on depression in elderly persons. *Journal of Health & Social Behaviors, 31*(2), 1442-1465.

Dellasega, C. (1998). Assessment of cognition in the elderly: Pieces of a complex puzzle. *Nursing Clinics of North America, 33*(3), 395-405.

DHHS (2003). The 2003 HHS poverty guidelines. *Federal Register, 68*(26), 6456-6458.

Diener, E., Emmons, R. A., Larsen, R. J., & Griffin, S. (1985). The satisfaction with life scale: A measure of life satisfaction. *Journal of Personality Assessment, 49,* 71-75.

Fabricatore, A. N., Handal, P. J., & Fenzel, L. M. (2000). Personal spirituality as a moderator of the relationship between stressors and subjective well-being. *Journal of Psychology & Theology, 28*(3), 221-228.

Fetzer Institute/National Institute on Aging (1999). *Multidimensional measurement of religiousness/spirituality for use in health research*: A report of the Fetzer Institute/National Institute on Aging working group. Kalamazoo, MI: John E. Fetzer Institute.

Fry, P. S. (2000). Religious involvement, spirituality and personal meaning for life: Existential predictors of psychological wellbeing in community-residing and institutional care elders. *Aging and Mental Health, 4*(4), 375-387.

Hays, J. C., Saunders, W. B., Flint, E. P., Kaplan, B. H., & Blazer, D. G. (1997). Social support and depression as risk factors for loss of physical function in late life. *Aging & Mental Health, 1*(3), 209-220.

Hertsgaard, D., & Light, H. K. (1984). Anxiety, depression, and hostility in rural women. *Psychological Reports, 55*(2), 673-674.

House, J. S., Umberson, D., & Landis, K. (1988). Structures and processes of social support. *Annual Review of Sociology, 14,* 293-318.

Idler, E. L., & Kasl, S. V. (1997). Religion among disabled and nondisabled persons I: Cross-sectional patterns in health practices, social activities, and well-being. *Journals of Gerontology: Series B: Psychological Sciences & Social Sciences, 52B*(6), S294-S305.

Jones, P. W. (1984). Aging as a spiritualizing process. *Journal of Religion and Aging*, *1*(1), 3-16.

Joseph, M. V. (1987). The religious and spiritual aspects of clinical practice: A neglected dimension of social work. *Social Thought*, *13*(1), 12-23.

Kaufman, A. V., Scogin, F. R., MaloneBeach, E. E., Baumhover, L. A., & McKendree-Smith, N. (2000). Home-delivered mental health services for aged rural home health care recipients. *Journal of Applied Gerontology*, *19*(4), 460-475.

Kendler, K. S., Liu, X. Q., Gardner, C. O., McCullough, M. E., Larson, D., & Prescott, C. A. (2003). Dimensions of religiosity and their relationship to lifetime psychiatric and substance use disorders. *American Journal of Psychiatry*, *160*(3), 496-503.

Koenig, H. G. (1995). *Research on religion and aging: An annotated bibliography.* Westport, CT: Greenwood Press.

Koenig, H. G., Cohen, H. J., George, L. K., Hays, J. C., Larson, D. B., & Blazer, D. G. (1997). Attendance at religious services, interleukin-6, and other biological indicators of immune function in older adults. *International Journal of Psychiatry in Medicine*, *27*, 233-250.

Koenig, H. G., George, L. K., Blazer, D. G., Pritchett, J., & Meador, K. G. (1993). The relationship between religion and anxiety in a sample of community-dwelling older adults. *Journal of Geriatric Psychiatry*, *26*, 65-93.

Koenig, H. G., George, L. K., & Siegler, I. C. (1988). The use of religion and other emotion-regulating coping strategies among older adults. *The Gerontologist*, *28*, 303-310.

Koenig, H. G., & Larson, D. B. (1998). Use of hospital services, religious attendance, and religious affiliation. *Southern Medical Journal*, *91*, 925-932.

Koenig, H. G., Siegler, I. C., & George, L. K. (1989). Religious and non-religious coping: Impact on adaptation in later life. *Journal of Religion and Aging*, *5*, 73-84.

Kraaij, V., Garnefski, N., & Maes, S. (2002). Joint effects of stress, coping, and coping resources on depressive symptoms in the elderly. *Anxiety, Stress, & Coping*, *15*(2), 163-177.

Krause, N. (1987). Satisfaction with social support and self-rated health in older adults. *Gerontologist*, *27*(3), 301-308.

Krause, N. (2002). Church-based social support and health in old age: Exploring variations by race. *Journal of Gerontology Series B Psychological Science and Social Sciences*, *57B*(6), S332-S347.

Levin, J. S. (1997). Religious research in gerontology, 1980-1994: A systematic review. *Journal of Religious Gerontology*, *10*(3), 3-31.

Levin, J. S., & Chatters, L. M. (1998). Religion, health, and psychological well-being in older adults. *Journal of Aging and Health*, *10*(4), 504-531.

Levin, J. S., Chatters, L. M., & Taylor, R. J. (1995). Religious effect on health status and life satisfaction among Black Americans. *Journal of Gerontology Social Sciences*, *50B*, S134-S163.

McFadden, S. (1993). Religion and well-being in aging person in an aging society. *Journal of Social Issues*, *51*(2), 145-160.

Mitchell, J., & Weatherly, D. (2000). Beyond church attendance: Religiosity and mental health among rural older adults. *Journal of Cross-Cultural Gerontology*, *15*(1), 37-54.

Moberg, D. O. (1990). Spiritual maturity and wholeness in later years. *Journal of Religious Gerontology, 7*(1/2), 5-24.

Morris, D. C. (1997). Health, finances, religious involvement, and life satisfaction of older adults. *Journal of Religious Gerontology, 10*(2), 3-17.

Newsome, J. T., & Schulz, R. (1996). Social support as a mediator in the relation between functional status and quality of life in older adults. *Psychology & Aging, 11*(1), 34-44.

Oman, D., & Reed, D. (1998). Religion and mortality among the community-dwelling elderly. *American Journal of Public Health, 88*(10), 1469-1475.

Pargament, K. I., Ensing, D. S., Falgout, K., Olsen, H., Reilly, B., Van Haitsma, K., & Warren, R. (1990). God help me: I. Religious coping efforts as predictors of the outcomes to significant negative life events. *American Journal of Community Psychology, 18,* 793-824.

Pargament, K. I., & Rye, M. S. (1998). Forgiveness as a method of religious coping. In E. L. Worthington, Jr. (Ed.), *Dimensions of forgiveness: Psychological research and theological perspectives* (pp. 59-78). Philadelphia: Templeton Foundation Press.

Radloff, L. S. (1977). The Center for Epidemiological Studies Depression scale: A self-report depression scale for research in the general population. *Applied Psychological Measurement, 1,* 385-401.

Rajagopal, D., Mackenzie, E., Baley, C., & Lavizzo, M. R. (2002). Effectiveness of a spiritually-based intervention to alleviate subsyndromal anxiety and minor depression among older adults. *Journal of Religion & Health, 41*(2), 153-166.

Rogers, C. C. (2002). The older population in 21st century rural America. *Rural America, 17*(3), 25-35.

St. George, A., & McNamara, P. H. (1984). Religion, race and psychological well-being. *Journal for the Scientific Study of Religion, 23*(4), 351-363.

Thomas, M. E., & Holmes, B. J. (1992). Determinants of satisfaction for Blacks and Whites. *Sociological Quarterly, 33*(3), 459-472.

Wethington, E., & Kessler, R. C. (1986). Perceived support, received support, and adjustment to stressful events. *Journal of Health and Social Behavior, 27,* 78-89.

Yoon, D. P., & Lee, E. O. (2004). Religiousness/spirituality and subjective well-being among rural elderly Whites, African Americans, and Native Americans. *Journal of Human Behavior in the Social Environment, 10*(1), 191-211.

Zimet, G. D., Davlem, N. W., Zimet, S. G., & Farley, G. K. (1988). Multidimensional scale of perceived social support. *Journal of Personality Assessment, 52,* 30-41.

Zinnbauer, B. J., Pargament, K. L., Cole, B., Rye, M. S., Butter, E. M., Belavich, T. G., Hipp, K., M., Scott, A. B., & Kadar, J. L. (1997). Religion and spirituality: Unfuzzying the fuzzy. *Journal for the Scientific Study of Religion, 36*(4), 549-564.

doi:10.1300/J083v48n03_01

Spirit of Aging Rising:
Cross-Cutting Thematic Modules
to Enrich Foundation Graduate
Social Work Courses

Connie Saltz Corley, PhD, LCSW
Pamela Davis, MSW
LaTina Jackson, MSW
Marlena Stuart Bach, MSW

SUMMARY. To enrich an urban generalist MSW program serving a diverse aging community, an innovative approach was initiated. A team of students, faculty and a field instructor collaborated in creating and evaluating 3 sets of cross-cutting thematic modules. An overview of the thematic modules (addressing elder abuse, family caregiving, and mental health), integrated across multiple curriculum areas (Human Behavior and the Social Environment, Macro/Policy, Practice and Research), is presented along with results of a faculty focus group evaluating the process of coordinating module content for one full week of class per foundation area (one topic per quarter). doi:10.1300/J083v48n03_02 *[Article copies available for a fee from The Haworth Document Delivery Service:*

This article was presented at the first National Gerontological Social Work Conference, Atlanta, GA, March 1, 2003. Funding was provided by the Geriatric Enrichment Program, a program of the John A. Hartford Foundation funded through the Council on Social Work Education.

[Haworth co-indexing entry note]: "Spirit of Aging Rising: Cross-Cutting Thematic Modules to Enrich Foundation Graduate Social Work Courses." Corley, Connie Saltz et al. Co-published simultaneously in *Journal of Gerontological Social Work* (The Haworth Press, Inc.) Vol. 48, No. 3/4, 2007, pp. 299-309; and: *Fostering Social Work Gerontology Competence: A Collection of Papers from the First National Gerontological Social Work Conference* (ed: Catherine J. Tompkins, and Anita L. Rosen) The Haworth Press, Inc., 2007, pp. 299-309. Single or multiple copies of this article are available for a fee from The Haworth Document Delivery Service [1-800-HAWORTH, 9:00 a.m. - 5:00 p.m. (EST). E-mail address: docdelivery@haworthpress.com].

1-800-HAWORTH. E-mail address: <docdelivery@haworthpress.com> Website: <http:// www.HaworthPress.com> © *2007 by The Haworth Press, Inc. All rights reserved.]*

KEYWORDS. Social work education, geriatric enrichment

INTRODUCTION

Issues arising from demographics of aging are increasingly drawing attention within the field of social work due to the dramatic growth of the older adult population in the United States, especially among the oldest (over 85) age segment. Average life expectancy has surpassed 75 years, and many older adults are part of four and even five generational families (Administration on Aging [AoA], 2003). The aging of the population affects all generations, e.g., the rise in kinship care and the pressing needs of adults in mid-life who are caring both for older family members as well as children. The aging population is increasingly diverse, with minority and ethnic subgroups of the older population increasing (Hooyman & Kiyak, 2002; McInnis-Dittrich, 2002).

In recognition of the challenges facing older Americans and the need for a professional response, the Council on Social Work Education generated *A Blueprint for the New Millennium* (CSWE/SAGE-SW) as part of a project funded by the John A. Hartford Foundation (Strengthening Aging and Gerontology Education for Social Work). In this report it is noted that in 1987 fewer than 30,000 social workers were engaged in full- or part-time work with older adults, but by the end of the first decade in the new millennium over twice as many social workers with expertise in gerontology/geriatrics will be needed. By 2030, as the peak of the Baby Boomers reach age 65, at least 20% of the population will be eligible for a variety of programs and services that social workers must be prepared to deliver.

As part of a multi-program initiative called the Geriatric Social Work Initiative, the John A. Hartford Foundation funded a 3-year program called the Geriatric Enrichment Program also called the GeroRich Program (Robbins & Rieder, 2002). According to the GeroRich website: "Our goals are to ensure that gerontology pervades students' learning experiences across the curriculum and to create transformative changes within social work curricula that are sustainable" (University of Washington, 2003). Reported here is the major accomplishment of one of 67 GeroRich programs, funded to the California State University Los Angeles (CSULA) with matching support from the Edward R. Roybal Institute of Applied Gerontology at CSULA. A team of faculty and students, complemented by a cadre of area faculty and community agency representatives who are experts in aging and cross-cultural issues, worked together to imbue the "Spirit of Aging Rising" (SOAR) into the foundation MSW curriculum. The two symbols for SOAR are blended from CSULA logos which together form the image of the eagle, representing wisdom, flying at sunrise. By imbuing the spirit of aging throughout the foundation year of the MSW program, SOAR endeavors to promote positive images of aging and creative solutions to critical issues experienced in aging across the life course, for ALL students enrolled in a graduate social work program.

THE CONTEXT AND PROCESS OF "GERIATRIC ENRICHMENT"

Based on a model of optimal team functioning (Damron-Rodriguez & Corley, 2002), the context and process of enriching the CSULA foundation year curriculum with aging content (one of several emphases of SOAR, which include recruitment strategies and advanced year enrichment) is now described.

The graduate MSW program at CSULA is based on an urban generalist model. Historically, it offered only a Children, Youth, Women and Families (CYWF) concentration in the advanced year. The first cohort of students to enroll in a second concentration, Aging and Families (AF), graduated in June, 2002. A Criminal Justice area of emphasis is also available to students in either concentration. A School of Social Work self-study process for the program's first re-accreditation was underway throughout the lifespan of the 3-year grant (through June, 2004), making it an ideal time to conduct a sustainable curriculum transformation.

A pyramid approach was used to identify the specific strategies for enrichment of aging content into the foundation curriculum, which is the "platform" of the pyramid. Three faces rising from the foundation guided the curriculum transformation process: (1) curriculum enhancement, (2) environmental modification and (3) issue-based action plans for an aging America.

The first face of the pyramid utilizes the curriculum enhancement strategies recommended by Scharlach, Damron-Rodriguez, Robinson and Feldman (2000) to "create and test model course outlines, curriculum modules, field experiences, and interdisciplinary training" (p. 531). In concert with the ongoing work of the School's Curriculum Committee and sequences (HBSE, Practice, Macro/Policy, Research and Field), course syllabi were reviewed to identify opportunities to enrich courses with aging content.

The second face of the pyramid addressed environmental modification strategies outlined by Kropf (2002), including promoting institutional collaboration and expanding community networks. Two grants funded in conjunction with the Edward R. Roybal Institute for Applied Gerontology at CSULA (elder abuse and family caregiving) provided a context in which to explore resources for the cross-cutting thematic modules.

The third face of the pyramid involved identifying issue-based action plans, using as a springboard "A Social Work Action Plan Addressing Issues of an Aging America" as outlined in *Social Work Response to the White House Conference on Aging* (Saltz, 1997). Target issues articulated at the 1995 White House Conference on Aging were examined. The combined expertise of all of those involved in SOAR spanned a variety of issues in the Action Plan, and combined with the interests of 3 students who were engaged in working with the team, three issues were chosen: elder abuse, family caregiving, and mental health.

STRUCTURE OF GERIATRIC ENRICHMENT

A team of students and faculty created/integrated a series of 3 cross-cutting thematic teaching modules, with the goal of simultaneous exposure to the content during one week each quarter to 9 foundation courses in the full-time program. Figure 1 shows the structure (Damron-Rodriguez & Corley, 2002) of the enrichment of 9 nine courses across the 3 themes: Elder Abuse, Family Caregiving, and Mental Health. Students worked with the PI and faculty Curriculum Committee representatives of the course foundation areas of Human Behavior in the Social Environment (HBSE), Practice, Macro/Policy and Research to create the modules. Pre/post-test surveys of knowledge and attitudes

FIGURE 1. Cross-Cutting Thematic Modules

	FALL 2002	WINTER 2003	SPRING 2003
CROSS CUTTING THEMES	ELDER ABUSE	FAMILY CAREGIVING	MENTAL HEALTH
COURSE SEQUENCES			
PRACTICE	√	√	
MACRO/POLICY	√	√	√
HBSE	√	√	√
RESEARCH			√

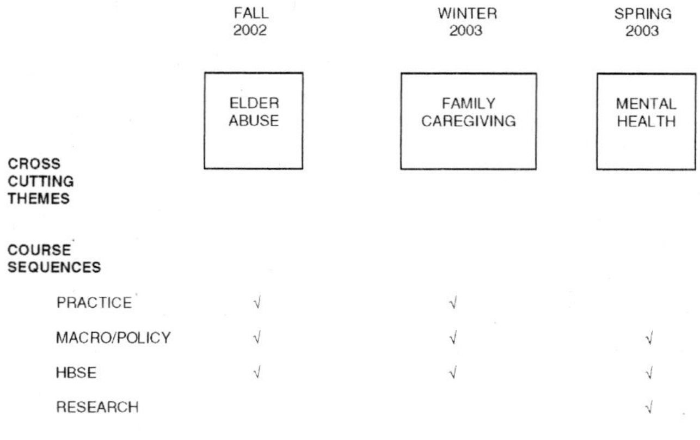

were administered each quarter. Full-time students in the foundation year (n = 35) were enrolled in all 9 courses. All students in the part-time program taking foundation courses (n = 82) were also exposed to the enriched content, although none of them were taking three foundation courses simultaneously in any given quarter.

Tables 1-3 detail the objectives by course for one module in each of the cross-cutting themes for 3 of the course sequences. Modules include case vignettes, outline of content, handouts, exercises, suggested readings and bibliographies. The cross-cutting thematic modules were presented at the first National Gerontological Social Work conference in March, 2003 and were highlighted as part of a presentation at the Gerontological Society of America in November, 2003. Following is an overview of the contents of all the modules, by theme:

Theme One: Elder Abuse and Neglect. All modules incorporate an overview of the needs of the growing population of elderly with an emphasis on the vulnerable older adult and elder abuse and neglect. The HBSE module includes content on biological changes of aging (normal and disease states) plus theories of aging, especially as they relate to abuse/neglect. Risk factors, geriatric assessment and ethical dilemmas are addressed in the Practice module. The Macro/Policy module builds upon the policies that were developed historically to reflect the needs of the elderly and focuses on the need for policy implementation and change to improve the quality of life of older adults.

Theme Two: Family Caregiving. The HBSE module addresses the diverse characteristics of family caregivers (including kinship care), stages/types/demands of caregiving, relevant theories (e.g., Exchange theory), and loss and recovery in the caregiving context. The Practice module includes the coverage of case management skills, comprehensive assessment and therapeutic intervention. In the Policy module, the initiation and implementation of the National Family Caregiver Support program is addressed, as well as advance directives, conservatorship and guardianship.

Theme Three: Mental Health. The HBSE module examines the diagnostic aspects of major mental health challenges among older adults. Cultural aspects of the manifestation and treatment of mental illness are addressed. The Practice module identifies issues related to diagnosis and also the challenges of diagnosis among diverse populations. The foundation Research course is the third module, and ties in with the issues already mentioned in terms of use of psychometric measures.

TABLE 1. Elder Abuse Module

Foundation MSW Courses	Knowledge/Skills/Values Content Identified for Each Course: Objectives	Resource/Materials/Methodologies Used
Macro/Policy; First quarter	1. To promote the empowerment of the older adult	Statement re: impact of macro perspective/policy on empowering older adults; history of attention to elder abuse in the U.S.
	2. To provide an overview of existing federal programs assisting the older adult	Overview of Social Security, Older Americans Act/Programs (including OAA 2000 provisions for the Prevention of Elder Abuse, Neglect and Exploitation Program)
	3. To gain a broader perspective of policy issues affecting the older adult	Definition and responsibilities of the mandated reporter
	4. Expand knowledge on responsibilities of the mandated reporter	Adult Protective Services Worker Training: http://calstatela.edu/dept/soc_work/ (click: APS Worker Training Program)
	5. To explore current and potential political trends regarding the older adult	Summary of suggested policy changes to address elder abuse
		List of definitions regarding elder abuse and neglect (from California Welfare and Institutions Code, Section 15610)
		HANDOUTS: List of Elder Abuse and Neglect websites plus other aging-related websites; Fact sheets on Medicare and Medicaid
		Reading: Wilber & McNeilly (2001), "Elder Abuse and Victimization"
		Case vignette; Bibliography

TABLE 2. Family Caregiving Module

Foundation MSW Courses	Knowledge/Skills/Values Content Identified for Each Course: Objectives	Resource/Materials/Methodologies Used
Parameters of Practice, Second Quarter	1. To understand gerontological case management and why it is an appropriate intervention for caregivers and care recipients	Overview of models, settings, and distinguishing features of case management for frail older adults
	2. To understand the special issues addressed by gerontological case management	Review of elements of care coordination: intake screening, comprehensive assessment; care planning; service arranging; case monitoring; reassessment; termination
	3. To identify the elements of care coordination	Use of case vignette: (a) to assess the caregiver as primary client; care recipient as primary client and (b) to identify services as part of a care plan using "Community Care Options" handout and identify other supports, strengths, areas for intervention, and ethical issues
	4. To apply the domains of comprehensive assessment	
	5. To create a care plan that demonstrates an understanding of the needs of both the caregiver and the care recipient and reflects an awareness of available community resources	Overview of therapeutic interventions including: problem-solving, supportive therapy, decision-making, education, crisis intervention, and life review Handout: caregiving websites and resources
	6. To identify the role of therapeutic intervention in a case vignette	Readings: Delmaestro, "Sharing Despair: Working with Distressed Caregivers" and Supiano, "Forming Relationships: The Key to Creative Care Management" Case vignette; Bibliography

TABLE 3. Mental Health Module

Foundation MSW Courses	Knowledge/Skills/Values Content Identified for Each Course: Objectives	Resource/Materials/Methodologies Used
HBSE, third quarter	1. Develop a basic understanding of biopsychosocial aspects of aging and their impact on one's mental health	Synopsis of factors impacting older adults which affect mental health
	2. Distinguish between normal and morbid changes in the psychiatric stability of older adults	Overview of psychological changes in normal functioning which can be precursors to cognitive/emotional decline
	3. Understand dominant theories on aging as they relate to mental health on the micro level	Synopsis of Disengagement Theory, Activity Theory, Continuity Theory, Life Course Perspective
	4. Identify the most common forms of morbidity in the psychological development of older adults	CHART: Summary of characteristics of delirium, dementia, depression, anxiety disorders, mania & psychotic disorders
	5. Identify signs, symptoms and treatment considerations for the most common mental illnesses in older adults	Exercise, "The Membership Exercise" (*Teaching Resource Kit* v. 2.0, Section 8.5, CSWE/SAGE-SW)
	6. Understand the importance of cultural impacts as they relate to mental health and aging	Summary of "Mental health: Culture, race and ethnicity" (http://www.surgeongeneral.gov/library/mentalhealth/cre/factsheet.asp)
	7. Understand the intergenerational impact of older adult mental health	Overview of intergenerational implications of mental health and aging
		Readings: Selections from Spring 2002 Generations issue on "Mental Health and Mental Illness in Later Life"
		Case Vignette; Bibliography

SUCCESSES AND CHALLENGES

The first significant outcome (Damron-Rodriguez & Corley, 2002) of SOAR is teamwork: 8 of the 10 full-time faculty members teaching courses and 2 part-time faculty members teaching in Year 2 integrated content from 3 thematic modules designed and evaluated by 3 graduate students into 9 foundation courses in the MSW program. Two additional full-time faculty members who did not teach foundation courses during the Implementation Year (Year 2), along with 2 new full-time faculty members, taught foundation courses in Year 3 (Evaluation and Dissemination) and incorporated module content into these courses. Hence, ALL full-time teaching faculty in Year 3 enriched foundation courses with aging content.

A focus group of the teaching faculty who participated in SOAR was held late in Year 2 to discuss the following: (a) the process of designing, implementing and evaluating cross-cutting thematic modules; (b) sustainability of curriculum changes; and (c) successful approaches for promoting interest in aging among students. Most of the discussion focused on the structure and implementation of the modules and "lessons learned." Faculty appreciated having content across the foundation courses for the topic being addressed. The modules included "ready to use" materials and are being revised and re-formatted for dissemination.

Implementation of the modules during the same time period (generally a week) across 3 classes at a time proved to be challenging and not always possible. This issue and some of the methodological issues related to the pre/post-tests were discussed at the focus group of SOAR teaching faculty. Clearly, to implement such an approach in the future would require much more advance planning per quarter, since in the case of 2 of the quarters materials were not available to faculty until after syllabi were prepared. More input from faculty would have also enhanced the completeness and in some cases the level and depth of content. It was also felt that for some topics, enrichment over more than one week of class time is preferable. Hence, module content continued to be incorporated during Year 3, but timing within a quarter or shifting topics across quarters to better fit a course sequence (e.g., Mental Health content in HBSE was covered in the first and third quarters) facilitated sustaining the incorporation of module content.

Other strategies for evaluating as an alternative to pre/post-tests of attitudes and knowledge were discussed by the SOAR teaching faculty in the focus group. For example, assessing knowledge of key concepts/terms at the beginning of the quarter then at the end of the quarter is one approach used. Another approach is having students examine a case study at the beginning of the quarter, then again at the end of the quarter. These and other strategies for evaluation are being considered in the module revisions.

Simultaneous presentation of content did not take place for students attending part-time since their coursework is taken over 3 years. Hence, more flexibility in incorporating module content is encouraged and supported via email updates, presentations at faculty meetings, and technical assistance to faculty teaching the target courses. Since CSULA faculty teach across both the undergraduate and graduate programs, faculty are also incorporating module content into undergraduate courses and this will be monitored in Year 3 of the grant.

A second major accomplishment in the Implementation Year (Year 2) was the involvement of students in the advanced full-time year concentrating in Aging and Families in the project. Three students focused their thesis research on aspects related to SOAR (two examined pre/post measures of two of the cross-cutting thematic modules, and one on student interest in working in the field of aging). These three students and the PI prepared a poster presentation for the first National Gerontological Social Work Conference in Atlanta (March 2003) and were among the few students participating as presenters. Two of these students and a third student in Aging and Families concentration (all of whom have now graduated) participated in a Recruitment Project in conjunction with their field placements affiliated with the Geriatric Social Work Education Consortium (GSWEC), a Practicum Partnership Program funded by the John A. Hartford Foundation to Partners in Care Foundation (Burbank, CA). The findings of this project were presented at the GSWEC annual meeting (April 2003).

CONCLUSION

Graduate social work programs face the challenge of educating all students to be prepared to work for a burgeoning aging population. To address this challenge, an urban generalist master of social work program enriched foundation coursework using a team approach to create cross-cutting thematic modules addressing elder abuse, family caregiving, and mental health in older adults. Faculty teaching in the Implementation Year of this program funded under one of the John A. Hartford Foundation's Geriatric Social Work Initiatives have shown a commitment to sustain the incorporation of module content into graduate courses and some are also using content to enrich undergraduate courses at CSULA. The "Spirit of Aging Rising" project successfully incorporated a team approach and engaged students in aging in leadership roles in the process.

REFERENCES

Administration on Aging [AoA] (2000). *A Profile of Older Americans* [Online] Available: <www.aoa.gov/aoa/stats/profile/default.htm>.

CSWE/SAGE-SW (2001). *Strengthening the Impact of Social Work to Improve the Quality of Life for Older Adults & Their Families: A Blueprint for the New Millenium.* Alexandria: VA: Council on Social Work Education. [Online]. Available: <www.cswe.org/sage/sw/>.

Damron-Rodriguez, J.A., & Corley, C.S. (2002). Social work education for interdisciplinary practice with older adults and their families. *Journal of Gerontological Social Work, 39*, 37-55.

Hooyman, N., & Kiyak, H.A. (2002). *Social gerontology: A multidisciplinary perspective.* Sixth edition. Needham Heights, MA: Allyn & Bacon.

Kropf, N.P. (2002). Strategies to increase student interest in aging. *Journal of Gerontological Social Work, 39*, 57-67.

McInnis-Dittrich, K. (2002). *Social work with elders: A biopsychosocial approach to assessment and intervention.* Boston: Allyn & Bacon.

Robbins, L.A., & Rieder, C.H. (2002). The John A. Hartford Foundation Geriatric Social Initiative. *Journal of Gerontological Social Work, 39*, 71-89.

Rosen, A. L., Zlotnik, J.L., & Singer, T. (2002). Basic gerontological competence for all social workers: The need to "gerontologize" social work education. *Journal of Gerontological Social Work, 39*, 25-36.

Saltz, C. Corley (1997). From issues to actions. In C. Corley Saltz (ed.), *Social work response to the White House Conference on Aging,* New York: The Haworth Press, Inc.

Scharlach, A., Damron-Rodriguez, J.A., Robinson, B., & Feldman, R. (2000). Educating social workers for an aging society: A vision for the 21st century. *Journal of Social Work Education, 36*, 521-538.

University of Washington (2003). Geriatric Enrichment Program. Available: <www.depts.washington.edu/gerorich/hartford/gerorich.shtml>.

doi:10.1300/J083v48n03_02

A Dual Process Model of Grief Counseling: Findings from the Changing Lives of Older Couples (CLOC) Study

Virginia E. Richardson, PhD

SUMMARY. This paper tests Stroebe and Schut's Dual Process Model of Bereavement using data from the Changing Lives of Older Couples (CLOC), a prospective study of 1,532 married persons over the age of 65. This analysis focused on a weighted sample of 104 widowers and 492 widows at six months, 18 months, and four years later. Bradburn's Affect Balance Scale was used as the dependent variable, and the independent variables were based on Stroebe and Schut's bereavement model. The multiple regression analyses revealed that loss- and restoration-oriented activities were important throughout bereavement. Implications for bereavement counseling are discussed. doi:10.1300/J083v48n03_03 *[Article copies available for a fee from The Haworth Document Delivery Service: 1-800-HAWORTH. E-mail address: <docdelivery@haworthpress.com> Website: <http://www.HaworthPress.com> © 2007 by The Haworth Press, Inc. All rights reserved.]*

The author would like to thank members of the CLOC team, especially Deborah Carr, Becky Utz, Margaret Stroebe, Randy Nesse, Amiram Vinokur, and Emanuelle Zech for assisting with this research and for providing funding for these analyses. The Changing Lives of Older Couples study was supported by grants from the Nancy Pritzer Research Network and the National Institute of Aging (P01-AG05561-01).

[Haworth co-indexing entry note]: "A Dual Process Model of Grief Counseling: Findings from the Changing Lives of Older Couples (CLOC) Study." Richardson, Virginia E. Co-published simultaneously in *Journal of Gerontological Social Work* (The Haworth Press, Inc.) Vol. 48, No. 3/4, 2007, pp. 311-329; and: *Fostering Social Work Gerontology Competence: A Collection of Papers from the First National Gerontological Social Work Conference* (ed: Catherine J. Tompkins, and Anita L. Rosen) The Haworth Press, Inc., 2007, pp. 311-329. Single or multiple copies of this article are available for a fee from The Haworth Document Delivery Service [1-800-HAWORTH, 9:00 a.m. - 5:00 p.m. (EST). E-mail address: docdelivery@haworthpress.com].

KEYWORDS. Bereavement, widowhood, grief counseling, older adults

INTRODUCTION

Many clinicians, researchers, and scholars beginning with Lindemann (1944) and Kubler-Ross (1969), who identified stages that terminally ill persons undergo, have conceptualized several grief stages that people typically experience during bereavement. More recently, researchers have questioned the applicability of stage models, and proposed alternative conceptualizations of bereavement that take into account circumstances of deaths and other factors that affect how people grieve. In this paper, I test a contemporary model of bereavement, specifically, Stroebe and Schut's (1999) Dual Process Model of Bereavement, using data from a national longitudinal study of widows and widowers. First, I review traditional theories of grief. Then I explain my methodology and findings. Finally, I apply these results to grief counseling for social workers.

Traditional Theories of Bereavement

Traditional theories of bereavement have emphasized "grief work," which involves focusing on the circumstances of the loss, the bereaved person's relationship to the deceased, and on feelings about the loss (Bowlby, 1980; Lindemann, 1944). Individuals must "work through" their painful feelings of loss to successfully resolve the loss, according to those theories. Those who avoid grieving and deny their feelings are at higher risk for "complicated grief reactions."

Stage theorists, e.g., Kübler-Ross (1969), Bowlby and Parkes (1970), have identified phases that people experience during mourning. Kübler-Ross identified four phases (denial, bargaining, despair, resignation, and acceptance) that people with terminal illnesses undergo. Although Kübler-Ross intended these phases for dying persons, others have applied her model to bereaved persons. Worden (1991) outlined tasks of grieving, which included accepting the reality of the loss, experiencing the pain of grief, redefining the relationship with the deceased, adjusting to the environment from which the deceased is missing, and finally withdrawing emotional energy and reinvesting in other relationships.

Most stage models of grief include three phases: an initial period of shock, disbelief, and denial, which sometimes last for weeks; an acceptance of the reality of the loss, which is an acute phase of mourning characterized by intense feelings of sadness, despair, anxiety, loneliness, and anger, and which may last for months; and a restitution or acceptance phase, when the intense feelings of grief subside, the bereaved person's feelings stabilize, and they reinvest in new relationships and activities.

Experts, e.g., Parkes (2001), have become increasingly skeptical about stage models of grief. They propose that people's grief reactions vary depending on the circumstances of the death, the cultural, social, and economic context, the survivor's attachment style, and the quality of the previous relationship with the decedent (Carr, Nesse, & Wortman, 2005; Bonanno et al., 2002). People can experience different phases simultaneously or at different times, or even take respites from intense grieving by visiting with friends, neighbors, and family members. People also differ in the intensity with which they grieve, and certain feelings are more intense than others at different times. While some bereaved individuals feel extreme panic or anger, others focus more on positive experiences they had with the deceased (Ong, Bergeman, & Bisconti, 2004). Still others may feel relief after a spouse dies especially if they have been engaged in extensive caring. Cultural variations also influence how people manifest grief and experience bereavement.

Contemporary Models of Bereavement

New models of bereavement that take into account these individual and cultural variations have replaced these traditional stage theories of grief. Although many theories have emerged recently, those that have garnered the most attention include the stress paradigm, the attachment model, and the Dual Process Model of Bereavement, which is the focus of this paper.

The stress paradigm emphasizes the circumstances surrounding deaths and the coping approaches that people use when loved ones die (Folkman, 2001). Proponents of this perspective argue that people react differently to the loss of a loved one depending on the circumstances of the death, including their degree of preparation, the presence of chronic stressors, such as caregiving, and whether the loss led to new stressors (Ong et al., 2004). For example, widows who must learn how to manage household expenses for the first time have more problems adapting to their new lifestyles than women who always paid bills and kept track of family finances. Similarly, widowers whose wives made all their social arrangements risk social isolation and loneliness after their spouses die. Researchers who have operationalized this stress and coping model have found that longstanding personality indicators have less influence on bereavement outcome than how bereaved persons coped (Meuser & Marwit, 2000; Ong et al., 2004). These results underscore the importance of taking into account bereaved persons' coping strategies.

Attachment theorists have expanded their ideas to bereavement. Attachment theory became prominent from the work of John Bowlby (1980), who studied the dynamics and processes involved in bonding, forming attachments, and separating; he found that people's responses to loss grow out of their earlier attachments with parental figures. Bowlby and others, e.g., Parkes and Weiss (1983), observed that the responses of many adults who lose a significant attachment figure resemble the reactions of infants' early "protest" phase of separation, characterized by anxiety, anger, and denial, after an initial numbing or disbelief. If the separation continues, the person enters a phase of "despair," marked by preoccupation with the lost person and feelings of intense yearning, a core reaction to loss and separation from a loved one. During this phase, people are vigilant for the possible return of the lost person, and they despair when this does not occur. Over time, when the lost persons are never recovered, bereaved persons enter the phase of "detachment" (later called reorganization), in which they reinvest in new activities and relationships.

Bowlby (1980) and Ainsworth, Blehar, Waters, and Wall (1978) identified two types of attachments: secure attachment relationships and insecure attachment relationships. In secure attachments people perceive that they can rely on their caretakers as an available source of comfort and protection if the need arises. When threats of separation arise, people in secure relationships direct attachment behaviors (including approaching, crying, seeking contact, and seeking to maintain that contact) to their caretakers, and they take comfort in the reassurance they offer. Secure attachments promote exploration and mastery of the environment. People with these attachments feel certain that their caretakers will respond sensitively to their needs, so they develop comfortable relationships, and confidently interact with others. Insecure or anxiously attached persons lack this confidence in their caretakers. They distrust whether these persons will respond with comfort and reassurance when needed, and feel anxious and angry when a caretaker is inaccessible.

Parkes (2002) and others, e.g., Stroebe et al. (2002), have tried to link attachment styles to bereavement outcomes. Preliminary studies suggest that people who began with secure attachments developed secure attachments with significant others later. They responded with typical yearning reactions during bereavement and while grieving. They experienced less grief and less distress than those who were insecurely attached. This latter group more often clung to parental figures during childhood and manifested significant separation distress during bereavement.

In an attempt to integrate traditional models with recent research Stroebe and Schut (1999) proposed the Dual Process Model of Coping with Bereavement. This model is organized around three concepts: loss-oriented coping, restoration-oriented coping, and oscillation. Loss-oriented coping occurs most often during the early stages of bereavement when people concentrate on, deal with, and process some aspect of the loss experience itself. Loss-orientation resembles "grief work" and involves focusing on the deceased person, the circumstances of the loss, and negative feelings, such as yearning, despair, and painful longing. Restoration-oriented coping comprises what needs to be dealt with (e.g., social loneliness) and how it is dealt with (e.g., by avoiding solitariness), and not with the result of this process (e.g., restored well-being and social reintegration). It includes attending to life changes, doing new things, distracting oneself from grief, and establishing new roles, identities, and relationships. Oscillation refers to the "alternation between loss- and restoration-oriented coping, the process of juxtaposition of confrontation and avoidance of different stressors associated with bereavement" (Stroebe & Schut, 1999, p. 215). This back-and-forth process between loss-oriented and restoration-oriented coping helps people adjust to loss without grieving continually. According to Stroebe and Schut (1999), people preserve their physical and mental health by periodically taking time off from grieving to participate in activities, such as socializing with friends and family or taking part in church or community events. Both loss-oriented and restoration-oriented coping co-exist and are expressed intermittently, but people engage in more loss-oriented actions during the early stages of bereavement and more restoration-oriented activities later. In addition, they usually experience more negative affect in the beginning, but they eventually feel better when they socialize more and meet new people.

In a previous study with 200 bereaved men, Richardson and Balaswamy (2001) examined the impact of loss and restoration factors at earlier and later stages of bereavement, and found that the early bereaved expressed more negative affect and less positive affect than the later bereaved widowers. In addition, both loss-oriented and restoration-oriented activities were important early and later in bereavement. Although the circumstances surrounding the loss (e.g., whether husbands had provided medical care to wives, and whether their wives died at home or in a hospital setting) influenced negative feelings, restoration-oriented interactions (e.g., involvement with neighbors) also affected a widower's well-being during early stages of bereavement. Widowers who dated later during bereavement experienced higher levels of positive affect than those who were not dating. I replicated Richardson and Balaswamy's earlier study by used a longitudinal sample that included older men and women who were tested at 6 months, 18 months, and 48 months after the death of their spouses. The results from these analyses are presented below.

METHOD

Participants

The Changing Lives of Older Couples (CLOC) study is a prospective study of a two-stage area probability sample of 1,532 married individuals from the

Detroit Standard Metropolitan Statistical Area (SMSA). To be eligible for the study, respondents had to be English-speaking members of a married couple in which the husband was aged 65 or older. All sample members were not institutionalized and were capable of participating in a 2-hour interview. Approximately 65% of those contacted for an interview participated, which is consistent with the response rate from other Detroit area studies. Baseline face-to-face interviews were conducted from June 1987 through April 1988.

The CLOC researchers monitored spousal loss by reading the daily obituaries in three Detroit-area newspapers and by using monthly death record tapes provided by the State of Michigan. The National Death Index (NDI) was used to confirm deaths and obtain causes of death. Of the 319 respondents who lost a spouse during the study, 86% (n = 276) participated in at least one of the three follow-up interviews, which were conducted 6 months (Wave 1), 18 months (Wave 2), and 48 months (Wave 3) after the death. The primary reasons for nonresponse were refusal to participate (38%) and ill health or death at follow-up (42%). Controls from the original sample of 1,545 were selected to match the widowed persons along the dimensions of age, race, and sex. The matched controls were reinterviewed at the three follow-up interviews at roughly the same time as their corresponding widowed persons (Carr et al., 2001).

I focused on bereaved persons at six months, Wave 1 (N = 250), 18 months, Wave 2 (N = 210), and four years after the loss of the spouse, Wave 3 (N = 106), for this investigation. Women were oversampled originally to maximize the number of respondents who would experience bereavement during the project. As a result, the sample included 35 men and 215 women at Wave 1 and 29 men and 181 women at Wave 2. The data on the widowers, who were analyzed separately from the widows, were weighted to adjust for unequal probabilities of selection and differential response rate at baseline. This resulted in 59 men at Wave 1 and 45 men at Wave 2. Only widows were analyzed at Wave 3. At Waves 1, 2, and 3, 83, 200, and 102 matched non-bereaved persons, respectively, were used as controls. About 80% of the respondents agreed to participate. Non-participants tended to be older, more anxious, and to own their homes at Wave 1 (Carr, 2001).

Measures

Dependent Variables. Bradburn's (1969) Affect Balance Scale (ABS) was used to measure the psychological well-being of respondents. Although this scale is a two-factor model, it generates three scores: quantity of positive affect, quantity of negative affect and ratio of positive to negative affect. The ratio of positive to negative affect measures overall psychological well-being. Many researchers have successfully used the ABS to measure psychological well-being (see Richardson and Balaswamy, 2001 for a more detailed discussion of the ABS).

The items that comprised negative affect included: (1) During the past week, I felt depressed about everything. (Did you feel this way hardly ever, some of the time, or most of the time?) (2) During the past week I felt lonely (same coding scheme). (3) During the past week, I felt that people disliked me. (4) During the past week, people were unfriendly. (5) How much have you felt so restless you couldn't sit still? (Did you feel this way not at all, a little bit, or extremely?)

The positive affect scale included: (1) Tell me how often you have felt particularly excited or interested in something during the past week. (always, often, sometimes, rarely, or never) (2) How often have your felt pleased about having accomplished something (same coding scheme)? (3) How often have you felt that things were going your way (same coding scheme)? (4) How often have you felt proud because someone complimented you on something you had done (same coding scheme)? (5) How often have you felt on top of the world (same coding scheme)?

These items comprised the negative and positive affect scales at the baseline measure, at six months following the death of the spouse, at 18 months follow-up, and at 48 months follow-up. Overall well-being was coded as positive affect subtracted by negative affect (PA-NA). A reliability analysis for the negative and positive affect measures was conducted at baseline and at each wave. In this paper, I focus on overall well-being although predictors of positive and negative affect often differ (Richardson & Balaswamy, 2001).

Despite moderate reliability coefficients, researchers use the ABS for several reasons. First, they prefer that it is an indirect measure of well-being and, thus less susceptible to social desirability. Second, they consider respondents' combined answers to several different items more valid than responses to one or two questions (Bradburn, 1969). Third, the Bradburn scale has demonstrated strong associations with other measures of negative affect, specifically anxiety and worries. Stacey and Gatz (1991) found it had convergent validity with the CES-D (Center for Epidemiological Studies Depression Scale).

Independent Variables. The independent variables comprised loss-oriented measures and reinvestment or restoration-oriented indices based on Stroebe and Schut's Dual Process Model of Bereavement. In addition, I included variables based on results from an earlier study (Richardson & Balaswamy, 2001). Several variables representing tasks related to a spouse's death, death circumstances, and other variables related to the loss were included as independent variables. These and the restoration-oriented variables, along with how they were coded, are listed in Table 1.

TABLE 1. Description of Independent Variables

Loss-Oriented Variables		Restoration-Oriented Variables	
Death Influences	M (SD)	Social Activities	M (SD)
Spouse's Condition was Painful (very true, some true, little, not true)	.94 (1.35)	Visit Friends (# week or month from 1 to 5 or never)	2.24 (1.23)
Spouse was Aware of Dying (yes, don't know, no)	43% yes	Friends/Relatives Total Support	.52 (.86)
Spouse Died from Ongoing Condition (suddenly, short notice, ongoing)	54% ongoing	Confidante (yes, no)	87% yes
		Contact with Children	1.34 (.72)
		Dating (yes, no)	3% yes
How Often went to Cemetery (a lot, little, none)	1.9 (1.1)	Attend Religious Services # Times Wk/Mo (5 categs)	2.7 (1.38)
Drawn to Places Spouse Went (never, rarely, some, often)	2.38 (1.37)	Attend Meetings (<1X-WK, 1X-WK, 1-3X-Mo, <1X-Mo, Never)	3.5 (1.47)
		Volunteer Work-12 mos (yes, no)	29% yes
Frequency Talked About Death (several times daily, daily, few Xs week, 1 a week, <1wk, never)	3.53 (1.36)	How Much Take Walks/Drive (a lot, little, never)	1.6 (.80)
Go Over and Over What Happened (never, rarely, some, often)	2.34 (1.2)	Hobbies (<1X-WK, 1X-WK, 1-3X-Mo, <1X-Mo, Never)	2.6 (1.6)
		Sports/Exercise (Often, sometime, rarely, never)	3.1 (1.2)
		Moved (yes, no)	93% no
		Changed Jobs (yes, no)	94% no

RESULTS

Sample Characteristics

The characteristics of the sample are described in Table 2. Few gender differences were statistically significant except for the respondent's age (men were older), age of the spouse at death (men were younger than women), whether the spouse lived in a nursing home prior to death (more women died

TABLE 2. Characteristics of Participants

	Women (n = 151)		Men (n = 59)	
	M or %	SD	M or %	SD
Warning Time Indicators				
No warning time before death	0.373	0.485	0.319	0.47
6 or more months warning time	0.287	0.454	0.288	0.457
Warning time, months	5.09	8.00	5.95	9.3
Death Context				
Spouse's age at death	77.1	6.42	72.56	7.3**
Spouse in ns. home before death	0.015	0.123	0.138	0.347**
Provided care to spouse in 6 mos prior to death	0.502	0.502	0.436	0.5
Communication About Death				
R and spouse discussed how R will cope with death	0.196	0.398	0.116	0.323
R was with spouse at death	0.397	0.491	0.536	0.503*
Demographic Characteristics				
Age, baseline	69.43	6.99	73.46	5.92***
Years of education	11.33	2.69	11.11	3.44
Own home, baseline	0.898	0.304	0.966	0.182
Income, baseline	20,480	16,380	22,511	16,745
Natural log of income	1.29	0.523	1.37	0.522
Months between baseline and Wave 1 interviews	36.55	18.15	35.83	19.21
Baseline Well-Being				
Depression, baseline (standardized)	0.128	1.05	−.089	0.736
Anxiety, baseline (standardized)	0.152	1.09	−.205	0.715*
Fair or poor health, baseline	0.299	0.459	0.409	0.497

Notes: t tests were used to assess significant gender differences between means. *Ns* are weighted *Ns*.
*p ≤ .05; **p ≤ .01; ***p ≤ .001.

in nursing homes than men), and whether the respondent was with the spouse at death (more men than women reported that they were with the spouse at the time of death) (Carr, 2001).

Changes in Well-Being Over Time

In Figure 1, the well-being of widows is compared to the controls at Wave 1, Wave 2, and Wave 3. The scores on the well-being scale for widows were 7.7, 8.5, and 8.6 at Waves 1, 2, and 3, respectively, while the well-being scores for the controls were 10.3, 9.9, and 9.2, respectively, for this same period. Note that widows and controls differed most at Wave 1 and became more similar by Wave 3; however, this was partly due to the decline in well-being among the non-bereaved from Wave 1 to Wave 3. These findings corroborated previous studies that have suggested that bereavement is especially stressful during the first year (Wilcox et al., 2003).

Multiple regression analyses were also conducted for the well-being scale at Wave 1 and Wave 2, separately for men and for women. Because of the small number of widowers at Wave 3, only women were analyzed at the four year follow-up. The results from these analyses are presented in Table 3.

Several conclusions can be drawn from these analyses. First, both loss and restoration variables influenced affect throughout bereavement, which supports Stroebe and Schut's (1999) Dual Process Model of Bereavement. For example, engaging in hobbies increased well-being for both men and women at Wave 1 and again for women at Wave 3. Interactions with friends, and especially confidantes among women, also influenced well-being at all phases of

FIGURE 1. Bradburn Effect Over Time Among Widows and Controls

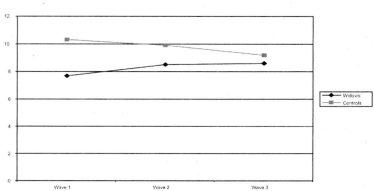

TABLE 3. Summary of Predictors of Well-Being

Wave 1		Wave 2		Wave 3	
Men	Women	Men	Women	Men	Women
Cemetery ($B = -.419***$)	Cemetery ($B = -.125*$)				Talk About ($B = -.210*$)
Don't Go Over ($B = .207*$)	Don't Go Over ($B = -.323***$)	Don't Go Over ($B = -.322***$)	Don't Go Over ($B = -.187*$)		Time Caring (mos.) ($B = -.281**$)
Sudden Death ($B = -.342***$)					
Hobbies ($B = -.357***$)	Hobbies ($B = -.338***$)	Religion ($B = -.541***$)	Religion ($B = -.202*$)		Hobbies ($B = -.341***$)
Friends ($B = -.361***$)	Confidante ($B = -.185**$)	Mtgs ($B = -.530***$)	Friends ($B = -.255*$)		Friends ($B = -.261*$)
	Mtgs ($B = -.175**$)	No Move ($B = -.711***$)	Job Chg ($B = -.168*$)		Confidante ($B = -.258*$)
					Moved ($B = -.347**$)
N = 59[+] R² = 67%	N = 215 R² = 33%	N = 45[+] R² = 83%	N = 181 R² = 17%		N = 96 R² = 32%

[+]*Notes: Ns* for men are weighted *Ns.*
$*p \leq .05; **p \leq .01; ***p \leq .001.$

bereavement. Yet circumstances of the death, such as whether one died from an ongoing condition or more suddenly, which significantly influenced bereaved men at Wave 1 (men whose wives died from an ongoing condition had lower well-being than men whose wives died suddenly), and how long one cared for one's spouse, which was significantly associated with well-being among widows at Wave 3 (widows who spent more months caring for their husbands had higher levels of well-being than widows who spent less time in these activities), also influenced well-being.

One of the most consistent predictors of well-being was how often widowed persons went over and over what happened. This was inversely related to well-being at Waves 1 and 2 for both men and women. Bereaved persons who ruminated more about the circumstances of their spouses' deaths demonstrated lower levels of well-being than those who rarely thought about what happened.

Religion was an important buffer for both men and women, and some significant gender differences emerged. For example, while widows who moved and changed jobs had higher well-being than women who did not experience these life changes, widowers who moved experienced lower well-being at Wave 2.

Although loss and restoration-oriented activities emerged as relevant throughout bereavement suggesting that people oscillate between these tasks or concomitantly deal with them, bereaved persons were more likely to engage in some activities during the early stages of bereavement and others in the later stages. Attending religious services may have buffered the initial pain of loss more during the early stages of bereavement than at the later stages. Visiting the cemetery was also more important during the early stages of bereavement than four years later. Social interactions, especially with friends, bolstered bereaved persons' affect throughout bereavement. Friendships, including interactions with confidantes, are especially needed for both widows and widowers to enhance well-being.

DISCUSSION

These findings support Stroebe and Schut's principles that bereaved persons engage in loss- and restoration-oriented activities throughout bereavement and corroborate Richardson and Balaswamy's findings among bereaved men. The significant associations between well-being and religious and social involvements resemble findings from other studies that demonstrate the buffering effects of religion and social support on grieving (Siegel & Kuykendall, 1990; Stroebe, Stroebe & Abakoumkin, 1999).

The significant inverse association between well-being and going over and over what happened suggests that practitioners need to help widowed persons differentiate constructive from destructive grief activities. While many widows and widowers benefit from visiting cemeteries and thinking about their loved ones, those who dwell excessively on the circumstances of a spouse's death might compromise their mental health. The direction of causality is unclear here, but others, e.g., Nolen-Hokesema (2002), have shown significant associations between rumination and depression. Practitioners should carefully assess how bereaved persons' grieving styles enhance or threaten their well-being. The significant differences in levels of well-being between the widows and controls in this study also attest to the significance of this life event many years later.

This investigation contains several limitations. One is unable to generalize these findings to subsequent cohorts of older widowed persons because they pertain to a particular cohort. The small number of widowers in the sample is another limitation. More in-depth studies of bereaved men with larger samples are needed to better understand older widowers' grief reactions. Future analyses of longitudinal samples should also focus on changes over time. In addition, several results in this research suggest that while some resources, such as friends and confidantes or religious involvement, mitigate the negative effects of losing a spouse, others, such as whether a spouse died suddenly or required long term care, can exacerbate grieving. The implications of these findings for grief counseling and social work practice are discussed below.

Grief Counseling

Grief counseling works best for those who seek help, who are in high distress, and, most importantly, who are at risk for complicated grief (Schut et al., 2001). Grief counseling can have adverse effects if it is administered preventatively with people who have not asked for help. When grief counseling is offered before bereaved persons' natural support systems have responded, friends and family members sometimes withdraw their support, especially if they sense that a bereaved person has alternatives (Schut, Stroebe, van den Bout, & Terheggen, 2001).

Clients vary in what they find useful during counseling. Some clients simply appreciate knowing that help is available, whether or not they use it. Others are glad to learn that their feelings are normal and that the acute pain of grief will eventually subside. One widow might learn how to manage her bills, while another gains new interpersonal skills or coping strategies. Some bereaved persons benefit from self-help groups; others need individual counseling (see Richardson, 2005, for a more in-depth discussion of bereavement interventions and services). The conclusions from reviews of the efficacy of bereavement counseling underscore the importance of assessment. Social workers can more effectively individualize grief counseling by comprehensively evaluating a bereaved client's context, circumstances, and personality. The tremendous variability in people's grieving indicates the need for comprehensive assessments and integrated, holistic approaches to bereavement counseling. Social workers who are sensitive to bereaved clients' needs and unique trajectories throughout bereavement will more effectively help bereaved persons find benefits from their experiences.

The Dual Process Model of Bereavement Counseling

The results from this research suggest that the circumstances of bereavement, such as whether a spouse died suddenly or after a long illness, and the extent to which someone emphasizes loss- or restoration-oriented coping, influence older persons' adjustments to widowhood. Many complicated grief reactions result from bereaved individuals' over-reliance on loss-oriented tasks or cognitions and from neglect of restoration types of involvements, such as attending religious services or interacting with friends and family members (Stroebe et al., 2002). These people need help bolstering their restoration-oriented skills and behaviors.

Stroebe and Schut (1999) recommend that bereaved persons accept not only the reality of loss, but also the reality of a changed world; experience the pain of grief and take time off from the pain of grief; and while they must adjust to life without the deceased they must concomitantly master a changed environment. Many widows and widowers continue to talk about their loved ones and maintain strong bonds with them but nevertheless move on to new jobs and different living arrangements. The bereaved persons who often visited the cemetery but avoided ruminating about what happened experienced higher levels of well-being than those who avoided the ceremony or dwelled on what happened, according to the findings from this research. Those who spent time with friends and confidantes and engaged in hobbies also adjusted more easily to the loss of a spouse than those who infrequently socialized with close companions. Widowed persons who overemphasize either loss or restoration-oriented coping need help balancing these activities.

Meaning-Making and Personal Growth

Bereaved persons who find meaning from grieving typically adjust better than those who avoid these existential concerns (Neimeyer, 1998). Meaning is comprised of two processes: finding meaning and finding benefit (Davis and Nolen-Hoeksema, 2001). Finding meaning involves making sense of the loss and focuses on maintaining or rebuilding a threatened worldview. The other process–finding benefit–consists of maintaining or rebuilding a threatened sense of self. Clinicians can help bereaved persons reestablish more control and meaning in their lives by helping them accept some outcomes and focus on areas that they can control, whether at a job or on a project or in relationships. Various obstacles prevent bereaved persons from successfully finding meaning and achieving control. Some losses are also easier to recover from and make sense of than others. Suicides and violent deaths are especially disturbing and difficult to grieve. People who think irrationally, avoid examining circumstances, and rigidly adhere to certain beliefs struggle more to find meaning than those who openly reflect about their situations (Thompson, 1998). According to Harvey, Orbuch, Weber, Merbach, and Alt (1992), it could take as long as 200 hours to resolve bereavement issues and achieve some closure to the loss. In addition, bereaved persons must feel comfortable talking about and focusing on the death and remain open to alternative conceptualizations of events.

The search for meaning is most beneficial to bereaved persons during the first few months following the death, but later, as the death becomes more remote, this process is less therapeutic, according to Davis and Nolen-Hoeksema (2001). Calhoun and Tedeschi (2001) also caution clinicians that some clients dread exploring the meaning of events. In these instances, clinicians should not pressure clients to "find meaning." Meaning-making can exacerbate bereaved persons' distress when they believe that what happened to them was senseless and random (Davis and Nolen-Hoeksema, 2001). These bereaved persons will benefit less from finding meaning and more from finding benefit, i.e., focusing on personal value or significance to the event, i.e., discovering how they may have grown or developed new strengths as a result of their experiences.

Finding benefit can be manifested in growth of character, change in life perspective, or strengthened relationships with others. Although clients should direct the discussions about finding benefit, social workers can facilitate the process in various ways. Gamino, Sewell, and Easterling (2000) found four factors that predicted positive outcomes and personal growth: seeing some good resulting from the death, having a chance to say goodbye to the loved one, intrinsic spirituality, and spontaneous positive memories of the decedent. They suggested that clinicians could facilitate positive growth by helping mourners recast their stories of death and loss in positive ways that can still include sorrowful aspects. In instances where bereaved persons missed opportunities to communicate prior to a death, clinicians can help grieving persons find symbolic ways to say goodbye, such as writing letters or visiting gravesites. Bereaved persons who have a religious affiliation might find comfort by becoming more involved with their organizations by finding alternative spiritual resources. Finally, instead of avoiding reminders of the deceased, clinicians can help bereaved clients visit cemeteries and celebrate special memories, which often strengthens people's connections to their loved ones. Most bereaved persons comment that they achieved the most personal growth after the intense grieving period subsided, when they felt ready to reinvest in life and strong enough to try out new activities and relationships.

Personal growth can emerge from transformations independent of the deceased. For example, some older widows who for the first time learn to manage their bills, attend to home repairs, and fix their cars feel empowered when they master new skills. Many bereaved women from this cohort often feel self-sufficient for the first time in their lives. Widows who moved and acquired new jobs experienced higher levels of well-being than those who avoided changes in this study. Personal growth occurs when an individual's social resources, coping skills, or personal resources are enhanced after bereavement (Shaefer & Moos, 2001). The majority of widows and widowers, regardless of the circumstances of their loved one's death, will find benefit and derive meaning from their grief.

Those who suffer from complicated bereavement need specialized treatments based on careful assessments. Unresolved issues, such as problems with dependency, often underlie chronic grieving and exacerbate these persons' anxieties, fears, and feelings of yearning for their deceased loved ones. Many circumstances contribute to complicated grief. Although many experts agree that complicated grief disorders exist, they have not yet agreed on how best to treat these disorders. Social workers should learn more about normal grieving, the different patterns of bereavement, and complicated grief reactions, including traumatic grief, which Prigerson and Jacobs (2001) have discussed, as well as chronic grief and chronic depression, which Bonanno et al. (2002) and Bonanno, Nesse, and Wortman (2004) have identified. Social workers should also remain abreast of innovative interventions created to help bereaved persons who seek help with normal grieving and of recent treatments designed to help those struggling with complications from grief.

NOTE

1. A previous version of this paper was presented at the First National Gerontological Social Work Conference, Atlanta, Georgia, February 28, 2003.

REFERENCES

Ainsworth, M. D. S., Blehar, M., Waters, E., & Wall, S. (1978). *Patterns of attachment: A psychological study of the strange situation.* Hillsdale, NJ: Erlbaum.

Bonanno, G. A., Wortman, C. B., & Nesse, R. M. (2004). Prospective patterns of resilience and maladjustment during widowhood. *Psychology and Aging, 19,* 260-271.

Bonanno, G. A., Lehman, D. R., Tweed, R. G., Haring, M., Wortman, C., Sonnega, J., Carr, D., & Nesse, R. M. (2002). Resilience to loss and chronic grief: A prospective study from preloss to 18-months postloss. *Journal of Personality and Social Psychology, 83,* 1150-1164.

Bowlby, J. (1980). *Attachment and loss: Volume 3.* New York: Basic Books.

Bowlby, J., & Parkes, C. (1970). Separation and loss within the family. In E.J. Anthony & C. M. Koupernik (Eds.). *The child in his family* (pp. 197-216). New York: Wiley.

Bradburn, N. M. (1969). *The structure of psychological well-being.* Chicago: Aldine.

Calhoun, L., & Tedeschi, R. (2001). Posttraumatic growth: The positive lessons of loss. In R. Neimeyer (Ed.) *Meaning reconstruction and the experience of loss* (pp. 157-172). Washington, DC: American Psychological Association.

Carr, D., Nesse, R. M., & Wortman, C. B. (2005). *Widowhood in late life: New directions in theory, research and practice.* New York: Springer Publishing Company.

Carr, D., House, J., Wortman, C., Nesse, R., & Kessler, R. (2001). Psychological adjustment to sudden and anticipated spousal loss among older widowed persons. *Journal of Gerontology: Social Sciences 56B,* S237-S248.

Davis, C. (2001). The tormented and the transformed: Understanding response to loss and trauma. In R. Neimeyer (Ed). *Meaning reconstruction and the experience of loss* (pp. 137-155). Washington, DC: American Psychological Association.

Davis, C. G., & Nolen-Hoeksema, S. (2001). Loss and meaning: How do people make sense of loss. *American Behavioral Scientist 44,* 726-741.

Folkman, S. (2001). Revised coping theory and the process of bereavement. In M. S. Stroebe, R. O. Hansson, W. Stroebe, W. & H. Schut (Eds). *Handbook of bereavement research: Consequences, coping, and care* (pp. 563-584). Washington, DC: American Psychological Association.

Fraley, R. C., & Shaver, P. R. (1999). Loss and bereavement: Attachment theory and recent controversies concerning "Grief Work" and the nature of detachment. J. S. Cassidy and P.R. Shaver (Eds.). *Handbook of attachment: Theory, research, and clinical applications* (pp. 735-739). New York: Guilford Press.

Gamino, L., Sewell, K., & Easterling, L. (2000). Scott and White grief study–phase 2: Toward an adaptive model of grief. *Death Studies, 24,* 633-640.

Harvey, J., Orbuch, R. L., Weber, A. L., Merbach, N., & Alt, R. (1992). House of pain and hope: Accounts of loss. *Death Studies, 16,* 99-124.

Jacobs, S. (1999). *Traumatic grief: Diagnosis, treatment, and prevention.* Philadelphia: Brunner/Mazel.

Janoff-Bulman, R., & Berg, M. (1998). Disillusionment and the creation of value: From traumatic losses to existential gains. In J. H. Harvey (Ed). *Perspectives on loss: A sourcebook* (pp. 35-47). Philadelphia: Taylor & Francis.

Kubler-Ross, E. (1969). *On death and dying.* New York: Springer Publishing Company.

Lindemann, E. (1944). Symptomatology and management of acute grief. *American Journal of Psychiatry, 101,* 141-148.

Meuser, T., & Marwich, S. (1999/2000). An integrative model of personality, coping and appraisal for the prediction of grief involvement in adults. *Omega: Journal of Death and Dying, 40,* 375-393.

Neimeyer, R. (1998). *Lessons of loss: A guide to coping.* New York: McGraw-Hill.

Nolen-Hoeksema, S. (2002). Stress and coping in bereavement. Presentation delivered at the Changing lives of older couples: Exploring bereavement among older adults workshop. Ann Arbor: University of Michigan.

Ong, A. D., Bergeman, C. S., & Bisconti, T. L. (2004), The role of daily positive emotions during conjugal bereavement. *Journal of Gerontology: Psychological Sciences, 59B,* P168-176.

Parkes, C. M., & Weiss, R. (1983). *Recovery from bereavement.* New York: Basic Books.

Parkes, C. M. (1985). Bereavement. *British Journal of Psychiatry, 146,* 11-17.

Parkes, C. M. (2001). A Historical overview of the scientific study of bereavement. In M. S. Stroebe, R.O. Hansson, W. Stroebe & H. Schut (Eds.) *Handbook of bereavement research: Consequences, coping, and care* (pp. 25-45). Washington, DC: American Psychological Association.

Parkes, C. M. (2002). Grief: Lessons from the past, visions for the future. *Death Studies, 26*, 367-385.

Prigerson, H., & Jacobs, S. (2001). Traumatic grief as a distinct disorder: A rationale, consensus criteria, and a preliminary empirical test. In M. Stroebe, R.O. Hansson, W. Stroebe & H. Schut (Eds.) *Handbook of bereavement research: Consequences, coping, and care* (pp. 613-637). Washington, DC: American Psychological Association.

Reisman, A. (2001). Death of a spouse: Illusory basic assumptions and continuation of bonds. *Death Studies, 25*, 445-460.

Richardson, V. E., & Balaswamy, S. (2001). Coping with bereavement among elderly widowers. *Omega: Journal of Death and Dying, 43*, 129-144.

Richardson, V. E. (2005). Implications for public policies and social services: What social workers and other gerontology practitioners can learn from the CLOC. In D. Carr, R. M. Nesse, and C. B. Wortman (Eds.). *Widowhood in late life: New directions in theory, research and practice.* New York: Springer Publishing Company.

Schaefer, J., & Moos, R. (2001). Bereavement experiences and personal growth. In M. Stroebe, R. O. Hansson, W. Stroebe, W. & H. Schut (Eds.). *Handbook of bereavement research: Consequences, coping, and care* (pp. 145-167). Washington, DC: American Psychological Association.

Schut, H. A., Stroebe, M. S., van den Bout, J., & Terheggen, M. (2001). The efficacy of bereavement interventions: Determining who benefits. M. S. Stroebe, R. O. Hansson, W. Stroebe, & H. Schut (Eds.) *Handbook of bereavement research: Consequences, coping, and care* (pp. 705-737). Washington, DC: American Psychological Association.

Shaver, P. R., & Brennan, K. A. (1992). Attachment styles and the "Big Five" personality traits: Their connections with each other and with romantic relationship outcomes. *Personality and Social Psychology Bulletin, 18*, 536-545.

Siegel, J., & Kuykendall, D. (1990). Loss, widowhood, and psychological distress among the elderly. *Journal of Consulting and Clinical Psychology, 58*, 519-524.

Stacy, C., & Gatz, M. (1991). Cross-sectional age differences and longitudinal change on the Bradburn Affect Balance Scale. *Journal of Gerontology, 46*, P76-P78.

Stroebe, W., Stroebe, M., & Abakoumkin, G. (1999). Does differential social support cause sex differences in bereavement outcome? *Journal of Community and Applied Social Psychology, 9*, 1-12.

Stroebe, M., & Schut, H. (1999). The dual process model of coping with bereavement: Rationale and description. *Death Studies, 23*, 197-224.

Stroebe, M., Schut, H., Stroebe, W., van den Bout, J., Zech, E., Gergen, M., & Gergen, K. (2002). Coping with attachment in bereavement: Toward better outcome prediction. Presentation delivered at the Changing lives of older couples: Exploring bereavement among older adults workshop. Ann Arbor: University of Michigan.

Thompson, S. (1998). Blockades to finding meaning and control. In J. Harvey (Ed.) *Perspectives on loss* (pp. 21-34). Philadelphia: Brunner/Mazel.

Wilcox, S., Aragaki, A., Mouton, C., Evenson, K., Wassertheil-Smoller, S., & Loevinger, B. L. (2003). The effects of widowhood on physical and mental health,

health behaviors, and health outcomes: The Women's Health Initiative. *Health Psychology, 22,* 1-10.

Worden, W. (1991). *Grief counseling and grief therapy: A handbook for the mental health practitioners.* New York: Springer Publishing Company.

Wortman, C., & Silver, R. C. (1989). The myths of coping with loss. *Journal of Consulting and Clinical Psychology, 57,* 349-357.

doi:10.1300/J083v48n03_03

Spiritual Assessment in Aging:
A Framework for Clinicians

Holly Nelson-Becker, PhD, LCSW
Mitsuko Nakashima, PhD
Edward R. Canda, PhD

SUMMARY. Older adults may benefit from clinical conversations about the role of spirituality in their lives, but social workers and other helping professionals often do not have an understanding of where to proceed beyond initial questions of whether spirituality and/or religion are important and if so, what religious preference is held. Much has been written about definitions of spirituality and religion, but the literature has not yet provided a clear focus on ways to assess whether these are integrated positively or negatively in the lives of older adults. This article identifies eleven domains in spirituality that might be assessed. Within each domain an explanation is provided as well as a brief discussion of the rationale for including it in the classification. Sample interview questions and an illustrative vignette are included. Together these eleven domains build an important framework and resource for spiritual assessment with older adults. doi:10.1300/J083v48n03_04 *[Article copies available for a fee from The Haworth Document Delivery Service: 1-800-HAWORTH. E-mail address: <docdelivery@haworthpress.com> Website: <http://www.HaworthPress.com> © 2007 by The Haworth Press, Inc. All rights reserved.]*

[Haworth co-indexing entry note]: "Spiritual Assessment in Aging: A Framework for Clinicians." Nelson-Becker, Holly, Mitsuko Nakashima, and Edward R. Canda. Co-published simultaneously in *Journal of Gerontological Social Work* (The Haworth Press, Inc.) Vol. 48, No. 3/4, 2007, pp. 331-347; and: *Fostering Social Work Gerontology Competence: A Collection of Papers from the First National Gerontological Social Work Conference* (ed: Catherine J. Tompkins, and Anita L. Rosen) The Haworth Press, Inc., 2007, pp. 331-347. Single or multiple copies of this article are available for a fee from The Haworth Document Delivery Service [1-800-HAWORTH, 9:00 a.m. - 5:00 p.m. (EST). E-mail address: docdelivery@haworthpress.com].

Available online at http://jgsw.haworthpress.com
© 2007 by The Haworth Press, Inc. All rights reserved.
doi:10.1300/J083v48n03_04

KEYWORDS. Spirituality, religion, aging, assessment, social work

INTRODUCTION

Assessment with older adults assists social workers and other geriatric professionals to identify how therapeutic and rehabilitative services can maintain or restore a satisfying quality of life. Social work has a tradition of providing geriatric evaluations as part of a healthcare team, but a gerontological social work assessment has a broader scope than one limited to helping older adults cope with disability. Because of the profession's commitment to understand human experiences from a holistic perspective, assessment and intervention involve not only considering physical, social, and psychological levels of functioning from the perspective of the client and significant others, but also factors related to spiritual support and distress. The goal of this paper is to discuss important domains in spiritual assessment that have particular relevance for older adults.

Research in religion and spirituality among different disciplines such as medicine, nursing, psychology, and social work has recently benefited from renewed interest, especially as the healthcare field has begun to explore whether religious beliefs and practice have any correlation with improved health outcomes (Koenig, 2002a; Koenig, McCullough & Larsen, 2001; Jackson, Chatters & Taylor, 1993). Health is identified by minority older adults who reside independently as a major life challenge second only to loss of family and friends; religious resources are their primary means of coping (Nelson-Becker, in press). Health generally is a concern of all older adults, but especially those who manage chronic illness and declining physical reserves (Kahana, Redmond, Hill, Kercher, Kahana, Johnson, & Young, 1995). Because gerontology enfolds large percentages of older adults who subscribe to the importance of religion, practitioners who work with older adults are strongly encouraged to develop assessment and intervention skills that address clients' religious/spiritual issues.

Existing research has shown that spirituality and religion play a significant role in the lives of older adults and their ability to cope with various hardships that accompany the aging process (Ramsey & Blieszner, 1999). For example, researchers have found a salient connection between religion and older adults' ability to cope with chronic illnesses (Mackenzie, Rajagopal, Meibohm & Lavizzo-Mourey, 2000), grief (MacKinlay, 2002), and facing their own mortality during the final stage in life (Herman, 2001; Nakashima, 2002).

Spirituality encompasses that which is regarded as sacred. Spirituality has been defined as connections with a power, purpose, or idea that transcends the self

(Canda, 1988; Joseph, 1988). It is the "search for significance in ways related to the sacred" (Pargament, 1997, p. 34). Caroll (2001) proposes a distinction between possible key interpretations centered in the word spirituality. It may be but one dimension among the many aspects of being (i.e., bio-psycho-social-spiritual) or it may be viewed alternately as the core or essence of the person. Spirituality is the motivational and emotional foundation of the quest for meaning. The transpersonal dimension of human experiences (i.e., states of consciousness that reach beyond the ordinary waking state such as a dream state or mystical experiences) is an important aspect of spirituality as it can often offer opportunities for spiritual transformation.

The most common uses of the terms spirituality and religion are that spirituality is concerned with the universal "aspect of what it is to be human, to search for a sense of meaning, purpose, and moral guidance for relating with self, others and ultimate reality" (Canda & Furman, 1999, p. 37) while religion involves a community's formalized, institutional pattern of beliefs, practices, and values that focus on spiritual concerns (Canda, 1997; Nelson-Becker, 1999). Therefore, in this article when we use the term spirituality, we include religious and nonreligious expressions.

SPIRITUAL ASSESSMENT IN THE CONTEXT OF SOCIAL WORK PRACTICE

Spirituality for social work is perceived as an overarching dimension that includes religion as one expression among many others. An operational model of spirituality is proposed by Canda and Furman (1999) who suggest that spirituality may be manifested in six interrelated domains including spiritual drives, spiritual experiences, functions of spirituality, spiritual development, content of an individual's or group's spiritual perspective, and for many people, religious expressions. Different types of spiritual manifestation in older adults' lives, whether single or combined with religion, can be explicitly identified and used in a manner to lead older adults to access resources that support coping and to integrate new understandings as they respond to change.

Spiritual domains have particular relevance for older adults who were often raised against the backdrop of a religious context in the United States. A recent Gallup poll confirmed that 58% of respondents assessed religion as very important while 68% hold membership in a religious organization (Princeton Religious Research Center [PRCC], 2001). This may carry different meanings for such older adults as a Catholic widow who seeks companionship and religious satisfaction through attending daily mass, an African-American man who relies on the African Methodist Episcopal church as a base of life continuity and extended friendships, a German-American woman from the Amana Colonies in Iowa who has lived with a religious minority history woven distinctively into community life patterns, or a Jewish Holocaust survivor who embraces spiritual concerns with meaning but does not participate in religion. The diversity of spirituality in aging ranges, for example, from the committed born-again Christian to the nominal Christian, from the Jewish Holocaust survivor who embraces spirituality only to the Orthodox Jew, or from the Laotian American who is a devoted practitioner of Theravada Buddhism to the Laotian American who is a convert to Christianity.

Spirituality should be explored with older adults whenever they identify that it is significant in their lives and relevant to their goals for the helping process. Older adults may seek social services for a number of reasons. Social workers need to be alert and proactive in helping older adults utilize spiritual resources to strengthen their resiliency. Some of the challenging circumstances that might call for careful examination of older clients' spirituality include but are not limited to the following: depression; relocation; chronic or terminal illness; anxiety about death; bereavement; caregiving; substance abuse; crisis of faith; abuse/neglect; and any trauma, difficult life event, or condition. Spirituality might also be examined for positive reasons such as when the client mentions it is central to his/her identity, gives a profound sense of meaning and purpose, shapes a positive outlook on mortality and death, or provides important resources of support via religious communities or spiritual friends and mentors.

The purpose of spiritual assessment for older adults is to clarify the role of spirituality in daily life. What are the values that the older individual assigns to his/her own spiritual practices, if any? What positive and negative associations does the older adult have with his/her religious background and history of religious affiliations? Questions about an older adult's spirituality help the social worker understand client worldview and context, facilitate client self-exploration, explore religion and spirituality as client resources, ascertain the degree of helpfulness in the client's belief system, uncover religious or spiritual problems, and determine appropriate helping activities (Frame, 2003).

Although assessment is a collaborative process, older adults may not voice spiritual concerns and interests unless the practitioner provides supportive space in the interaction for that to explicitly occur. For example, in one study (Nelson-Becker, 1999), older adults indicated they only discussed their religious coping strategies when specific questions about it were presented. Because religion and spirituality hold somewhat personalized positions in our culture, older adults will not usually initiate discussion in these areas unless directly asked, even when it may be the basis for their help-seeking behavior.

It is important to ascertain the client's interest before pursing spirituality. Even if the issues of religion/spirituality may not become a focal point of the immediate intervention with clients, the social worker will have further information on which to base possible interventions. If spiritual assessment is determined to be desirable, Olson and Kane (2000) suggest that the next task is to decide how to accomplish this and what particular aspects should be considered in the assessment process. In the following section, important domains of spiritual assessment will be identified and discussed.

A GERONTOLOGICAL SPIRITUAL ASSESSMENT FRAMEWORK

A few social workers (Bullis, 1996; Canda & Furman, 1999; Hodge, 2001) as well as gerontologists and other allied professionals have suggested different models for exploring spirituality with clients (Fitchett, 1993; Koenig, 2002a; Koenig, 2002b; Sulmasy, 2002). These are helpful because they suggest ways to begin a conversation on this topic and to determine areas to consider beyond the initial question of what role, if any, spirituality may have in a client's life. Canda and Furman (1999) recommend that assessment be done in the context of a collaborative relationship with the client based on a sense of respect for client self-determination and the client's particular spiritual perspective.

The proposed framework incorporates salient components from various existing frameworks (Canda & Furman, 1999; Hodge, 2001; Fitchett, 1993; Koenig, 2002a; Olson & Kane, 2000) and distinguishes eleven domains that, when assessed, will provide a comprehensive understanding of an older individual's relationship to spirituality. It can also help determine whether a need exists for counseling, referrals, or other work in this area. These domains are not necessarily mutually exclusive and questions from each domain do not need to be explored with all clients. Rather, these domains incorporate a fairly complete range of aspects of spirituality and religion that could have clinical benefit in a therapeutic interaction. Social work practitioners could begin with prefatory (initial) questions about perceived importance of spirituality and, depending on that response, move to discuss affiliations, belief, behavior, and emotion, if relevant. Other domains can be investigated to build understanding and a clear focus for treatment.

The spiritual assessment domains include: (1) spiritual affiliation; (2) spiritual belief; (3) spiritual behavior; (4) emotional qualities of spirituality; (5) values; (6) spiritual experiences; (7) spiritual history; (8) therapeutic change factors; (9) social support; (10) spiritual well-being; and (11) extrinsic/intrinsic spiritual focus. For each area, a definition, sample interview questions, and an illustrative vignette relevant for practice is provided.

Prefatory Questions

The following questions might be used to begin exploring spirituality with clients, to determine whether further questions in this area are welcome or have potential import, and what related terms are preferred by the client.

- Is spirituality, religion, or faith important in your life?
- What terms do you prefer? Please explain.

Affiliation

Affiliation lists the formal religious and spiritual groups, if any, with which an individual identifies or holds membership and includes discussion of how this may affect daily life. Ellison (1999) and others have suggested that a question related to religious preference is fundamental in assessment. In fact, questions related to affiliation and whether an individual prays have historically been the single two dimensions used to measure religiosity in the General Social Survey and others. It is important to note that some people affiliate with or incorporate aspects of multiple spiritual groups and perspectives (Canda & Furman, 1999).

Assessment Questions:

- Do you belong to any spiritual group(s)?
- What does membership in this group(s) signify to you?
- Do you express your spirituality outside of participation in religious or spiritual support group?

Vignette. Ann Murphy is an 83-year-old Irish-American member of a Catholic parish. She has attended the same parish for almost 50 years. When her house became too hard to maintain after her children left home and her husband died, she moved to a smaller condominium that was within walking distance of the parish. She continues to participate in daily mass. She finds comfort in singing familiar hymns and participating in familiar rituals in the company of friends she has known many years. She reports that attending church gives her life meaning and perspective, grounds her in routine, but also keeps her aware of the need for social action through the work of a parish social justice committee that she supports financially.

Spiritual Beliefs

Beliefs include the cognitive content of the spiritual perspective such as ideas about an afterlife, the existence of an ultimate or transcendent power, and whether this power or God can be active in one's life for good or misfortune. What an older adult believes can be a sustaining force in times of sadness, but equally, belief may contribute to despair when what one believes comes into conflict with what one feels. Many national and local sample surveys assess whether one believes in God and other types of religious belief (PRCC, 2001; Joseph, 1988).

Assessment Questions:

- What religious or spiritual beliefs give you comfort or hope? Describe.
- What religious or spiritual beliefs upset you? Describe.
- Do you believe in God, a Transcendent Power, or Sacred Source of Meaning?
- Describe your vision of who God or this Transcendent Power is?
- Do you believe in an afterlife? What does this mean for you now?

Vignette. Letha Jones is a 66-year-old European American who had been a member of a Baptist church most of her life. She believes in a God who is active in the world and also helps her when she tries to treat others well. Her image of God also includes a prescription of right behavior towards God: God is a Being one can never question. Miss Jones suffers from Rheumatoid Arthritis and has been confined to a wheelchair and institutional living for about 15 years. When she received a new diagnosis of cancer, she was angry with God. She had lived her life as well as she could, but now she faced a new disease. God had failed her and she was angry, but how could she be angry with God when her belief in respect for God contradicted her feeling of anger towards Him/Her? The social worker normalized Miss Jones' feelings and phoned her minister with her permission. The minister met with her and provided support and reassurance of God's love.

Spiritual Behavior

Behavior comprises the practices or actions in which older adults may engage such as attending a faith community, praying alone or with others, meditating, reading, or using scripture or spiritual writings. Spiritual behavior or practices include both organizational or public behavior and nonorganizational or private behavior (Levin, 2000). Organizational behavior includes attending church, synagogue, or other formal religious community-based services while nonorganizational spiritual behavior might include private prayer, meditation, or taking a walk in the woods in an intentionally spiritual way.

Assessment Questions:

- What religious or spiritual behaviors do you engage in?
- How often do you engage in these religious or spiritual behaviors?
- What about these behaviors do you find nourishing or undermining?

Vignette. Nancy Arnold, a 92-year-old African American, lives in an urban high rise housing facility, but is no longer able to go out of the building very often due to heart disease and other ailments. Although she often experiences physical pain, she prays both for herself and for others, especially for friends who live in the same building and who share their concerns with her about troubles family members face. One neighbor has a son in jail for murder; another neighbor has a daughter trying to support three children as a single mother. Mrs. Arnold prays about all of these needs. She indicates that she also never fails to thank God for the daily gifts that come to her: a phone call from a distant family member or seeing the birds at her window. The act of prayer lifts her up and helps her feel her actions can still make a difference despite her frequent pain.

Emotions

Emotion considers feelings evoked by spiritual activities/experiences such as relying on one's faith in times of stress. However, it also addresses the role of spirituality in causing one to feel joy, awe, mystery, and hope; eliciting anxiety, shame, or guilt related to belief; or engendering active and passive types of coping. Schleiermacher (1821/1928) viewed emotion as being the essence or source of religion. Even James (1902/1961) believed emotion carried immediacy and thus a type of authority. It is the object of the emotions that defines whether an experience is spiritual, religious, or neither.

Assessment Questions:

- Have you recently experienced an emotion such as anger, sadness, guilt, or joy in the context of religious or spiritual experience?
- What significance if any did this have for you? Or if a client is describing an experience, one can ask, What feelings did you have in response? (To better clarify the meaning of the experience for this person.)

Vignette. Humberto Reyes, a 72-year-old Hispanic male, attended church regularly with his grandmother when he was young. In his teens he gradually stopped attending because none of his other friends went and his parents had little interest. He was diagnosed with a form of Multiple Sclerosis in his twenties and needed a wheelchair for mobility by his mid-thirties. In his sixties, a neighbor invited him to attend a church service with her. He agreed and was surprised by the powerful emotions of awe and joy that swept over him as he sang a hymn he had sung years before. He felt fully alive and understood this experience as an indication that he could benefit from renewing a church relationship. He continues to attend with this neighbor and was also able to release his guilt that perhaps the reason for his disease was God's displeasure with him. The social worker understands Mr. Reyes pays attention to his emotions and has learned to cue her helping activities to his needs.

Spiritual Experiences

Spiritual experiences detail private or shared experiences that convey a sense of special meaning about life and death, inspiration, personal encounters with transcendent or sacred forces, or significant altered states of consciousness (e.g., God, angels, deceased loved ones, out of body near-death experience) (Numbers & Amundsen, 1986/1998).

Assessment Question:

- Have you had any spiritual experiences that communicate special meaning to you? If so, please describe.

Vignette. The husband of Bessie Hausmann, an 81-year-old Jewish woman, died in an auto accident after they had been married 51 years. She grieved over not being able to say good-bye to her lifetime lover. One night she dreamed she saw him on a train platform. He didn't say anything, but he waved to her and smiled as he got on the train and departed. She remembers the look of love in his eyes and perceives the dream as his way of saying good-bye and bringing her comfort. She believes this was an actual experience of her husband rather than simply a dream.

Values

Values explore the moral principles and ethical guidelines rooted in spirituality that provide guidance for older persons as they negotiate life changes and challenges. For example, though they may appreciate the concerns of their adult children, older adults sometimes make decisions that might place themselves at risk financially or physically (Idler, 1999; Koenig, 1994; Koenig, 2001). Important spiritual values to some older adults may include maintaining friendships and social activities, preserving solitary time for reflection, seeking wisdom or inner harmony, and finding peace in nature. Values also address moral positions on such acts as use of life sustaining measures and religious motivations for leaving behind financial benefits for loved ones or society generally.

Assessment Questions:

- What are the guiding moral principles and values in your life?
- How do these principles guide the way you live life?

Vignette. Celia Anderson is an 81-year-old European American who lives in a rural community. Although becoming a widow ten years earlier, she continues to value her independence and her daily walks in the fields nearby where she feels close to her ancestry, God, and the beauty of nature. Four months ago, she fell and broke her arm. While this fracture healed well, her daughter was very concerned and put pressure on her mother to move into an assisted living complex. Celia spoke with her daughter about how moving into a city would "kill her soul" and the daughter finally understood how much her mother's environment mattered to her. As a compromise, a home care aide was hired to do light housekeeping and check in on Mrs. Anderson weekly.

Spiritual History

Spiritual history asks about the developmental path over time including gradual growth or pivotal times of crisis and life change an individual has experienced in relation to religion and spirituality. This incorporates both problematic or difficult experiences and affirming, insightful spiritual expressions. For example, Koenig (2002a) encourages medical professionals to complete a spiritual history that includes asking about spiritual and religious coping, involvement in a supportive spiritual community, troubling spiritual questions, and spiritual beliefs that might influence treatment. The value of creating a spiritual and religious biography across the life span is detailed by George (1999) who suggests this may include asking about loss of faith as well as growth and change in spiritual understanding.

Tools that may assist in this process include developing a spiritual genogram or a timeline marking an individual's spiritual journey. Canda and Furman (1999) suggest that this timeline can be associated with important aspects of all the domains, thus putting such things as spiritual mentors or pivotal spiritual experience in a developmental context.

Assessment Questions:

- Were you raised in a spiritual or religious tradition? Do you now practice in the tradition in which you were raised? Describe early experiences and parental involvement.

- •. In what decades of your life were you involved in spiritual practices? Would you rate your involvement as low, medium, or high for each? Were there any change points?
- • What events in your life were especially significant in shaping your spirituality?
- • Who encouraged your spiritual or religious practices?

Vignette. Bill Carlotti, a 69-year-old European American male, has pancreatic cancer and is in hospice care. His parents were not religious, yet he became interested in a neighborhood community church and was a regular church attendee in elementary school. His parents, though they did not encourage this, also did not object. He recounted an event that had a powerful impact on the development of his spirituality. When he was a senior in high school, a fellow classmate died in a tragic auto accident. The minister who led the funeral said she would not be "saved" because she was never baptized. A week later, a man died after years of battling alcoholism and abusive treatment of his family. The same minister told the congregation that this man would "go to Heaven" because he had been baptized years ago. Mr. Carlotti was dismayed at this injustice and never went to church again. However, as he aged he began to explore spiritual texts and affirmed that he thought "Something loving" was in the universe although he didn't know exactly what it was. This belief in a loving power leads him to show his love for others by giving dinner parties for his friends where the only taboo topic is his illness. As long as he is able to, he plans to enjoy these lively evenings and give his friends the gift of fine memories.

Therapeutic Change

Therapeutic change refers to particular individual strengths and resources that are harnessed for healing, growth, and overall well-being over time, as well as the strategies for transformative helping fostered by spiritual support groups and rituals. For example, a person may overcome an unwanted personality trait through meditative self-reflection, or promote healing from a severe illness through a rite of anointment or laying on of hands. On a larger level, it can involve concerns about social or world conditions and lead one to invest time or money in supporting altruistic causes (Bellah, 1991; Dossey, 1993; Niebuhr, 1932).

Assessment Questions:

- • What might be an object or image that symbolizes/represents your spiritual strengths?

- Could you tell me a story of how spirituality helped you cope with difficulties in the recent past?
- How do you see this particular spiritual strength as being able to help you in your current problems?
- What spiritually-based strategies, rituals, or actions have helped you to cope with times of difficulty or to experience healing or growth?

Vignette. David Lester is a 78-year-old European-American male who grew up in a rural Midwestern area. He identifies himself as Christian but does not belong to a particular denomination in his adult life. He developed a special affinity with nature, which he identifies as a core strength of his spirituality, during his youth years. He returned to his birthplace after retiring from a state administrative position for environmental protection. He continues to be very passionate on environmental protection issues and is very proud of his accomplishments. He suffers from depression after developing a debilitating spinal stenosis that caused paralysis in his lower body because he had to drastically limit his social activities. However, he has excellent communicative skills. Using e-mail, he continues lobbying activities for environmental protection. Through this social engagement, he has restored a sense of self-worth and well-being.

Social Support

Consideration of social environmental support has been a critical part of social work assessment from a person-in-environment perspective. The existence and degree of spiritual support from other individuals and groups is an essential element of spiritual assessment (Koenig, 2002a; Krause, 2002; Fitchett, 1993). Social support includes exploration of the types of support provided by fellow spiritual group members and the ways in which that is helpful or problematic for the older adult.

Assessment Questions:

- When you have religious/spiritual concerns and problems, who do you talk to?
- In the past, what types of supports have you received from these people that you have just described?
- If you belong to a religious or spiritual group, what types of support do you receive or provide to them? To what extent are you satisfied? Explain.

Vignette. Jose Martinez is an 86-year-old Mexican American who is a hospice patient. His hospice social worker learned that he had been an active member of a local Catholic church, St. John. When he lost his wife, he received a series of grief counseling sessions from Father Jim and he was very comfortable talking to him about his own dying. While Father Jim visits Jose every other week, Jose now feels a need to talk more about issues of mortality from other perspectives. He wants someone with whom he can speak in Spanish, his native language.

Well-Being

Spiritual well-being refers to the individual's subjective sense of happiness and overall life satisfaction related to his/her spirituality. The National Interfaith Coalition on Aging (1975) defined spiritual well-being as the quality of life through a relationship with God, self, community, and environment that nurtures and celebrates wholeness in human beings. Assessing the spiritual dimension of quality of life is especially important for individuals whose physical and mental capacity has declined due to chronic and life threatening illnesses (Byock & Merriman, 1998; Cohen et al., 1997). They frequently experience diminished sense of self-worth, so social workers need to tune into clients' subjective sense of spiritual well-being as it often becomes the central quality of life domain supporting frail older adults.

Assessment Questions:

- How worthwhile do you find living your current life? Can you tell me more about it? How does this relate to your spirituality?
- How does your spirituality help you to find meaning in your life?
- How strongly do you feel connected to God/Higher Power/Spirit/ Universe?

Vignette. Harry Kim is a 65-year-old Korean male. He is a hospice patient with a terminal lung disease. He claims no affiliation to any particular religious or spiritual groups or orientations. According to him, he left Christianity when he was young because of his mistrust in church authority. However, he calls himself a "spiritual seeker" as he has studied different types of spiritual teaching including Eastern philosophy. His hospice social workers explored some spiritual questions to get a sense of his level of spiritual well-being. Harry states that he finds his life meaningful and worthwhile as he is a part of the big mystery of the Universe. Without any particular object of worship, he feels a strong sense of connection with the Higher Power which he calls "Spirit" or the "Universe."

Extrinsic/Intrinsic Spiritual Propensity

Extrinsic/intrinsic spiritual propensity refers to a preferred relationship pattern for the way an older adult chooses to involve spiritual elements in his/her life. Intrinsic and extrinsic religiosity were first described by Allport (1967) to assess the reasons that people became involved in religious and spiritual practice. Intrinsic religiosity referred to cultivating an inner relationship with a divine power, internal self-determination, while extrinsic religiosity referred to joining a church to gain social standing or meet other external needs in accord with group norms. In the broader concepts of extrinsic or intrinsic spiritual propensity, there is no judgment implied. Rather it addresses two dimensions of spiritual life: intrinsic (self-directed or inward) and extrinsic (outer-directed and group based). These could be complementary or a person might emphasize one over the other (Canda & Furman, 1999).

Assessment Questions:

- Do you find the teachings and values of your spiritual groups similar or different from your own? Please explain.
- How integrated are your spiritual practices with your daily life apart from spiritual group participation?

Vignette. Lydia Thomas is a 72-year-old African-American woman who became Buddhist in midlife. She enjoys occasional participation in a gospel church similar to the one in which she was raised. While she practices with a Sangha regularly and values being with other meditation practitioners, she also practices daily meditation at home. She exhibits a well-integrated extrinsic and intrinsic spiritual propensity.

CONCLUSION

Spirituality is an area that many older adults find personally meaningful, yet social workers are often not well trained in addressing this aspect of human behavior. This paper has attempted to address a gap in the literature by moving beyond definitions of what spirituality is to exploring with older clients how it functions in their lives. Spiritual assessment in social work with older adults is beginning to enter a new phase of expansion as helping professionals start to explore its many facets as well as its capabilities for both support and distress.

This article has provided a detailed framework for spiritual assessment by describing eleven domains, sample questions, and vignettes. Our hope as authors is that this will serve as a guide for social workers who would like to address this area, but feel limited by lack of formal training about spiritual assessment.

REFERENCES

Allport, G. R. (1967). Personal religious orientation and prejudice. *Journal of Personal and Social Psychology, 5*, 432-443.

Bellah, R. N. (1991). Beyond belief: Essays on religion in a post-traditional world. Berkeley, CA: University of California Press.

Bullis, R. K. (1996). Spirituality in social work practice. Washington, D.C.: Taylor & Francis.

Byock, I. R., & Merriman, M. P. (1998). Measuring quality of life for patients with terminal illness: The Missoula-VITAS quality of life index. *Palliative Medicine, 12*, 231-244.

Canda, E. R. (1988). Conceptualizing spirituality for social work: Insights from diverse perspectives. *Social Thought, 14*(1), 30-46.

Canda, E. R. (1997). Spirituality. In R. L. Edwards (Ed.), Encyclopedia of social work 19th Edition Supplement (pp. 299-309). Washington, D.C.: National Association of Social Workers.

Canda, E. R., & Furman, L. D. (1999). Spiritual diversity in social work practice. New York: The Free Press.

Caroll, M. (2001). Conceptual models of spirituality. *Social Thought, 20*, 5-22.

Cohen, S. R., Mount, B. M., Burera, E., Provost, M., Rowe, J., & Tong, K. (1997). Validity of the McGill quality of life questionnaire in the palliative care setting: A multi-centre Canadian study demonstrating the importance of the existential domain. *Palliative Medicine, 11*, 3-20.

Dossey, L. (1993). Healing words: The power of prayer and the practice of medicine. San Francisco: Harper.

Ellison, C. (1999). Religious preference. In Fetzer Institute (Ed.), Multidimensional measurement of religiousness/spirituality for use in health research (pp. 81-84). Kalamazoo, MI: The Fetzer Institute/NIA.

Fitchett, G. (1993). Assessing spiritual needs: A guide for caregivers. Minneapolis, MN: Augsburg Press.

Frame, M. W. (2003). Integrating religion and spirituality into counseling: A comprehensive approach. Pacific Grove, CA: Brooks/Cole.

George, L. K. (1999). Religious/spiritual history. In Fetzer Institute (Ed.), Multidimensional measurement of religiousness/spirituality for use in health research (pp. 65-70). Kalamazoo, MI: The Fetzer Institute/NIA.

Hermann, C. P. (2001). Spiritual needs of dying patients: A qualitative study. *Oncology Nursing Forum, 28*, 67-72.

Hodge, D. R. (2001). Spiritual assessment: A review of major qualitative methods and a new framework for assessing spirituality. *Social Work, 46*(3), 203-214.

Idler, E. (1999). Values. In Fetzer Institute (Ed.), Multidimensional measurement of religiousness/spirituality for use in health research (pp. 25-30). Kalamazoo, MI: The Fetzer Institute/NIA.

Jackson, J., Chatters, L., & Taylor, R. (1993). Aging in Black America. Thousand Oaks, CA: Sage.

James, W. (1902/1961). The varieties of religious experience. New York: Collier Books.

Joseph, M. V. (1988). Religion and social work practice. *Social Casework, 60*(7), 443-452.

Kahana, E., Redmond, C., Hill, G., Kercher, K., Kahana, B., Johnson, J. R., & Young, R. F. (1995). The effects of stress, vulnerability, and appraisals on the psychological well being of the elderly. *Research on Aging, 17*(4), 459-489.

Koenig, H. G. (1994). Aging and God: Spiritual pathways to mental health in midlife and later years. New York: Haworth Press.

Koenig, H. G. (2002a). Spirituality in patient care: Why, how, when, and what. Philadelphia: Templeton Foundation Press.

Koenig, H. G. (2002b). A commentary: The role of religion and spirituality at the end of life. *The Gerontologist,* 42(Special Issue III), 20-23.

Koenig, H. G., McCullough, M. E., & Larson, D. B. (2001). Handbook of religion and health. New York: Oxford University Press.

Koenig, T. L. (2002). Ethical dilemmas faced by women as caregivers of frail elders: A qualitative study (Doctoral Dissertation, The University of Kansas, 2002). *Dissertation Abstracts International, 38*(01), 2002, No. 23.

Krause, N. (2002). Church-based social support and health in old age: Exploring variations by race. *Journals of Gerontology Series B: Psychological and Social Sciences, 57*(6), S332-S348.

Levin, J. (2000). Religion. In G. L. Maddox (Ed.), The encyclopedia of aging: A comprehensive resource in gerontology and geriatrics, Vol 2 (3rd ed.), (pp. 866-869). New York: Springer Publishing.

Mackenzie, E. R., Rajagopal, D. E., Meibohm, M., & Lavizzo-Mourey, R. (2000). Spiritual support and psychological well-being: Older adults' perceptions of the religion and health connection. *Alternative Therapies, 6*(6), 37-45.

MacKinlay, E. (2002). Health, healing and wholeness in frail elderly people. *Journal of Religious Gerontology, 13,* 25-34.

Nakashima, M. (2002). A Qualitative Inquiry into the Psychosocial and Spiritual Well-Being of Older Adults at the End of Life. (Doctoral Dissertation, The University of Kansas, 2002). *Dissertation Abstracts International, 38*(3), 2002, No. 1141.

National Interfaith Coalition on Aging. (1975). Spiritual well-being: A definition. Athens, GA: National Interfaith Coalition on Aging.

Neibuhr, R. (1932). The contribution of religion to social work. New York: Columbia University Press.

Nelson-Becker, H. B. (1999). Spiritual and religious problem-solving in older adults: Mechanisms for managing life challenge. (Doctoral Dissertation, The University of Chicago, 1999). *Dissertation Abstracts International, 35*(4), 1999, No. 1620.

Nelson-Becker, H. B. (in press). Meeting life challenges: A hierarchy of coping styles in African American and Jewish American older adults. *Journal of Human Behavior in the Social Environment.*

Numbers, R. L., & Amundsen, D. W. (1986/1998). Caring and curing: Health and medicine in the Western religious tradition. Baltimore, MD: Johns Hopkins University Press.

Olson, D. M., & Kane, R. A. (2000). Spiritual assessment. In R. L. Kane and R. A. Kane (Eds.), Assessing older persons (pp. 300-319). New York: Oxford University Press.

Pargament, K. I. (1997). The psychology of religion and coping. New York: Guilford Press.

Princeton Religious Research Center (PRCC). (2001). Importance of religion. PRRC Emerging Trends. Princeton, N. J.

Ramsey, J., & Blieszner, R. (1999). Spiritual resiliency in older women. Thousand Oaks, CA: Sage Publications.

Richards, P. S., & Bergin, A. E. (1997). A spiritual strategy for counseling and psychotherapy. Washington, D.C.: American Psychological Association.

Schleiermacher, F. D. (1928). The Christian faith. Edinburgh, Scotland: T. & T. Clark.

Sulmasy, D. P. (2002). A biopsychosocial-spiritual model of the care of patients at the end of life. *The Gerontologist*, 42(Special Issue III), 24-33.

doi:10.1300/J083v48n03_04

Providing Mental Health Services to Older People Living in Rural Communities

Allan V. Kaufman, PhD
Forrest R. Scogin, PhD
Louis D. Burgio, PhD
Martin P. Morthland, MPhil
Bryan K. Ford, MSW

SUMMARY. Rural dwelling elders who experience mental health problems often have difficulty finding help since rural communities often lack adequate mental health service providers. This paper reports on the initial phase of a 5-year, interdisciplinary clinical research study that is testing the effectiveness of providing a home delivered, therapeutic psychosocial intervention, aimed at improving the emotional well-being and the quality of life of medically frail elders who live in rural communities. In the early phases of this study, the clinical research team encountered a number of interesting and often unanticipated challenges as it attempted to recruit study participants and provide services to them. In this article, we examine these challenges and share what we

This study was supported by a grant from the National Institute on Aging (1RO1 AG16311-01). A version of this paper was presented at the First National Gerontological Social Work Conference, Atlanta, February, 2003.

[Haworth co-indexing entry note]: "Providing Mental Health Services to Older People Living in Rural Communities." Kaufman, Allan V. et al. Co-published simultaneously in *Journal of Gerontological Social Work* (The Haworth Press, Inc.) Vol. 48, No. 3/4, 2007, pp. 349-365; and: *Fostering Social Work Gerontology Competence: A Collection of Papers from the First National Gerontological Social Work Conference* (ed: Catherine J. Tompkins, and Anita L. Rosen) The Haworth Press, Inc., 2007, pp. 349-365. Single or multiple copies of this article are available for a fee from The Haworth Document Delivery Service [1-800-HAWORTH, 9:00 a.m. - 5:00 p.m. (EST). E-mail address: docdelivery@haworthpress.com].

have learned so far about providing mental health services to elderly persons living in rural environments. doi:10.1300/J083v48n03_05 *[Article copies available for a fee from The Haworth Document Delivery Service: 1-800-HAWORTH. E-mail address: <docdelivery@haworthpress.com> Website: <http://www.HaworthPress.com> © 2007 by The Haworth Press, Inc. All rights reserved.]*

KEYWORDS. Rural environments, mental health services, psychosocial intervention, interdisciplinary

INTRODUCTION

The growth of our older population during the past century has been dramatic. Since 1900, the percentage of Americans aged 65 and older has tripled and in 2000 this group comprised 12.4% (35 million) of the total population. It is expected that the number of persons 65 years of age and older will continue to grow rapidly and will more than double by the year 2030. At that time, it is estimated that those 65 and over will number approximately 70 million and will comprise 20% of the total population of the United States (Administration on Aging, 2003).

It is important for policy makers, practitioners, service providers and researchers to consider the diversity of our older population, and to not treat this segment of our society as one large homogeneous group. Whether we look at such characteristics as gender, race, ethnicity, or socioeconomic status, it is clear the older population is composed of different subgroups which experience special challenges or concerns. One often overlooked and therefore underserved subgroup of older persons is composed of those who reside in rural areas. Twenty-three percent of the older population in this country lives in non-metropolitan communities (Administration on Aging, 2003). This translates into 8 million persons 65 years of age or older who live in rural America. Over the past two decades, the percentage of older persons living in such areas has been steadily growing due to the overall increase in the number of persons reaching old age, combined with the continued flight of younger persons out of rural communities.

The provision of human services to rural elders has not kept up with the need for such services because of a "lack of financial and human capital, urban biases in government funding and reimbursement mechanisms ... a shortage of trained practitioners, and a culture of individual self-reliance that leads individuals to eschew formal services for informal supports" (Krout, 1998, p. 247). Elders who live in rural communities and who experience problems in mental health or cognitive functioning are a particularly disadvantaged group when it comes to finding help. for such problems since there is a general lack of adequate mental health services in such communities (Buckwalter, Smith, Zevenbergen, & Russell; 1991; McCulloch & Lynch, 1993; Scheidt, 1985; Rathbone-McCuan, 2001).

This paper reports on the initial phase of a 5-year, interdisciplinary clinical research study that is testing the effectiveness of providing a home delivered, therapeutic psychosocial intervention, aimed at improving the emotional well-being and the quality of life of medically frail elders who live in rural communities. In the early phases of this study, the clinical research team encountered a number of interesting and often unanticipated challenges as it attempted to recruit study participants and provide services to them. In this article, we examine these challenges, share what we have learned so far about providing mental health services to elderly persons living in rural environments, and discuss their implications for social work practice and research. Future articles will report the treatment findings of this study as they become available.

THE MENTAL HEALTH OF OLDER PERSONS IN RURAL AREAS

Emotional well-being is one of the primary dimensions that must be considered when measuring the quality of life of older persons (Stewart & King, 1994). There is evidence that as a group, older people, compared to younger adults, have a lower prevalence rate of most mental health disorders (Bourdon, Rae, Locke, Narrow, & Regier, 1992; Regier, Boyd, & Burke, 1988; Meyers et al., 1984). However, there is also evidence that significant numbers of older individuals suffer from emotional problems associated with anxiety disorders, mood disorders, phobias, obsessive-compulsive disorders and severe cognitive impairment associated with Alzheimer's Disease and other related dementias (Blazer, Hughes, & George, 1987; Cohen, 1990; Junginger, Phelan, Cherry, & Levy, 1993; United States Department of Health and Human Services, 1999; Mott, Dean, Wang & Wood, 1992). It has been estimated that approximately 20% of persons aged 55 and over suffer from some type of the above mentioned mental health problems, and it is also believed that there has been a significant underreporting of the incidences of such mental health problems among members of our older population (Department of Health and Human Services, 2001).

Treatment of Mental Health Problems in Rural Areas

Many physicians who treat community dwelling elders have little specialized training in diagnosing or treating the most common mental health problems of older people. Symptoms of older individuals' underlying mental health problems are often either ignored, misdiagnosed, or simply attributed to the inevitability of the "aging process" and then left untreated (Butler, Lewis, & Sunderland, 1998). Where specialized mental health resources for the elderly do exist, they tend to be concentrated in more densely populated cities and suburban areas.

People living in rural communities are often faced with significant challenges associated with poverty, geographic and social isolation, and the lack of a service infrastructure capable of helping rural residents with needs related to transportation, housing and medical care (Bull, 1998; Krout, 1998; Rubinstein, 1995). Providers of human services in rural areas face challenges such as maintaining client confidentiality and working with clients who may be culturally or religiously different from them (Boyle, Jacobsen, & MacNair, 1994; Bull, 1998; Helge, 1981; Rubinstein, 1995/96).

Parish and Landsberg (1984) note that when providing outreach mental health services to rural elders, such persons are "... often [found to be] isolated and homebound and transportation [is] frequently inaccessible or nonexistent" (p. 76). Geographic barriers and poor or even nonexistent roads may make it difficult for service providers to reach people living in isolated areas making travel expensive and services difficult to deliver in a timely fashion. This geographic isolation may lead to the social isolation of certain rural residents and may contribute to feelings of fear, suspicion or stigmatization about accepting mental health services (Lawrence & McCulloch, 2001).

Culture, Religion, and Use of Mental Health Services

The cultural and religious beliefs, traditions, and value systems of some younger and older residents of rural communities may act as barriers to their use of available human services (Boyle et al., 1994; Helge, 1981 & 1984; Krout, 1998; Rubinstein, 1995/96). Both aged and non-aged people who live in rural communities, and who could benefit from the receipt of mental health and other types of services may often be unwilling to step outside of local traditional community norms regarding the acceptance of help or the utilization of formal services from service providers who are not native to a particular local community (Abraham & Neese, 1993; Heard-Mueller et al., 1994; Helge, 1981 & 1984; Krout, 1998; Parish & Landsberg, 1984; Rich & Dalton, 1995; Rubinstein, 1995/96; Van Hook & Ford, 1998).

Therefore, knowledge of community belief systems, values, and traditions is critically important in trying to provide mental health services to rural residents, especially if they are members of ethnic or racial minority groups who have experienced the types of oppression that may have affected their trust and willingness to accept help from persons not from their community. "... [r]eligion and spirituality are strong influences in the lives of people who feel the effects of oppression ... [and] social workers who ignore fundamentalist belief systems may forego any possibility of effective communication with their client families ... racial and cultural sensitivity is critical for effective practice in rural areas" (Boyle et al., 1994, pp. 7-8).

INCOME

Poverty is often a prevalent problem in rural communities and can be a significant factor governing older residents' quality of life (Abraham & Neese, 1993; Bull, 1998; Heard-Mueller et al., 1994; Helge, 1984). Lack of adequate income can contribute to or exacerbate the mental health problems of older persons, and can provide serious challenges and obstacles to the provision or use of mental health services. Poverty can influence elders' economic choices regarding what needs should be met and how. Basic needs for food, shelter and other necessities may have to take precedence over costly mental health care. Payments for recommended medications or psychosocial treatments that might improve their emotional well-being may not be realistically affordable for many low income rural dwelling older persons (Bull, 1998; Bull & Bane, 1993; Glasgow & Brown, 1998; Krout, 1998). Poverty does not only provide challenges for rural elders and their families, its effects are often also felt in the mental health service infrastructures of the communities in which these persons live. Poor rural communities often lack the diversity of mental health service programs and resources needed to respond to the mental health problems of their residents. A lack of available mental health services in many rural communities constitutes a major barrier affecting the ability of the residents of such communities to access needed mental health treatment (Lawrence & McCulloch, 2001; Rathbone-McCuan, E., 2001).

Project to Enhance Aged Rural Living

The Project to Enhance Aged Rural Living (PEARL) is a 5-year interdisciplinary research study, funded by a grant from the National Institute on Aging. The study is using a delayed treatment control design to test the effectiveness of providing cognitive behavioral therapy (CBT) to medically frail, cognitively intact persons, 65 years of age or older, who live in rural areas of Alabama, and who are experiencing diminished emotional well-being and diminished quality of life. The research design calls for the provision of 16 to 20 treatment sessions, provided by trained clinical social workers, delivered without charge, in the participants' homes. One of the unique aspects of the study is the recruitment and training of an informal caregiver who helps to facilitate the treatment process by assisting the primary subject with the completion of "homework assignments" that take place between scheduled therapy sessions. Participating caregivers are also taught general problem solving skills to enable them better to cope with problems encountered in their own lives.

Primary subjects recruited to the study are randomly assigned to either the immediate treatment condition or the delayed treatment condition. Those in the delayed condition receive a full course of treatment after a waiting period of 3 months. The delayed treatment control design allows PEARL to offer treatment to every primary subject recruited for the study, including those participants assigned to the control condition.

Because of the demographics of the older population of rural Alabama, it is expected that most of the study participants will be widowed women with less than a high school education, who live alone, and who have annual incomes of less than $10,000. A recruitment goal of the study is to have an equal number of white and African American elders make up the study sample of 90 participants. Since the primary participants will all be medically frail, it is expected that in addition to their problematic health conditions, most of the participants will need some degree of assistance with one or more of the basic or instrumental activities of daily living.

In addition to the Masters' level social work practitioners who conduct the CBT with the primary participants and the problem solving training with their caregivers, the field staff includes baccalaureate level research assistants whose responsibilities include screening potential study participants to determine if they meet specific eligibility criteria, and who conduct a series of pre and post treatment assessments with each participant (elders and caregivers). The social workers and the research assistants also have responsibility for a variety of ongoing project recruitment activities designed to maintain a steady flow of participants coming into the study. It is important to note that all primary participants and caregivers receive modest financial incentive payments for taking part in the study. These payments are linked to the assessment process, so that primary participants and their caregivers receive a payment after the completion of each of the scheduled assessments.

Recruitment of potential primary study participants (medically frail elders), depends heavily upon the continuing active involvement and close cooperation of staff members from a variety of health and human service agencies located in the rural areas served by PEARL that have agreed to act as referral sources for the study. The nurses and social workers at these agencies first identify agency clients who appear to meet eligibility criteria for inclusion in the study and then provide information about PEARL to these individuals. Those agency clients who indicate a potential interest in participating in PEARL and who agree to be referred, are contacted by one of the research assistants who provides a full explanation of the study, including all of the information associated with the informed consent process. If the potential participant then indicates a willingness to join the study, the research assistant administers a brief screening protocol to determine initial eligibility. Those persons for whom the brief screen and a second, more extensive screening assessment process confirms that they meet inclusion criteria, are then invited into the study and are assigned to either the immediate treatment or the delayed treatment control condition.

STUDY IMPLEMENTATION CHALLENGES

A weekly group staff meeting is held with all field staff to review and discuss any clinical or research issues that emerge as part of ongoing project responsibilities. A portion of each of these meetings is devoted to examining challenging methodological or treatment delivery issues that require special attention by the research team. The material presented below, regarding the challenges we have encountered so far in conducting our clinical gerontological research study, was gathered during these meetings and from additional, focused, semi-structured interviews conducted individually with each member of the field staff.

Recruitment

So far, the most difficult aspects of mounting this clinical study have been linked to the recruitment process. The ability to recruit a sufficient and steady flow of participants into clinical mental health related research studies has been a challenge reported by other researchers (Kelleher & Long, 1994) regardless of whether the geographic setting is rural or urban. While some of the recruitment issues that have been encountered in our study are not unique, others appear to be directly related to normative, cultural and educational factors associated with the rural Alabama communities that serve as catchment areas for the project.

Despite the initially high level of enthusiasm about PEARL that we received from potential cooperating agencies with whom we had discussed participant referrals, and the stated expectations of those agencies that many referrals would be forthcoming, the actual numbers of referrals provided have been somewhat low and have been provided on a rather sporadic basis. We try to keep up a steady level of communication with the direct service staff of these agencies who are in the best position within these organizations to make potential referrals. This has been a very challenging process since we do not want to "pester" these staff members to the point that we would alienate them, yet our experience has been that if we do not keep up a steady level of contact, little or no referrals occur. We think that while these personnel are truly supportive of the project, the realities of the day-to-day demands of working in these agencies leave staff little time for the "extra" efforts required to participate in the referral process. While this problem is probably not unique to developing cooperative clinical research arrangements with human service agencies in non-rural communities, the agencies in the rural communities that make up the PEARL catchment area tend to be constantly struggling to obtain the scarce resources needed to adequately serve their clients. Most agencies report that they are severely understaffed and that their staff members have very high caseloads. A number of the agencies that had agreed to cooperate with us are public or proprietary home health care service providers and these agencies have been particularly hard hit over the last several years by cuts in federal and state level reimbursement rates for their services. Another factor that may be related to the rural nature of the communities served by these agencies which appears to be negatively influencing the referral process is the cautious and sometimes suspicious attitudes of the clients served by these agencies regarding their participation in a clinical research project. It is probably safe to speculate that because of the cultural and normative characteristics of the agencies' clients, staff members from these agencies are finding that the process of explaining PEARL to their clients, and gaining their agreement to allow an initial referral, is a more complex and time consuming process than they first anticipated.

As a result of the challenges associated with generating sufficient agency referrals, we have made several changes in the project's recruitment protocol. We have expanded the original number of rural catchment areas of the study and we have reached out to a larger number of potential referral agencies than originally planned. This has resulted in devoting more PEARL staff time than originally allocated to developing and maintaining working arrangements with community agencies, and has also increased the project's anticipated travel expenses and expenses related to promotional materials. We have also modified the recruitment process to try to attract referrals from a wider range of community gatekeepers such as clergy and physicians, and we began to solicit self-referrals to the project through a variety of publicity efforts in our targeted rural communities.

We have learned that successful recruitment of our primary participants is often dependent on the support of their immediate family, especially those family members who provide some level of care or assistance to the older person. These family members tend to function as gatekeepers with regard to obtaining access to these frail elders. Our experience has been that the elder is often reluctant to make a decision about entering the study without first discussing the matter with a particular member of the family, and then, making their decision based on that person's level of support or enthusiasm about the elder's participation in the study. These family members tend to be most concerned about whether study involvement might be too physically or emotionally demanding for the elder. It is interesting to note that some of the rural areas served by PEARL are located in geographic proximity to the city of Tuskegee, Alabama, home of the infamous Tuskegee studies, which have become widely known to many African American and white residents of the area, and which may explain, in part, some of the caution and concerns expressed by some residents of the area with regard to their involvement with our study.

In addition to continuing challenges involved in recruiting primary participants, it has also been somewhat difficult to recruit caregiver participants into the study. Competing time demands and just a general lack of interest have been the most frequently stated obstacles to recruiting such individuals. Accommodating the scheduling issues of potential caregiver participants has forced field staff to develop very flexible approaches to scheduling assessments and in-home therapeutic sessions, resulting in some sessions being conducted evenings or weekends. These scheduling challenges have created some difficult travel issues that have added to the time and monetary costs associated with the study.

Delivery of Treatment

For the social workers, the most challenging and frustrating aspects of carrying out their project responsibilities have been the delivery and completion of scheduled therapy sessions. They spend much time traveling to participants' homes to conduct these sessions and it is not unusual for them to travel an hour to a participant's home for a scheduled appointment only to discover that no one is there, or that the older person is not feeling well enough to participate in a treatment session. Often, the reason given for a participant not being at home for a scheduled appointment is related to some type of acute medical crisis that has required an emergency trip to a doctor's office or the hospital. At times, though, the social workers have learned that non-emergency family matters or other competing time demands have resulted in the participants not being at home for their scheduled appointments. Some of the social workers have remarked that it appears as if part of the culture of the participants' rural communities involves an attitude or conception of "time" that treats time related matters more casually or less precisely than might be the case in urban environments. One social worker stated that one particular study participant "… thought I was coming only just down the road, and not traveling from an hour away. She didn't understand why I just couldn't stop by to see her on my way back from another appointment."

The field staff has developed several approaches that have helped to overcome missed appointments. They continually discuss with participants and their caregivers the importance of keeping scheduled appointments or contacting the staff person if appointment times need to be changed, and doing so as far in advance as possible. Written appointment notes are provided to the participants, and participants are encouraged to utilize appointment calendars to keep track of appointment dates. Field staff members try telephoning participants just before leaving the office to make home visits in order to confirm that participants are expecting them and will be at home when they arrive. A toll free telephone number has been established so that participants who need to reschedule appointment times can call the project's program office, without cost to them, from anywhere in the state. However, despite all of the attention that has been focused on the appointment process, broken appointments continue to be a challenge affecting the management and flow of staff time and the use of travel resources, and continuing work to improve this problem area is ongoing.

A second challenging aspect of conducting either the in-home assessments or therapeutic sessions relates to the variety of distractions or interruptions that field staff members have encountered trying to complete these visits. Occasionally the sessions or assessments are conducted under less than ideal conditions, possibly compromising the integrity of the session. Examples of such situations include unexpected visits of friends, relatives, or other service providers who just happen to arrive during a scheduled cognitive behavior therapy session. In some instances the therapeutic session can be completed by the social worker and the client moving to another part of the house that offers privacy and that is free from distraction. In other cases, however, the session has to be ended abruptly and rescheduled for another time.

The geographic locations of some of the participants' homes have provided some challenging travel issues for PEARL staff. We have found that travel to the homes of many of our participants generally involves negotiating poorly marked roads that are often unpaved, making for less than ideal driving conditions, especially when a staff person encounters inclement weather. Staff members have reported potential safety issues in traveling in some of the unfamiliar rural areas served by the project, and they carry a personal cellular telephone with them for safety reasons. We have found that cellular telephones are particularly important aids for rural travel since many rural area streets and roads are not marked with name or number signs and travel directions are generally given using descriptions of landmarks rather than the provision of street names. Typical directions to a participant's house might be given as "Across from the church that burned down last year," or "Turn when you see an old barn and then it's the third green house on the right." In such situations it is easy for field staff to get hopelessly lost on their way to a home visit and being able to call the person being visited by cellular phone is often a significant help in finding a particular address, as well as a significant time saving aid. It is recommended that researchers considering projects in rural areas requiring extensive travel make budget provisions for cellular telephone service to facilitate staff communication and safety. Unfortunately, because cellular service is lacking in some rural areas, this strategy is not always an available option.

A factor that has introduced challenges in conducting cognitive behavioral therapy with some of our participants has been their degree of religiosity. Some of the more religious participants appear to be reluctant to verbally express and work on the alleviation of feelings of worry, anxiety, despair or other negative emotions regarding such matters as their personal health or family issues, because expressing such emotions might be seen as a "lack of faith." When some of these participants discuss potentially emotionally charged issues, it is not unusual to hear them make a statement such as: "I'll just turn that over to God." Therefore, since "God" is now going to help them deal better with a particular issue or problem, they have no further need to discuss it in their therapy sessions. One social worker reported that she deals with this type of therapeutic challenge by encouraging such participants to use those traditional coping tools that have worked for them in the past, like their religious faith, but she also encourages these older persons to view the CBT process as another helpful coping tool to supplement their spiritual beliefs. "Once a participant can be helped to understand the cooperative nature of the CBT process, rather than viewing CBT as something that we are going to 'do' to them, we can usually make good therapeutic progress."

Most of our rural participants have had limited formal education, and, as a result, many have limited vocabularies and low levels of literacy. The educational limitations of some participants have challenged our field staff to creatively adapt aspects of the project's methodology related both to the administration of assessment instruments, and the conduct of CBT sessions. The research assistants have become skilled at reframing items from the study's assessment instruments, or interpreting the meaning of words contained in certain items. The social workers have incorporated the use of aids such as audio playing/recording devices and picture charts to take the place of some of the written materials and procedures generally used in traditional approaches to the delivery of CBT. Field staff members have also learned the importance of slowing down the pace of interview and therapy sessions to ensure that participants more fully understand the material that is being discussed. Because of the need to adapt procedures to the educational limitations of some of the study's participants, the amount of time originally planned to complete participant assessments and to conduct therapeutic sessions has had to be extended. This has necessitated the modification of staff workload and scheduling expectations, which in turn, has had implications for the project's overall time planning and management processes.

A factor that has influenced both participant recruitment and the delivery of CBT to study participants is the generally negative stigma that is often attached to mental health issues and terminology by many residents in the rural communities served by PEARL. The field staff has learned the necessity of avoiding the use of psychological jargon with participants and their caregivers. Avoiding the use of jargon, and substituting instead non psychological terms to discuss the variety of emotional issues with which participants are struggling, has been an important factor in helping field staff to develop rapport with participants, and has facilitated the development of therapeutic alliance between PEARL social workers and participants. Although the issue of stigma has been discussed before as a treatment issue in the mental health and aging literature (Roskes, Feldman, Arrington & Leisher, 1999; Russell, 1997; Segal, Silverman & Temkin, 1993; Sirey et al., 2001), it seems to be a particularly salient issue for the rural participants in our study, and one that our staff members have become particularly sensitive about.

The apparent poverty of some of our rural study participants sometimes presents challenging issues for the field staff. Some participants are in such desperate need of material resources that their inability to secure them creates a crisis situation in their lives. Since funding for PEARL does not provide for the provision of services designed to help participants secure material assistance, staff are sometimes faced with the challenge of helping these folks get assistance for these kinds of needs while not losing the focus of the clinical intervention they are engaged in. We have found that it is often a difficult task to motivate people who are beset with concrete resource issues to devote the time and psychic energy needed to also participate in a therapeutic process designed to help them examine troublesome thoughts and feelings.

The run-down and potentially dangerous housing conditions that project staff have encountered in the course of making home visits has sometimes tested their comfort levels and their ability to conduct therapeutic interviews in some very challenging situations. One social worker described visiting a bed-bound participant to conduct a CBT session and being asked to retrieve a treatment manual from under the participant's bed only to be startled as a swarm of roaches, which the participant called "homies," ran in all directions. Another social worker recalled a situation in which she was engaged in a CBT session and began to notice a growing number of flying insects swarming around the room. The social worker tried to ignore the insects as best she could, occasionally swatting at them to keep them off of her head. At this point, the participant's caregiver entered the room and remarked about the number of termites covering the ceiling. The CBT session was temporarily halted as the caregiver covered the participant with a sheet and sprayed the room with insecticide. The CBT session continued when the termite infestation had been cleared.

Culturally Sensitive Challenges

It was expected that in the rural communities in Alabama that PEARL would be focusing on as catchment areas, race would be a potentially influential variable in the manner in which relationships between participants and staff would be established, and that issues of race had the potential to affect the project's treatment outcomes. Several methodological approaches have been used to try to minimize these potential effects. One of the consultants involved with PEARL is a nationally recognized expert in research issues related to matters of diversity and has helped us to design our research methodology and our therapeutic intervention to be as culturally sensitive as possible. She has been fully involved in the training of our field staff and provides ongoing consultation to the study, including participation in regular staff meetings and case presentations. We have also been successful in our efforts to hire and maintain a racially diverse field staff of research assistants and social workers. And finally, as mentioned above, our recruitment goal is have an equal number of African American and white elders as participants in the study. At this point in the project, the field staff has reported few situations in which they attribute problematic treatment issues or problematic assessment issues to factors related to the racial background of participants or members of the field staff. Continuing attention will be paid to potential research and treatment issues and challenges related to cultural factors, and the potential effects of race on the study's outcome measures will be examined as part of the final data analyses.

DISCUSSION

We believe that what we have learned so far has the potential to inform social work practitioners who are planning to provide clinical mental health services to medically frail older persons who live in rural communities. Since most social workers, whether they practice in urban or rural settings, have not had specialized training in working with elders and their families, we would first encourage social work practitioners who work with this population to become as knowledgeable as possible about the mental health issues and problems that affect older persons in general, and to learn about the special challenges faced by such persons in securing needed care. In those rural communities which lack specialized mental health services for older persons, we encourage social workers to advocate for the allocation of resources that would facilitate the development of such services, so that older persons are not denied needed care. Furthermore, we encourage knowledgeable social workers in such communities to help educate and inform human service agencies and primary care medical practitioners about the mental health problems of older persons and about the types of mental health interventions that have been shown to be effective with this population.

Social workers in rural communities must be particularly sensitive to community and ethnic group values, norms and beliefs about mental health issues. The stigma often attached to mental illness and to the receipt of mental health treatment or services presents formidable barriers to providing help to older persons who are experiencing emotional problems, especially those who live in some rural communities. In this regard, social workers need to be knowledgeable about working with community and family gatekeepers and the key members of their older clients' informal social support networks. These networks can be extremely important in the lives of older persons, especially with those physically or medically frail elders who are heavily dependent upon members of these networks for needed care. The ability to develop rapport with influential family caregivers, and the ability to gain their confidence and support may be the most important factors in providing successful mental health interventions to older persons in rural areas.

Based on our experiences with PEARL, we offer several suggestions to gerontological social work researchers who plan to conduct mental health related research in rural communities. Before undertaking such research, it is important to understand and appreciate the existing cultural context in the communities in which you will be working. It is essential to carefully consider and understand the behavioral norms and belief systems of community residents, especially where they involve factors related to race, ethnicity, and socioeconomic level. It is critically important to learn community beliefs and values regarding mental illness, and the degree to which residents may be subject to community stigmatization for acknowledging that they are experiencing mental health problems or using mental health services. Other cultural factors that should be considered include sensitivity to possible suspicion or fear of "outsiders" and how such emotions may affect feelings of trust toward social work researchers, and the importance that religion may play in the day to day lives of elders and members of their informal social networks.

It is crucial for researchers to seek out and gain the support of knowledgeable and influential community gate keepers such as religious leaders, medical professionals, and human service personnel, who can help to obtain community acceptance of research projects, and can help to identify and recruit potential research participants. It is necessary to consider the educational experiences and attainments of community elders and where indicated, adapt research protocols such as data collection procedures and study instruments to best match the abilities of community residents so that the reliability and validity of study data are not compromised.

Finally, when planning to conduct field research in rural communities, it is essential to consider the budget impact of such research. Expense issues related to time management, travel, communications, and recruitment of participants can make many types of research studies, especially those involving some type of service delivery, more costly to conduct in rural areas than would be the case in urban or suburban communities. Careful budget preparation is a necessary aspect of all research planning, but this is especially the case for research in rural areas where hidden challenges may not become apparent until the research has actually begun, and where there is little literature available to provide guidance to perspective investigators.

Despite the challenges discussed above, we have been successful in recruiting participants and in implementing an evidence-based psychosocial intervention. Early data indicate that so far, for most of our older rural study participants, PEARL is having a positive impact on their emotional well-being and their quality of life. Should these encouraging early patterns prove to be reliable indicators of the final study outcomes, we believe that the results of this study could have importance for the delivery of gerontological mental health services. We think that the future successful development of mental health services for frail older adults, particularly those living in rural areas, is tied to the concept of accessible delivery. For many frail elders, this means service delivery in the home, whether through in-person interventions, or through the use of currently available or emerging electronic technologies. Though the provision of high-quality in-home mental health services for older persons can be relatively costly in the short term, we believe the payoff in the longer term will be improved quality of life for these individuals, at lower, overall costs to the health care system. Providing high quality mental health services for this population makes sense from a public health perspective based on the known relations between emotional well-being, quality of life, and functional status. If efficacious services can be provided to improve the mental health of older persons, costs associated with excessive disability and the use of traditional health care services can be reduced. We believe, however, that the real impetus to constitute the delivery of mental services under challenging circumstances for these vulnerable individuals should not be in relation to possible long term cost savings, but rather, because of the potential improvements that can be gained in their participative well-being and the quality of their lives.

REFERENCES

Abraham, I. L., & Neese, J. B. (1993). Outreach to the elderly and their families. *Aging, 365,* 26-32.

Administration on Aging (2003). *A profile of older Americans: 2002.* Retrieved August, 12, 2003, from http://www.aoa.gov/prof/statistics/profile/2002profile.doc.

Blazer, D., Hughes, D. C., & George, L. K. (1987). The epidemiology of depression in an elderly community population. *The Gerontologist, 27,* 281-287.

Bourdon, K. H., Rae, D. S., Locke, B. Z., Narrow, W. E., & Regier, D. A. (1992). Estimating the prevalence of mental disorders in U.S. adults from the epidemiologic catchment area survey. *Public Health Reports, 107,* 663-668.

Boyle, D. P., Jacobsen, M., & MacNair, R. H. (1994). Introduction to the special issue: The effect of culture on the delivery of human services. *Human Services in the Rural Environment, 17* (3/4), 7-8.

Buckwalter, K. C., Smith, M., Zevenbergen, P., & Russell, D. (1991). Mental health services of the Rural Elderly Outreach Program. *The Gerontologist, 31,* 408-412.

Bull, C. N. (1998). Aging in rural communities. *National Forum, 78* (2), 38-42.

Bull, C. N., & Bane, S. D. (1993). Growing old in rural America. *Aging, 365,* 18.

Butler, R. N., Lewis, M. I., & Sunderland, T. (1998). Aging and mental health (5th ed.). Boston: Allyn & Bacon.

Cohen, G. D. (1990). Prevalence of psychiatric problems in older adults. *Psychiatric Annals, 20,* 433-438.

Glasgow, N., & Brown, D. L. (1998). Older, rural, and poor. In R. T. Coward and J. A. Krout (Eds) (1998). *Aging in rural settings* (187-207). New York: Springer.

Heard-Mueller, B., Darville, R., & Watson, J. B. (1994). Health care utilization among rural elderly women. *Human Services in the Rural Environment, 17* (3/4), 34-41.

Helge, D. (1981). Problems in implementing comprehensive special education programming in rural areas. *Exceptional Children, 47,* 514-520.

Helge, D. (1984). Models for serving rural students with low-income handicapping conditions. *Exceptional Children, 52,* 313-324.

Junginger, J., Phelan, E., Cherry, K., & Levy, J. (1993). Prevalence of psychopathology in elderly persons in nursing homes and the community. *Hospital and Community Psychiatry, 44,* 381-383.

Kelleher, K., & Long, N. (1994). Barriers and new directions in mental health services research in the primary care setting. *Journal of Clinical Child Psychology, 23,* 133.

Krout, J. A. (1998). Services and service delivery in rural environments. In R. T. Coward and J. A. Krout (Eds). *Aging in rural settings.* New York: Springer Publishing Company, 247-286.

Lawrence, S. A., & McCulloch, B. J. (2001). Rural mental health and elders: Historical inequities. *Journal of Applied Gerontology, 20,* 144-169.

McCullogh, J. B., & Lynch, M. S. (1993). Barriers to solutions: Service delivery and public policy in rural areas. *Journal of Applied Gerontology, 12,* 388-403.

Meyers, J. K., Weisssman, M. M., Tischler, G. L., Holzer, C. E., Leaf, P. J., Orvaschel, H. et al. (1984). Six-month prevalence of psychiatric disorders in three communities: 1980-1982. *Archives of General Psychiatry, 41,* 959-967.

Mott, G. E., Dean, A., Wang, B., & Wood, P. (1992). Identifying clinical syndromes in a community sample of elderly persons. *Psychological Assessment, 4,* 174-184.

Parish, B., & Landsberg, G. (1984). Developing a geriatric mental health outreach unit in a rural community. *Journal of Gerontological Social Work 7* (3), 75-82.

Rathbone-McCuan, E. (2001). Mental health care provision for rural elders. *Journal of Applied Gerontology, 20,* 170-183.

Regier, D. A., Boyd, J. H., & Burke, J. D. (1988). One-month prevalence of mental disorders in the United States. *Archives of General Psychiatry, 45,* 977-986.

Rich, R. O., & Dalton, W. B. (1995/96). Preparing for managed mental health care in a rural environment: Impacts on the organization and delivery of mental health services in Northeastern Washington. *Human Services in the Rural Environment 19* (2/3), 14-19.

Roskes, E., Feldman, R., Arrington, S., & Leisher, M. (1999). A model program for the treatment of the mentally ill offenders in the community. *Community Mental Health Journal 35,* 461.

Rubinstein, P. G. (1995). The development of battered women's services in rural areas. *Human Services in the Rural Environment 19* (2), 29-33.

Russell, R. (1997). The senior outreach program of Park Ridge Mental Health: An innovative approach to mental health and aging. *Journal of Gerontological Social Work, 29,* 95.

Scheidt, R. J. (1985). The mental health of the aged in rural environments. In R. T. Cowart & G. R. Lee (Eds.). *The elderly in rural society* (pp. 105-127). New York: Springer.

Segal, S. P., Silverman, C., & Temkin, T. (1993). Empowerment and self-help agency practice for people with mental disabilities. *Social Work, 38,* 705-712.

Sirey, J. A., Bruce, M. L., Alexopoulos, G. S., Perlick, D. A., Raue, P., Friedman, S. J. et al. (2001). Perceived stigma as a predictor of treatment discontinuation in younger and older patients with depression. *The American Journal of Psychiatry, 158,* 479-481.

Stewart, A. L., & King, A. C. (1994). Conceptualizing and measuring quality of life in older populations. In R. P. Abeles, H. C. Gift, & M. G. Ory (Eds.), *Aging and Quality of Life.* New York: Springer, 27-54.

United States Department of Health and Human Services (1999). *Mental health: A report of the Surgeon General.* Rockville, MD: U.S. Department of Health and Human Services.

Van Hook, M. P., & Ford, M. E. (1998). The linkage model for delivering mental health services in rural communities: Benefits and Challenges. *Health & Social Work, 23,* 53-60.

doi:10.1300/J083v48n03_05

Using Collaboration to Maximize Outcomes for a John A. Hartford Foundation Geriatric Enrichment Project

Debra Fromm Faria, MSW
Virginia V. David, MSW
Jason Dauenhauer, MSW, PhD
Diane Dwyer, MSW

SUMMARY. Two institutions representing two BSW and one MSW program and a geriatric education center collaborated in a John A. Hartford geriatric enrichment project. Sharing the risks and benefits of a collaborative model, 75 percent of faculty participated in mini faculty fellowships, and bi-monthly dinner meetings with colleagues from each of the three programs, and actively engaged in the curricula revisions. Faculty report pervasive geriatric enrichment in each program's foundation content areas, and increases in students placed in geriatric enriched field practicum settings, from pre-project levels of 8.1 percent to a high of 24 percent. The features of the collaborative project include: respecting each program's autonomy while actively sharing ideas, resources and partnering with community's aging experts; and strengthening mutually

[Haworth co-indexing entry note]: "Using Collaboration to Maximize Outcomes for a John A. Hartford Foundation Geriatric Enrichment Project." Faria, Debra Fromm et al. Co-published simultaneously in *Journal of Gerontological Social Work* (The Haworth Press, Inc.) Vol. 48, No. 3/4, 2007, pp. 367-386; and: *Fostering Social Work Gerontology Competence: A Collection of Papers from the First National Gerontological Social Work Conference* (ed: Catherine J. Tompkins, and Anita L. Rosen) The Haworth Press, Inc., 2007, pp. 367-386. Single or multiple copies of this article are available for a fee from The Haworth Document Delivery Service [1-800-HAWORTH, 9:00 a.m. - 5:00 p.m. (EST). E-mail address: docdelivery@haworthpress.com].

reciprocal relationships among faculty and the gerontologic practice community. This model of shared risks and benefits also provides opportunities for innovation, diverse thinking, and shared decision making. doi:10.1300/J083v48n03_06 *[Article copies available for a fee from The Haworth Document Delivery Service: 1-800-HAWORTH. E-mail address: <docdelivery@haworthpress.com> Website: <http://www.HaworthPress.com> © 2007 by The Haworth Press, Inc. All rights reserved.]*

KEYWORDS. Geriatric enrichment, collaborative model, undergraduate education, graduate education

INTRODUCTION

The State University of New York (SUNY) College at Brockport and Nazareth College of Rochester, in conjunction with the Finger Lakes Geriatric Education Center (FLGEC) at the University of Rochester collaborated in a John A. Hartford Geriatric Enrichment Project to provide baccalaureate and masters-level social work (BSW and MSW) students from two academic institutions, comprising three social work programs, with geriatric learning opportunities to prepare them to meet the diverse needs of older adults and their families.

The strengths of this project included the combined resources and faculty expertise from two locally-based accredited BSW programs, one MSW program in candidacy with the Council on Social Work Education (CSWE), and one university-based federally-funded Geriatric Education Center specializing in the development and implementation of continuing geriatric education programs for multidisciplinary audiences. Each partner entered into this project having shared a rich history of successful collaborative partnership experiences. SUNY College at Brockport and Nazareth College of Rochester developed the Greater Rochester Collaborative MSW Program (GRC MSW), the first private/public university bi-institutional MSW program in the United States. Nazareth College has an already established formal relationship with FLGEC, collaborating to provide knowledge and skills focusing on culturally competent and cultural congruent health care for older adults from diverse backgrounds through a Multidisciplinary Ethnogeriatric Education Grant. By leveraging each respective institution's financial and intellectual resources, this project maximized the expansion of geriatric learning opportunities for a much larger group of social work students than could be accomplished by any one academic program.

NEED FOR GERIATRIC ENRICHMENT CURRICULA DEVELOPMENT

All three programs include gerontologic content in Human Behavior and the Social Environment (HBSE) life-span courses using a chronological age approach. The delivery of this content typically occurs at the end of the course, increasing the risk of short-changing gerontologic content due to course time constraints. For instance, information regarding child welfare and younger family systems is given much more attention than issues related to the unique needs of older adults and their families, or intergenerational family issues. The level of gerontologic content in other courses (practice, policy, diversity, etc.) is dependent upon the differential preferences and expertise of faculty members teaching those courses. A cursory review of the curricula vitae indicated that most faculty had negligible expertise in this arena. We also found that there were a limited number of gerontologic readings or assignments required in foundation courses.

SUNY College at Brockport offers a social work elective in gerontology, which can be taken for graduate or undergraduate credit. Additionally, both academic institutions offer undergraduate minors in gerontology that are interdisciplinary and consist of 18 credit hours. However, few students choose or are unable to take advantage of these opportunities. The Field Education component of each program's curriculum provides opportunities for students to integrate theory and knowledge into practice though skill development and skill refinement within the context of professional ethics. Although opportunities exist for students to select field practicum sites in agencies serving older adults and their families, relatively small number of students (11 of 135) from the collaborating institutions selected age-enriched social work field practicum sites in 2001. The small number of students (8.1 percent) selecting age-enriched field practicum sites directly affects the gerontologic exposure social work students glean from one another in to the practicum-based assignments, class discussions, and presentations.

The Greater Rochester Metropolitan area is fortunate to have a multitude of potential gerontologic focused field practicum sites. Many of these sites offer students opportunities to collaborate with multi-disciplinary teams. These sites exist in health care settings (nursing homes, hospitals, home-based care agencies), community settings (Office on Aging Programs, Adult Protective Services, day care programs and residential facilities), and to a lesser degree, acute care settings (geriatric evaluation, geriatric consultation services, geropsychiatric ward, and geriatric outpatient) (Lubben, Damron-Rodriguez, & Beck, 1992). Additionally, university-based and agency-based programs located in the Greater Rochester Metropolitan area have demonstrated leadership in development and implementation of innovative gerontologic programs including a Programs of All-inclusive Care for the Elderly (PACE) program, one of the first multi-disciplinary geriatric assessment clinics, innovative programs to prevent elder abuse, geriatric addictions and others. However, many students do not choose these field sites for placement during the practicum planning process. The programs collectively have affiliation agreements with approximately 30 aging service providers with the vast majority serving urban populations. The fact that so few students choose to intern in aging-related settings suggests that the lack of gerontologic course content, combined with negative ageist stereotypes, biases the selection process.

The lack of aging content in each of the collaborating institutions' social work programs reflects similar findings as described in the literature, which identify barriers to the incorporation of aging content into both undergraduate and graduate curricula. Researchers found these barriers include a lack of faculty with expertise in geriatrics, curriculum that is too full, fiscal constraints, low salaries for geriatric social workers, and ageist attitudes on the part of social work students and faculty (Lubben et al., 1992; Berkman, Damron-Rodriguez, Dobrof, & Harry, 1996).

OUR COLLABORATIVE PROJECT

Given the limited gerontologic content in the existing curricula, minimal expertise by the majority of faculty in aging related issues and the lack of infusion across the educational experience, three objectives were established to accomplish the goal of providing gerontologic education to BSW and MSW students. Objective 1: *infuse aging-enriched content into existing BSW generalist and MSW foundation year curricula following a comprehensive and critical review;* Objective 2: *provide didactic and experiential geriatric education for social work faculty to increase their knowledge of gerontologic issues*; Objective 3: *increase and enhance the number of aging service-provider field placement sites in both urban and rural settings by a minimum of ten percent (and increase by at least 25 percent the number of students who select these sites).*

Year One: Project Planning

To ensure the successful development, implementation, and evaluation of these objectives, the collaborating institutions constituted a series of six components in the planning phases from January 2002 to August 2002, including the: (1) creation of a memorandum of understanding between each of the collaborating partners outlining the responsibilities of each collaborator, (2) establishment of a monthly executive leadership committee meeting to manage the progression of the project, (3) development of a community-based multidisciplinary advisory committee to assist with curricular and field practicum development, (4) development and implementation of a faculty curriculum review committee, (5) creation of a gerontology education resource library for faculty use, and (6) utilization of a curricular consultant with a background in gerontology and geriatric social work education.

Project Infrastructure

The *Executive Leadership Committee* (ELC) worked collaboratively to plan, coordinate and implement project objectives. ELC members shared responsibility in providing direction and support to faculty, recruiting members for a community-based multidisciplinary advisory committee, co-managing faculty development opportunities and outcome assessment. Two ELC members (project co-directors) are chairpersons of social work departments and BSW program directors at their respective institutions; one member serves as project director and is director of field education for the MSW program, and the faculty consultant from FLGECC maintains linkages and networking opportunities through his position at the university. The structure of ELC ensures that each program is represented fully in the administration of the project from project design, management through evaluation. This model of shared leadership and responsibility is possible when working relationships are based on mutual trust, clear communication and a commitment to group process (Dougherty et al., 2000). ELC members have experience working collaboratively on other projects and funded grants. Through this model, ELC members share the project's risks and rewards. Each member has a stake in the outcome, which enhances meeting project goals and objectives in a sustainable manner in all three programs.

The *Faculty Curriculum Committee* (FCC) involves interested faculty from the three programs and has three roles: to review current courses and to identify where gerontologic content could be added; to identify barriers to geriatric enrichment opportunities in each program; and to identify and foster individual faculty interest in gerontologic social work issues.

Initially, we planned to identify and select a number of interested faculty from each program to form one FCC. However, as we began planning, we realized that to maximize the cross-fertilization opportunities among interested faculty, all interested faculty would be invited to all project events and meetings, and that each program's ELC member would coordinate specific enrichment strategies with faculty from her/his own program in FCC subcommittees. This approach ensured that each program had autonomy in choosing how to enrich identified courses across the foundation curriculum with gerontologic content, while offering faculty professional development programs and opportunities to meet together to share ideas, approaches, and experiences.

Multidisciplinary Advisory Committee (MAC) advisory in nature, with the goal that committee members would be a resource to faculty; assist with curricular and field practicum development; recommend items for the development of a geriatric education resource library, and assist ELC to develop a community-wide speakers' bureau of aging experts. It was our expectation that partnering with the community in this manner would further the development and utilization of MAC and would benefit this project by bringing best practice issues and expertise into the academic environment and foster the development of additional field practicum sites.

Year One Activities and Accomplishments

Multidisciplinary Advisory Committee: Eighteen potential participants were identified with letters of invitation mailed in February 2002. Several of the invitees had written letters of support for the grant application, and had expressed interest in participating. We were pleased that all of the individuals identified as perspective members agreed to serve on MAC. The committee is composed of five older adults, three of whom are family caregivers, and two retired social workers. Seven members are community social workers in gerontologic social work leadership and practice positions, and six members are aging specialists and service providers representing multidisciplinary perspectives. The advisory committee met twice during the planning year. The first meeting provided an overview of the project and a speakers' bureau. During the second meeting, the community advisory committee assisted the ELC in planning mini field shadowing experiences for faculty by offering to open their programs to faculty to spend time in their agencies, and in assisting the ELC in making connections with other service providers for faculty shadowing experiences.

FACULTY ENGAGEMENT

The development of faculty support or "buy in" for the project is the first step in promoting the overall project goal of achieving gerontologic pervasiveness and sustainability in the curriculum. We adopted a multi-pronged approach including collaborative engagement with program faculty and the practice community. The infrastructure design of the project provides a vehicle for this partnership to sustain project initiatives.

ELC met with faculty in each program in March and April 2002. Faculty meetings served as forums to: introduce faculty to the funded CSWE /Hartford geriatric enrichment project, introduce faculty to collaborative partners, provide project background information including copies of the project's executive summary, and introduce plans to support faculty with stipends for mini faculty fellowships and professional development support for conferences and trainings. In preparation for each meeting, ELC members talked informally with faculty colleagues about the project, a strategy we found helpful in keeping faculty interest in the project design before the initial faculty group meetings.

Surveys were distributed to all faculty with a 100 percent return rate. The survey design invited faculty comments regarding their assessment of foundation curriculum modifications needed to meet gerontologic enrichment goals in foundation curriculum. These data provided us with information about faculty perceptions of potential barriers, and the types of resources and topic areas of interest to faculty. Survey data were utilized to plan a two-day faculty development mini fellowship, and to develop strategies to engage faculty in curricula discussions. The survey results suggest that a majority of faculty in each program teaches limited age enriched content in foundation courses, and a correlation between the gerontologic content incorporated in foundation courses related to faculty interest, knowledge and comfort level with this material. These data reinforced our initial assessment that limited gerontologic course content is related to the minimal expertise by the majority of faculty in aging related issues and the lack of infusion across the educational experience.

These initial meetings provided a springboard for a *Faculty Curriculum Review Committee* that would bring faculty together to share ideas and resources for gerontologic course content enrichment across foundation curricula.

Mini-Faculty Fellowships

One of the primary methods to achieve faculty buy-in in relation to curricular infusion was the development and implementation of "mini-geriatric fellowships" for social work faculty. This initiative relates directly to Project Objective 2: *provide didactic and experiential geriatric education for social work faculty to increase their knowledge of gerontologic issues.* Because many faculty lack expertise and knowledge about aging issues, we thought it critical to provide geriatric education for faculty to increase their knowledge about aging in a way that was conducive to curricular integration.

Nearly all faculty (90%) surveyed expressed interest in learning how to infuse aging content. Recognizing that the mini-fellowships would occur when faculty were off contract in the summer and as an incentive to attend the program, faculty were offered a $300 stipend.

Offered on two consecutive days, an interactive program was attended by nearly 75% of all full-time faculty (n = 14) representing three social work programs, 50% of all adjunct faculty (n = 5) and three MAC members. Based on faculty interests, speaker availability, and project directors' experience, the program covered six topics: comprehensive geriatric assessment, end-of-life decision making/ethical issues, cultural competency and geriatrics, elder abuse, social security, and successful aging. Each session lasted approximately 1.5 hours and included time for discussion. A critical feature of this training was the use of the video, *To Be Old, Black, and Poor*, providing a case study presentation framework. In preparation for the training, each presenter viewed the video and incorporated relevant subject matter into her/his presentation. Faculty were given binders with content distributed by CSWE/SAGE-SW, including a CD-ROM with aging resources, a locally produced CD on elder abuse, an elder abuse identification flow chart, and a host of other important aging resources. "Ethnogeriatrics," developed and compiled by the Stanford Geriatric Education Center, was purchased on the behalf of each program as an additional faculty resource.

Evaluations from the didactic portion of the fellowship were highly positive with a mean score of 3.52 out of 4 points (4 = excellent). One of the few criticisms dealt with faculty who felt they knew much of the aging "basics" such as demographic as well as foundation information for some of the other topics. Essentially, they felt they could have skipped some of the introductory content for more detailed subject matter. However, in reviewing pre/post test results of the Palmore's *Facts on Aging Quiz*, faculty perception of knowledge and missed questions on the *Aging Facts Post Test* provide evidence that additional content on aging is needed to facilitate further knowledge development.

MOVING FROM PLANNING TO IMPLEMENTATION

At the close of the final session, participants were asked to complete a work plan for how they planned to infuse aging content in a particular course or course module. The project leaders discussed meeting together with faculty prior to the beginning of the next academic year to develop implementation strategies. To our surprise, fellowship participants strongly suggested scheduling a follow-up meeting sooner rather than later for group discussions. Faculty expressed interest in talking with colleagues to discuss course work plan ideas and requested that the meeting be scheduled within several weeks of the completion of the didactic portion of the mini faculty fellowship. Although this meeting took place over the summer when faculty were not on contract and were not compensated to participate in the follow up meeting, twelve faculty from three programs met together for a four-hour dinner meeting at one of the colleges.

ELC members used *Questions to Guide the Creation of Age-Rich Learning Opportunities* available on the www.gerorich.org web site. Faculty discussed the questions as a whole and then met separately by individual program to discuss ways to infuse aging content into their specific social work foundation. The larger group then reconvened and shared ideas with colleagues in the other programs.

Agency-Based Experiential Component

The second component of the fellowship was the geriatric field experience. Faculty received a $100.00 stipend for participating in eight hours of geriatric field experience. In conjunction with the community advisory board, twelve different "internships" were developed. Faculty selected a community-based service provider and a long-term care facility and spent at least four hours in each setting, meeting with and shadowing gerontologic social workers. Three rural settings were identified by the local Rural Area Health Education Center. Faculty choosing a rural setting received an additional $100.00 stipend from funding support from the Rural Area Health Education Center. In all, eight faculty participated in the geriatric field experience and four faculty spent some time in a rural geriatric setting.

Evaluations were highly positive with a number of faculty setting up site visits for their students (e.g., practice class). Many commented how their scope of knowledge about geriatric social work had expanded and was directly applicable to the courses they taught. Faculty also met with community geriatric practitioners and leaders, which informally led to invitations to guest lecture in 2002 classes. This unanticipated outcome was identified as the informal beginning of our speakers' bureau.

Year Two Implementation

Each program used existing mechanisms to incorporate generated ideas into curricula modifications (e.g., curriculum committee, faculty meetings). Faculty from each program (full-time, half-time, and adjunct faculty) were invited to dinner meetings in a popular local restaurant to mutually share implementation experiences. On average, 75% of full-time and 70% of adjunct faculty participated regularly in these dinner meetings, an indicator of faculty engagement with this project during the implementation stage. Through these meetings, faculty acquired new information directly applicable to their courses, developed relationships with colleagues teaching in other programs and further developed relationships with the multidisciplinary advisory committee members who periodically met with faculty at these dinners.

Year Two Implementation Outcomes (by Program)

Nazareth's BSW Program faculty developed enrichment strategies in multiple courses. Program faculty coordinated the enrichment activities to build on the knowledge, theories and skills incrementally. For example, in the social work introductory class, students visited a long-term care setting, met with a social worker at this setting and an older adult residing at the facility. In the junior level practice course, all juniors interviewed an older adult from their practicum setting or as arranged by the program. Students learned what "life was like" when the older adult was the same age as the student interviewer, what were their hopes and dreams, as well as the conventional views/attitudes/stereotypes that might have existed relative to older adults. Students were required to write reflective journals about their experiences with this assignment. Student reported positive experiences in meeting and interviewing an older adult. Faculty reported that this assignment provided students with opportunities to consider similarities and differences within an historical context and what influences and characteristics shape us. In addition, students in this course had several female caregivers speak in their classes and share their experiences as caregivers. In HBSE and Practice I, the video *Big Mama* was shown and HBSE and practice faculty developed concurrent assignments. The video *To Be Old, Black, and Poor* was used for a variety of course content areas; for example, the diversity course used this video to explore ageist attitudes and stereotypes. In the policy course, policy implications were identified and analyzed. Additionally, BSW seniors, as a college-wide requirement for all graduating students, completed a comprehensive examination demonstrating generalist knowledge and skills across the social work foundation content areas as well as the liberal arts, from the case study presented in the video.

The Nazareth College/SUNY Brockport GRC MSW Program enriched the foundation curriculum in the following ways: In the foundation practice course, a community collaboration project was developed in which students interviewed older adults regarding their attitudes toward front line health care workers. Videos with gerontologic content (*To Be Old, Black, and Poor* and *Big Mama*) were shown as case studies for in-class assessment exercises. Students were provided opportunities to connect with a community-based kinship care resource center to increase intergenerational attention in assessments. In the second practice class, readings were added to the syllabus related to community practice with older adults. In the first HBSE course, the life span was presented in reverse, beginning with end of life. An interdisciplinary panel participated gerontologic perspectives in a discussion related to ecosystems theory; and the video, *Growing Old Aging Well* presented positive views of aging. In the first research course, students complete a research ethics quiz to ensure that they understand human subject protection requirements. The instructor for Research I and Practice I partnered together, assisting students to make the connection between research and practice in the interview project with older adults. In Research II, gerontologic statistical data sets were used for SPSS lab practices. The foundation level policy course included content on policy issues affecting older adults including a class project involving policy research as an advocacy model to support an under-funded geriatric assessment clinic in the community. In the MSW concentration year interdisciplinary health policy course, students organized and presented a community forum featuring interdisciplinary experts on elder abuse. This forum was advertised in the community and well attended by a diverse audience. Additionally, a popular family law elective was enriched by including content on elder law, end-of-life decisions and elder abuse.

The SUNY Brockport BSW program also incorporated the video *Big Mama* in each section of the junior practice class. Faculty teaching other junior level courses related themes from this video to course content, providing students with a multiple opportunities to relate generalist social work principles to aging from a micro/mezzo/macro systems perspective. Junior level field students were encouraged to interview an older adult during their field practicum, thus identifying opportunities to explore intergenerational connections. In HBSE, an existing family role play assignment was modified to require at least three generations in each segment of the role-play as the family "ages" across the lifespan. In the junior year policy course, one of the first units presented is "Programs and Services for Older Adults." Later in the semester, after presenting child and youth welfare programs, the two are compared and contrasted. Faculty report themes presented in *Big Mama* lend themselves nicely to this analysis. In the research course, a study on aging was added to a unit on experimental designs (as an example of a longitudinal design), and students participate in a needs assessment project in a community senior center. This project incorporates a student service-learning component, in support of a new program initiative. Field seminar instructors report that they are more attentive in integrating concepts such as intergenerational family concerns, successful aging, elder abuse, cultural patterns of aging, and adolescent relationships with older adults in field seminar discussions.

SUPPORTING CONTINUED FACULTY DEVELOPMENT

Full-time faculty in each of the three programs were eligible to receive up to $600.00 for travel and conference costs for the first National Gerontological Social Work Conference (NGSWC) in Atlanta, Georgia. February 27-March 2, 2003. Requirements for this support included APM/NGSWC conference registration, completion of a conference summary form indicating sessions attended, and descriptions of plans to integrate new gerontologic enriched content into future courses. Sixteen percent of eligible faculty received support for attending NGSWC through this project; another 16% of faculty attended NGSWC sessions, but did not apply for project support for conference costs as other travel/conference support was available.

Co-Sponsored Geriatric Enrichment Events

Nazareth College's Annual Helen Guthrie Memorial Lecture held in spring semester 2003 had a gerontologic focus and was titled *Social Work and Gerontology: Aging Awareness and Advocacy.* Five panelists participated in a 2.5-hour presentation related to social work advocacy and empowerment in long term care settings, geriatric addictions, elder abuse services, and community services. Faculty, students, field instructors, and project community advisory members attended the lecture. This program provided gerontologic enriched didactic information, and opportunities for discussion, and community networking. Thirty-one percent of faculty attended this lecture.

During fall semester 2003, a session titled *Ethnogeriatric Issues and Trends in Social Work Practice* was presented. It was co-sponsored by our John A. Hartford geriatric enrichment project, the Nazareth College Multidisciplinary Ethnogeriatric Education project, NASW-GVD, and the Social Work Departments at Nazareth College and SUNY Brockport. Students, field instructors, faculty, advisory committee members, NASW members, and participants at the annual NYS Social Work Education Association Annual Conference were invited to attend this reception/program, which featured an expert on ethnogeriatric issues. This program represented an example of collaborating with other partners to sustain the efforts of this project.

CONCLUSION

We are in process of evaluating this geriatric enrichment project. Results from the year one didactic and experiential mini faculty fellowships were rated positively. Stipends served as a motivator and recognized the value of faculty involved in project activities. We found that faculty with little background in gerontology became excited about the material when it was presented in a logical and useful manner. Organizing the training so that information could be directly incorporated into coursework was a key to the success of the fellowship. The geriatric field experience, though selected by fewer faculty, was by all accounts a success as it provided faculty first-hand exposure to real-life issues being faced by social worker professionals and their constituents. The key to providing this type of education is timing. Perhaps if it were offered at a more convenient time of the year, more would have taken advantage of the opportunity. Also, faculty needed to contact and arrange a meeting time with the preceptor on their own. It is possible that some faculty were not interested in making these contacts due to other commitments during his or her summer break.

Most faculty (75 percent) participated in the didactic portion of the mini geriatric fellowship and year two bi-monthly dinner meetings. Faculty report positive student responses, which provided affirmative reinforcement of curricula enrichment. Faculty in each program report having a sense of ownership for the curricula changes. This appears related to faculty actively participating in the process and outcome. Faculty also report that the collaborative model adopted for this project provided multiple opportunities for cross-fertilization of curriculum enrichment ideas and opportunities to develop contacts with aging specialists in the community.

While we are very pleased with the support we received for project initiatives, we must also point out that 25 percent of faculty did not participate in project-supported initiatives regardless of the stipends, delicious meals, fellowship and lively discussions. However, some did enrich their courses with gerontologic content by adding readings and inviting guest speakers to classes. The follow up faculty survey will attempt to learn more from these faculty members about their perceptions and experience with curriculum enhancements and the project.

In reviewing field practica data collected for year one, and comparing this data to year two and to the partially collected data for year three, we find that the number of aging enriched field placement sites and students placed at these sites are increasing. For example, our 2001 baseline demonstrates 8.1 percent of students from all three programs were in aging enriched field sites; this was increased by 10% in the first year (averaging all three programs). In year two, 25% (N = 33) of the Nazareth BSW students, 16% (N = 66) of GRC MSW students and 10% (N = 40) of Brockport BSW students were placed in aging enriched placements. Year three data is in process of being collected. To date, the MSW program reports 24 percent of students are placed in aging enriched field sites. Our success in increasing the number of rural and urban field sites appears related to two key factors: (a) the relationships developing between faculty and members of MAC and (b) the use of a proactive stance to encourage students to consider a gerontologic or intergenerational internship.

Additional follow up with faculty during the 2003/2004 academic year is planned using several additional evaluation methods. A faculty survey developed by ELC will be distributed in fall semester 2003 (Appendix). In addition, content analysis of syllabi, review of course enrichment strategies and materials, review of evaluative data collected to date and a faculty focus group are planned. We are also tracking the unanticipated outcomes that have resulted from this project. For example, the Nazareth College co-director was named co-director of the Multi-Ethnogeriatric Education Grant at Nazareth College. The SUNY Brockport BSW program identified the opportunity to develop a service-learning project with the geriatric enrichment activity.

Through our collaboration, mutually reciprocal relationships are strengthened among faculty and the gerontological practice community. This model of shared risks and benefits provides opportunities for innovation, diverse thinking, and shared decision making (Dougherty, 2000). These features are vital in securing faculty support to enrich foundation curricula in a pervasive and sustainable manner.

REFERENCES

Berkman, B., Damron-Rodriguez, J., Dobrof, R., & Harry, L. (1996). The state of the art in geriatric social work education and training. In S. Klein (ed.), *A national agenda for geriatric education: White papers* (pp. 220-247). Rockville, MD: Health Resources and Services Administration.

Candy, D. & Gifford, R. (2002, Summer). Taking a closer look at community collaboration in *The Rosamond Gifford Community Exchange Forums: Community Collaboration.* Vol.1, Issue 2.

Dougherty, M. (2000). *Psychological consultation and collaboration: In school and community settings* (3rd ed.). Boston, MA: Brooks Cole.

Films for the Humanities & Sciences. (Producer). (2000). *Living longer aging well* [Motion Picture] (Available from Film for Humanities, PO Box 2053, Princeton, NJ 08543-2053).

Films for the Humanities & Sciences (Producer). (1993). *To be old, black and poor* [Motion Picture] (Available from Film for Humanities, PO Box 2053, Princeton, NJ 08543-2053).

Lubben, L.E., Damron-Rodriguez, J.A., & Beck, J.C. (1992). A national survey of aging curriculum in schools of social work. In J. Mellor & R. Solloman (Eds.), *Geriatric social work education,* 151-171. New York: The Haworth Press, Inc.

Seretean T. (Producer & Director), & McFerrin B. (Composer). (2000). *Big Mama* [Motion Picture]. (Available from California Newsreel, P.O. Box 2284, South Burlington, VT 05407).

University of Washington, Gerorich project (2001). *Questions to guide the creation of age-rich learning opportunities.* Retrieved June 9, 2002, from University of Washington, Gerorich project Web site: http://www.gerorich.org.

doi:10.1300/J083v48n03_06

APPENDIX

Geriatric Enrichment Faculty Survey

Introduction: The purpose of this survey is to assess the degree of faculty education and integration of aging content into existing curricula as result of the activities associated with the aging infusion grant from the John A. Hartford Foundation and Council on Social Work Education. The results of the survey will be used to identify faculty needs and barriers associated with the infusion of aging content and how to best meet these needs.

1. If you participated in any of the following activities developed as part of this geriatric education initiative, please rate how useful each of these programs were to <u>improving your knowledge about aging issues</u>. If you select *not useful* for any of the questions, please describe.

	Did Not Participate	Not Useful	Somewhat Useful	Very Useful
A. Geriatric 2-day fellowship (June, 2002)	❑	❑	❑	❑
B. Geriatric field experience (June/July 2002)	❑	❑	❑	❑
C. Any faculty lunch/dinner meetings to discuss aging content issues (June 2002-February 2003)	❑	❑	❑	❑

Comments: _____

_____

2. If you participated in any of the following activities developed as part of this geriatric education initiative, please rate how useful each of these programs were to <u>incorporating aging content into your courses</u>. If you select *not useful* for any of the questions, please describe.

	Did Not Participate	Not Useful	Somewhat Useful	Very Useful
A. Geriatric 2-day fellowship (June, 2002)	❑	❑	❑	❑
B. Geriatric field experience (June/July 2002)	❑	❑	❑	❑
C. Any faculty lunch/dinner meetings to discuss aging content issues (June 2002-February 2003)	❑	❑	❑	❑

Comments: _____

_____

APPENDIX (continued)

3. Which, if any, courses you teach have been modified (since June 2002) to incorporate aging content? Please list the course title and number and a brief description about the new material. Use the back of this form if necessary.

For the course(s) described in Q 3, is this new content reflected in the <u>course syllabi</u>? Please list the course(s) and check where in the syllabus the new information may be found.

A1. Course title/number: _____

B1. Content in syllabus: ❑ Yes   ❑ No

C1. Location in syllabus: (Please check all that apply)

❑ Objectives ❑ Readings ❑ Assignments (e.g., papers) ❑ Class activities/discussions

❑ Other (Please describe) _____

A2. Course title/number: _____

B2. Content in syllabus: ❑ Yes   ❑ No

C2. Location in syllabus: (Please check all that apply)

❑ Objectives ❑ Readings ❑ Assignments (e.g., papers) ❑ Class activities/discussions

❑ Other (Please describe) _____

A3. Course title/number: _____

B3. Content in syllabus: ❑ Yes   ❑ No

C3. Location in syllabus: (Please check all that apply)

❑ Objectives ❑ Readings ❑ Assignments (e.g., papers) ❑ Class activities/discussions

❑ Other (Please describe) _____

A4. Course title/number: _____

B4. Content in syllabus: ❑ Yes   ❑ No

C4. Location in syllabus: (Please check all that apply)

❑ Objectives ❑ Readings ❑ Assignments (e.g., papers) ❑ Class activities/discussions

❑ Other (Please describe) _____

A5. Course title/number: _____

B5. Content in syllabus: ❑ Yes   ❑ No

C5. Location in syllabus: (Please check all that apply)

❑ Objectives ❑ Readings ❑ Assignments (e.g., papers) ❑ Class activities/discussions

❑ Other (Please describe) _____

A6. Course title/number: _____

B6. Content in syllabus: ❏ Yes   ❏ No

C6. Location in syllabus: (Please check all that apply)

❏ Objectives ❏ Readings ❏ Assignments (e.g., papers) ❏ Class activities/discussions

❏ Other (Please describe) _____

4. This geriatric initiative developed the following resources to assist faculty with the infusion of aging content. Please tell us if you were aware of the tools, if you utilized them and how useful they were.

A. Speakers Bureau (Professionals with various aging expertise who are willing to present in your classes)

A1. I was aware of this resource	❏ Yes	❏ No
A2. I utilized this resource	❏ Yes	❏ No

If "Yes" to QA2,

A3. How useful was this resource to help you infuse new aging content?

❏ Not Useful   ❏ Somewhat Useful   ❏ Very Useful

B. Textbooks on aging topics

B1. I was aware of this resource	❏ Yes	❏ No
B2. I utilized this resource	❏ Yes	❏ No

If "Yes" to QB2,

B3. How useful was this resource to help you infuse new aging content?

❏ Not Useful   ❏ Somewhat Useful   ❏ Very Useful

C. PowerPoint presentations with aging content

C1. I was aware of this resource	❏ Yes	❏ No
C2. I utilized this resource	❏ Yes	❏ No

If "Yes" to QC2,

C3. How useful was this resource to help you infuse new aging content?

❏ Not Useful   ❏ Somewhat Useful   ❏ Very Useful

APPENDIX (continued)

D. Handouts on specific aging issues (e.g., social issues, policy issues, etc.)

    D1. I was aware of this resource   ❑ Yes   ❑ No

    D2. I utilized this resource   ❑ Yes   ❑ No

    If "Yes" to QD2,

    D3. How useful was this resource to help you infuse new aging content?

    ❑ Not Useful   ❑ Somewhat Useful   ❑ Very Useful

E. Aging-related video tapes

    E1. I was aware of this resource   ❑ Yes   ❑ No

    E2. I utilized this resource   ❑ Yes   ❑ No

    If "Yes" to QE2,

    E3. How useful was this resource to help you infuse new aging content?

    ❑ Not Useful   ❑ Somewhat Useful   ❑ Very Useful

G. Other (please describe): _____

    G1. I was aware of this resource   ❑ Yes   ❑ No

    G2. I utilized this resource   ❑ Yes   ❑ No

    If "Yes" to QG2,

    G3. How useful was this resource to help you infuse new aging content?

    ❑ Not Useful   ❑ Somewhat Useful   ❑ Very Useful

5. What other courses do you think may benefit from incorporation of aging content? *(Please list)*

6. What types of barriers exist in regards to enhancing the current curricula to include aging content? *(Please describe)*

7. What types of aging issues you would like to learn more about?
(*Please check which topics interest you*)

❑ Biology of Aging

❑ Comprehensive Geriatric Assessment

❑ Cultural Competence

❑ Dementia & Older Adults

❑ Developmental Disabilities and Aging

❑ Elder Abuse

❑ Ethical Decision Making/End of Life

❑ Grand parenting

❑ Informal/Family Caregiving

❑ Interdisciplinary Teams

❑ Poverty & Aging

❑ Programs & Services for Older Adults

❑ Psychology of Aging

❑ Successful Aging

❑ The Aging Family

❑ Other Topics: _____

_____

8. In what format would you be most likely to participate in continuing geriatric education?

	Very Likely	Somewhat Likely	Not At All
A. Day-long conference	❑	❑	❑
B. Half-day conference	❑	❑	❑
C. Lunch meeting	❑	❑	❑
D. Dinner meeting	❑	❑	❑
E. On-Campus	❑	❑	❑
F. Off-Campus	❑	❑	❑
G. Other: _____	❑	❑	❑

9. How likely would you be to participate in a geriatric field experience of your choice? (e.g., shadowing a social work professional for varying lengths of time)

	Very Likely	Somewhat Likely	Not At All
A. Day-long conference	❑	❑	❑
B. Half-day conference	❑	❑	❑
C. Lunch meeting	❑	❑	❑
D. Dinner meeting	❑	❑	❑
E. On-Campus	❑	❑	❑
F. Off-Campus	❑	❑	❑
G. Other: _____	❑	❑	❑

APPENDIX (continued)

	Yes	No
10.Would you participate in this field experience if it was unpaid?	❏	❏

	Not Knowledgeable	Somewhat Knowledgeable	Moderately Knowledgeable	Very Knowledgeable
11. Overall, how would you rate your knowledge of aging/geriatrics in the context of teaching your students?	❏	❏	❏	❏

	Not Knowledgeable	Somewhat Knowledgeable	Moderately Knowledgeable	Very Knowledgeable
12. Overall, how would you rate the knowledge of aging/geriatrics in the students you teach?	❏	❏	❏	❏

13. Please describe any ideas you may have about improving the aging competencies of social faculty and students.

Bringing the Community In: Partnerships for Aging Enrichment

Joy Swanson Ernst, MSW, PhD
Lynda Sowbel, LCSW-C, BCD

SUMMARY. Aging enrichment of undergraduate social work curricula ensures that program graduates will be prepared to practice with older adults. This article reports the results of focus group research that was designed to engage social workers from community agencies serving older adults in preparing students to become "aging-savvy" social workers. The workers highlighted the importance of wide-ranging exposure to older adults, the changing needs of older adults, and the importance of increasing students' comfort with self-determination. These findings informed the program's ongoing curricular transformation process through the incorporation of new assignments that enabled increased contact with older adults in a variety of settings. doi:10.1300/J083v48n03_07 *[Article copies available for a fee from The Haworth Document Delivery Service: 1-800-HAWORTH. E-mail address: <docdelivery@haworthpress.com> Website: <http://www.HaworthPress.com> © 2007 by The Haworth Press, Inc. All rights reserved.]*

The authors thank Angela Burrier and Tamre D. Swisher for their assistance with this project. They are grateful for the support of the Hood College Board of Associates Summer Research Institute and the Hartford Geriatric Enrichment in Social Work Education Project.

An earlier version of this paper was presented at the first National Gerontological Social Work Conference, Atlanta, Georgia, March 1, 2003.

[Haworth co-indexing entry note]: "Bringing the Community In: Partnerships for Aging Enrichment." Ernst, Joy Swanson, and Lynda Sowbel. Co-published simultaneously in *Journal of Gerontological Social Work* (The Haworth Press, Inc.) Vol. 48, No. 3/4, 2007, pp. 387-403; and: *Fostering Social Work Gerontology Competence: A Collection of Papers from the First National Gerontological Social Work Conference* (ed: Catherine J. Tompkins, and Anita L. Rosen) The Haworth Press, Inc., 2007, pp. 387-403. Single or multiple copies of this article are available for a fee from The Haworth Document Delivery Service [1-800-HAWORTH, 9:00 a.m. - 5:00 p.m. (EST). E-mail address: docdelivery@haworthpress.com].

KEYWORDS. Curricular change, social work education, teaching methods, focus groups

INTRODUCTION

In January 2002, the social work program at Hood College, a small college in Frederick, Maryland with a small undergraduate social work program, was one of 67 social work programs that received a Geriatric Enrichment in Social Work Education (GeroRich) grant from the Council on Social Work Education/John A. Hartford Foundation. This grant gave the program the opportunity to transform its foundation curriculum in order to graduate generalist social work practitioners with basic competencies related to aging. This article reports the results of focus group research that was designed to engage social workers from community agencies serving older adults in preparing students to become "aging-savvy" social workers. It also provides information on how those results informed the program's ongoing curricular transformation process. The engagement of community practitioners results from the goals and challenges faced by faculty of small undergraduate social work programs in bringing about meaningful change while managing the day-to-day concerns of the program.

Involvement in geriatric enrichment makes sense. Today's baccalaureate level social work graduates will likely work with older adults in almost any setting that employs them. Demographic statistics suggest that the proportion of the population who will be over 65 will steadily increase over the next 50 years and double to more than 70,000,000 by the year 2030 (Hartford Geriatric Enrichment in Social Work Education, 2003). According to population projections based on the 2000 Census and released by the Maryland Department of Aging, Frederick County, Maryland, the location of Hood College, will experience a 131% increase in its population aged 60 and older over the next 20 years and a 214% increase by 2030 (Maryland Department of Aging, 2003). Baccalaureate social work programs such as Hood's must make a more concerted effort to teach their students about aging and to graduate competent, well-prepared social workers.

THE NEED FOR COMMUNITY INPUT INTO CURRICULAR CHANGE

Cooperation and collaboration with multiple "communities" can help enrich small social work programs. In the process of curricular transformation, we considered a number of factors that influence the ability to successfully enrich the curriculum. Engaging the practice community in the program's gerontological education efforts occurred with the increasing awareness of the need to surmount certain barriers for the aging enrichment efforts to have some success. These barriers include program size, departmental "walls," and student resistance to working with older adults.

Program Size

Issues associated with running small social work programs are connected to the need to look to the community to assist with aging enrichment efforts. Similar to 45% (n = 103) of the respondents from small social work departments in a survey on autonomy and visibility in social work programs that were part of a multidisciplinary department in the college or university (Johnson & Hull Jr., 1992), Hood College has a small social work program in a small department of sociology and social work. The number of social work majors ranges from 25 to 40. The program struggles with resource constraints such as a small budget, limited faculty, and minimal support services. The program, like many small programs, has two full time faculty members, a Program Director and a Field Director, who both carry significant teaching and administrative responsibilities (Morrow, 2000). However, Hood's program is not unique. Currently, eighty-five accredited baccalaureate programs in the United States have 3 or fewer full-time faculty members (personal communication, CSWE, October 2002).

Hood's small baccalaureate social work program presents both strengths and challenges related to curriculum development and delivery. The faculty knows the student's strengths and weaknesses very well, provides individualized attention to the student; and has frequent, consistent contact with the practice community, especially the field instructors. We must perform many functions with minimal faculty. Consistent with research reported by Drumm and Suppes (2000), the program's strengths include individualized attention, quality of advisement, mentoring, and quality of interaction with students, although these strengths also consume a great deal of faculty time and energy at times. The strengths related to delivery of curriculum are also consistent with the findings of this research. The Field Director is a long-time practitioner in the community. Faculty members value the interaction with students in the classroom, the close working relationships with field instructors, and the relationships with the practice community, which have been strengthened throughout this process.

Intra- and Interdepartmental Relationships

The social work faculty peacefully co-exists with the members of the sociology faculty. Consistent with research results reported by Johnson and Hull

(1992), the social work program faculty finds the level of autonomy provided in this arrangement to be satisfactory. However, consistent with the same research results, faculty has sought visibility both on campus and in the community, in part to prevent isolation. Faculty from small social work programs must heed the advice given to political scientists at small colleges that faculty must open communications with colleagues in other disciplines in order to build a successful academic career (Durfee, 1999).

Three faculty members in the psychology department have extensive experience, in teaching and in clinical practice, in working with older adults and in dealing with death and dying among populations of all ages. They oversee the college's minor in gerontology and a master's degree in thanatology, and they already have a relationship with the aging practice community. The social work program is a part of the sociology department. Thus, disciplinary "walls" and physical distance between the two departments, the competing demands of other facets of the social work program administration (such as re-affirmation of accreditation), turnover among the social work faculty, and simple inertia had prevented much in the way of cooperation between the two groups in the past.

Student Resistance

Consistent with literature on bringing gerontology into social work programs, the faculty had noticed student resistance to working with the elderly (Kropf, Schneider, & Stahlman, 1993; Scharlach, Damron-Rodriguez, Robinson, & Feldman, 2000). During screening interviews for the program, students were much more forthright about saying "I don't want to work with old people," for example, than they were about any other population group served by social workers. Of the fourteen field preference forms filled out for the 2002-2003 school year, only one student expressed a preference for working with older adults, although seven were open to it. One student wrote the following in a paper written for her Methods I class during spring semester 2002: "I do have biases and prejudices against working explicitly with pedophiles, severe drug addicts, and what I refer to as the late life senior citizen population." Thus, she grouped older adults with some of the most difficult and stigmatized population groups served by social workers. While this student's opinion may seem extreme, other students expressed doubts as well.

Another student commented in a focus group about a field trip to an assisted living facility in her Introduction to Social Work class.

> I don't particularly like dabbling with the elderly population because I am more geared towards children and adolescents. Well, I'd never been

exposed to the elderly population ... I thought, man you know this is going to be boring ... but it opened my eyes.

Student resistance, as evidenced by these attitudes, raised awareness of the need to increase the students' knowledge and awareness of issues facing older adults and their willingness to consider settings that serve older adults as potential field placements and employment sites.

Research into the effects of social work curricular efforts to positively affect the attitudes of social work students and their willingness to work with older adults (gerontological content in foundation social work classes, structured intergenerational contact through agency visits, service learning or volunteer work, and skill building) has not been conclusive and is related to students' prior interest in and contact with older adults (see review in Cummings & Galambos, 2002, pp. 78-81).

Community Support and Input

Accreditation standards demand that social work programs have "ongoing exchanges with external constituencies" that include regular interaction with social work practitioners and social service agencies, among other entities (Council on Social Work Education, 2002). Hood College's social work program relies on the practice community to serve as field instructors and as supervisors for volunteer experiences. In addition, two practitioners serve on the Social Work Advisory Committee. Although little research exists on the extent to which community-based social service providers influence curricular content for particular social work programs, the research of Forte and colleagues suggests that the practice community welcomes the opportunity to provide input into decisions related to social work curricula (Forte & Mathews, 1995). However, the Hood College social work program previously had not asked a broad range of community professionals for their input on curricular content and desirable student learning outcomes in the area of services to older adults. The following section describes results of the survey and focus group and presents information on how some of the findings were implemented.

THE PROCESS AND FINDINGS: BRINGING THE COMMUNITY IN

The Field Director met with a number of community agencies that serve older adults in the spring of 2002 and the program faculty consulted with psychology faculty, who facilitated the contact with the head of the Department of Aging. Overall the explorations within the community yielded an expansion of gerontology field sites. During the 2002-03 year, four out of fourteen seniors were placed in agencies serving older adults including nursing homes, the Department of Aging, and the Department of Social Services' Senior Care Program.

Faculty also sought the expertise of the local gerontological social work community to find out how to make the transformed courses relevant for what practitioners see as the most pressing educational needs of the students. Through the initial contacts and through several directories of community services, a variety of agencies that provide a continuum of services and programs for older adults were identified. These ranged from the community centers to several acute-care settings. The desire for a greater connection with the aging service providers provided an impetus for the agency survey, the focus group, and the individual interviews. Two students worked with the project director during summer 2002 to carry out these tasks. They developed the focus group questions and conducted the individual interviews.

Survey

In June 2002, 82 social workers or other service providers at 54 agencies received the survey. Forty-four individuals from 35 agencies returned their surveys, for a 54% response rate. Nineteen (43.2%) worked for publicly funded agencies, such as the Department of Social Services and the Department of Aging; nine (20.5%) worked for private, non-profit agencies; and fifteen (34.1%) worked for private, for profit organizations. One respondent did not identify himself or his agency. The majority (43.2%) had a master's degree in social work or higher. Eleven (25%) had bachelor's degrees in social work, while 12 (27.3%) were non-social workers.

The survey asked the service providers to rank the top 35 gerontology competencies on a 5-point scale, with one being "very important" and five being "not at all necessary." The ten competencies with the mean correspond somewhat with the "Top Ten List of Aging Competencies for All Social Workers" provided by SAGE-SW (Council on Social Work Education, 2000, June), but there were differences as well. Table 1 compares the top ten competencies as ranked by experts in the field with the top ten ranked by the Hood College respondents.

Focus Group

Respondents to the survey could indicate if they were interested in participating in a focus group. Of the sixteen who initially expressed interest, eight participated in a focus group on July 18, 2002. Seven of the eight participants were either bachelors- or master's-level social workers. Three of the participants worked in a

TABLE 1. Comparison of Important Competencies for Social Workers–SAGE-SW and Hood College Survey Respondents

SAGE Top Ten	Hood College Top Ten
Assess one's own values and biases regarding aging, death and dying.	Accept, respect, and recognize the right and need of older adults to make their own choices and decisions within the context of the law and safety concerns
Educate self to dispel the major myths about aging.	Understand normal physical, psychological, and social changes in later life
Accept, respect, and recognize the right and need of older adults to make their own choices and decisions about their lives within the context of the law and safety concerns.	Use social work case management skills (such as brokering, advocacy, monitoring, and discharge planning) to link elders and their families to resources and services.
Normal physical, psychological and social changes in later life.	Knowledge about the availability of resources and resource systems for the elderly and their families
Respect and address cultural, spiritual, and ethnic needs and beliefs of older adults and family members.	Demonstrate awareness of sensory, language, and cognitive limitations of clients when interviewing older adults
The diversity of attitudes toward aging, mental illness and family roles.	Incorporate knowledge of elder abuse in conducting assessments and intervention with clients and families
The influence of aging on family dynamics	Assist families that are in crisis situations regarding older adult family members
Use social work case management skills (such as brokering, advocacy, monitoring, and discharge planning) to link elders and their families to resources and services.	Evaluate safety issues and degree of risk for self and older clients
Gather information regarding social history such as: social functioning, primary and secondary social supports, social activity level, social skills, financial status, cultural background and social involvement.	Gather information regarding social history such as: social functioning, primary and secondary social supports, social activity level, social skills, financial status, cultural background and social involvement.
Identify ethical and professional boundary issues that commonly arise in work with older adults and their caregivers, such as client self-determination, end-of-life decisions, family conflicts, and guardianship.	Collaborate with other health, mental health, and allied health professional in delivering services to older adults

nursing home setting, one worked for a home health agency, one was in private practice with a focus on older adults, one worked for the Department of Social Services, one worked in a local agency that serves individuals of all ages with chronic mental illness, and one worked for the Department of Aging. The student researchers also conducted three individual interviews with social workers in long-term care settings and a group interview with staff representatives from the Frederick County Department of Aging.

The focus group and interview questions covered the following topics:

- Accommodating and providing services to baby boomers;
- How and what to teach about aging;
- Involving older adults in teaching social work students;
- Ethical issues and professional boundaries;
- Important policy issues related to aging.

Participants in the focus groups and individual interviews underscored many of the competencies that had been rated as "very important" by the majority of the respondents. The themes that emerged in some cases supported the ideas about curricular change, while other findings caused us to think in new ways about the teaching approaches. Analysis of the focus group and interview transcripts revealed themes related to the importance of exposure to and contact with a range of older adults, the changing needs and characteristics of older adults, and the need for students to understand the nuances and ramifications of client self-determination as it relates to older adults. These themes guided many of the new learning activities that have been implemented, which are described below.

Contact and Exposure

One theme that arose out of the focus groups was the importance of giving the students exposure to many different types of older adults, in many different situations. As one social worker stated, "It is important for students to get out and see older adults in their own surroundings." The same worker suggested that students have a focus group with seniors at a senior center, or to "Go and visit and have lunch with them, stay for whatever meeting they are having afterwards and interact with them and watch them interact with each other and see what they talk about, get involved with them." Students need "many and varied experiences" of seniors to appreciate the diversity of older adults, the diversity of their problems, and to bring together multi-faceted dimensions of the knowledge needed to practice social work. A worker from the Department of Social Services related how her clients would reuse adult diapers, even though the department supplied them with all they need: "They still use them over because they don't waste things and some of it has to do with the Depression–and some of it has to do with being depressed." This idea highlights the broad array of knowledge that including various historical contexts as well as empirical data related to psychiatric diagnosis and symptoms that a social work student must acquire.

Changing Needs of Aging Adults

Due to the influence of history and cohort effects, the needs of the aging adult will change as the aging adults change. The focus group participants responded to the question about the possible needs of aging baby boomers with a great many ideas about the amenities they will demand, the need to have programs and services to meet the boomers' lifestyles, and the fact that baby boomers will "ask for what they want" in care as they age. In contrast, today's older adults are "more accepting." Students will need to be aware of these cohort influences. Family composition is changing in ways that have implications for elder care. There are more single parent families, lesbian and gay families, and families with no children. Families are smaller, children and other family members live farther away, and the children of the "old old" are aging themselves.

Comfort with Self-Determination

The composition of the focus groups, which included several workers from health care or nursing home settings, may have driven home one recurring theme, which related to self-determination. Many workers mentioned the importance of being able to understand what advanced directives are and how to communicate about them with elders. The focus group participants felt strongly that bachelor's level students should have the sensitivity and skills needed to ask detailed questions about what is important to people as they make end of life decisions, and to recognize how difficult it is for many seniors to face this issue. The service providers suggested that students must learn to allow older adults to make up their own minds, in spite of their personal feelings or values. Advanced directives provide a context for learning about self-determination and the elderly, a topic that the service providers emphasized in relation to many different topic areas. Self-determination creates challenges for students; as one worker stated, "The students need to know that adults are permitted to make stupid choices or what we think are stupid choices." This worker felt that, especially for young students, this particular area was difficult.

The social worker's commitment to the core social work value of self-determination also emerged as a theme related to the social worker's role as part of a team in health care or medical settings. A social worker in private practice stated that the "medical community doesn't understand the whole idea of self-determination" and that doctors will speak disparagingly about "you idiot social workers" whose concern for the self-determination of the older person makes decision-making processes related to the older person's health care more complicated. Social workers with older adults must also become knowledgeable about medical terms, procedures (invasive or otherwise), and diseases, because "You can't talk to a frail elderly person if you know less about their diseases than they do."

In addition to these knowledge and skill areas elaborated above, the service providers also brought up several areas where other problem areas are intersecting with issues related to aging. For example, students may have particular difficulty in discussing or even considering sexuality in later life. The providers spoke of difficult situations related to dementia and sexuality, AIDS in the elderly, and domestic violence in assisted living centers as examples of issues that they had encountered. They emphasized how public policy areas such as Medicare, Medicaid, prescription drugs, and Social Security influence the planning, decision-making, and choices available to older persons in need of care. They raised issues of fairness and equity (such as the question of whether low-income elders are welcomed into senior centers) and called attention to the great diversity of older adults. On the whole, the service providers offered the program valuable insights into what they saw as the most important knowledge for students. They also acknowledged that their wisdom was the result of many years of experience, and so, as a counterbalance, underscored the need for realistic knowledge goals, and a regimen that includes life-long learning.

STRATEGIES USED, BRIDGES BUILT, AND PRELIMINARY OUTCOMES

Based upon this feedback from community providers, the social work program began the process of using members of the community in new ways. Many of the practitioner's recommendations have been incorporated into the curriculum. Feedback from students and others regarding these activities suggests that "bringing the community in" has positive results for students, faculty, and the program as a whole. Infusion of material–rather than merely adding it to an already bulging curriculum–remains a challenge. Student evaluations of specific learning activities suggest that the efforts to infuse have not been entirely successful, although the program faculty has made subsequent improvements. The next section describes some of the activities that were incorporated into the curriculum that most directly relate to the first focus group theme, which is the importance of exposure and contact with older adults across many settings. These include field trips, volunteer and field placements, and the increased use of guest speakers from the aging community.

Exposure to Older Adults Through Classroom Activities and Assignments

Because of the emphasis on exposure to older adults as one way of overcoming student fears and resistance, a number of classroom activities that allow students to have face-to-face contact with older adults were added to the curriculum. First, in the "Communication Skills" unit of the Introduction to Social Work class, students spent one class period at a local senior citizen continuing care community talking with the older residents of independent living, assisted living, and skilled nursing units of the facility. Second, several students chose to interview older adults for an assignment for their Methods I class that required that they do three interviews, a process recording, and a psychosocial assessment.

Fourteen introductory social work students participated in the field visit to the senior citizen community. The continuing care facility was located in an idyllic, semi-rural setting and served a population of mostly white seniors with sufficient resources to pay for their housing and care. This setting enabled the students to focus on their communication skills and not upon extreme poverty or substandard living quarters. The residents who participated were recruited by the facility's social worker; she told them that they were being asked to help train beginning social workers.

Eight of eight students who responded to the evaluative survey rated this activity as "helpful" and stated that it should be continued. Some reasons for the favorable ratings included that, "It got the class out of the classroom and into an environment where the social work skills learned can be utilized," and that the activity "provided an atmosphere with little pressure regarding performance, yet it gave us the opportunity to practice communication skills with receptive people."

Other students commented that it was interesting to hear the elders' stories, but one student felt that she did not have enough issues to discuss. When asked how the activity should be improved, four of the eight students who responded suggested that more time be allotted to the activity and that more background on the center be provided before the visit. In subsequent years, the activity has been expanded to give students a choice of whether to go to an assisted living facility or to a senior center. The instructor now allots more time to the visits and includes a self-assessment sheet that will allow students to evaluate the communication skills used.

The Methods I class, a course that focuses on the planned change process and practice with individuals, has assigned a series of practice interviews for the past several years. The assignment includes three interviews, a process recording and a psychosocial assessment. In spring 2002, with the incentive of "extra credit," approximately 50% of the class chose an older person to interview for this assignment. Two students who specifically mentioned the older adults as a group they wanted to avoid, on an initial about their personal prejudices or biases in working with clients, chose to interview elderly women for this assignment. In spring 2003, the seven students in this class were required to interview a person older than sixty.

While the students that participated in this assignment did not have uniformly positive experiences, the comments of one student, who initially professed her resistance to working with the elderly, suggest useful learning outcomes and beneficial effects of exposure via an assignment such as this one. In her final critique of her three interviews with a 74 year-old woman, this student wrote that after the initial meeting:

> I also felt relieved that I was not as frustrated or as nervous as I was during the first session. These experiences made me more confident in my abilities with older adults.

This student described her need to accommodate to her client's physical losses:

> The time during the sessions that I felt most uncomfortable is when the client began crying when speaking about her loss of vision.
>
> More importantly, I considered the background information that I had on my "client," especially the fact that I knew she was legally blind, and made preparations for slightly altering my interviewing methods since she would not be able to see my facial expressions. For example, I knew that I would have to use more extreme nonverbal cues to show her that I was actively listening to her such as nodding my head or moving my hands ... I also had to keep in mind that the client might be highly sensitive to any movements that I made since it is difficult for her to see much else.

On the question of diversity, the student expressed her uncertainty regarding the large age difference between them. The client's description of her childhood presented a new historical context for the student, with associated different belief systems that the student had only read about in books. The student described her skill of eliciting clarification frequently as an important strategy for dealing with the differences. She summed up her interviewing experience with the following thoughts.

> I learned a great deal about myself and my abilities as a social worker through these interviews. First, I learned that I am capable of working with older adults and that it can be quite rewarding. I never thought that I would get so much enjoyment from hearing about someone's childhood during a time period so different from the one in which I grew up! Similarly, I learned that I am capable of applying the methods that I learn in class to actual situations.

Exposure Through Volunteer and Field Work

The number of volunteer placement and field placement settings that serve older adults has increased. The instructor of the Introduction to Social Work class, which requires 40 hours of volunteer work in a social agency, urged students, in class and in the syllabus, to choose a volunteer setting that involves older adults. In 2002, six of fourteen students (43%) chose to do so. In 2003, six of 24 (25%) students have chosen to volunteer in settings where older adults are the primary clients. Comments from volunteer experience papers from 2002 suggest that this exposure–40 hours of volunteer work over the course of the semester–offers a low-stress way to introduce the students to the population of older adults.

In 2002, three students, all "traditional age" college juniors (20 to 21 years old) did their volunteer work in nursing homes. These placements helped the students deal with their fears and stereotypes about working with older adults in nursing home settings. In reflective papers, two students noted how apprehensive they were at first, but realized that older adults appreciated having younger people with whom to converse, that they had interesting stories to tell, and that their negative views had been proved wrong. A third student touched upon one area that causes some students anxiety in working with older adults:

> When you choose to be a social worker working with the elderly population you must be ready to accept death as a part of life. Working at [the nursing home] taught me how to handle my emotions about death, and it also forced me to be more comfortable with the inevitable (Hood College junior, age 20, who experienced the death of one of the residents with whom she had developed a relationship).

The experiences of two "non-traditional" aged students revealed both rewards and frustrations of working with older adults. The student who worked in the telephone reassurance program for seniors noted that the "resiliency and strength" of her clients contradicted "the numerous stereotypes associated with aging" and noted "what a loss it is for the many students who avoid this population as a result of inaccurate stereotypes and fears related to aging and dying" (Hood College junior, age 31). The student that worked for the Senior Care program, a 55-year-old grandmother, wrote eloquently of the passion and dedication with which the social workers there served their clients. She also expressed frustration with the system and limited resources that resulted in long waiting lists and strict eligibility guidelines, and expressed doubts about whether she would be able to work in that setting.

The results of the focus groups suggested that students and field instructors might benefit from hearing from those with expertise on particular topics and experiences related to aging. This led us to request funds to support honoraria for guest speakers who spoke to social work classes. Speakers have included a worker from adult protective services, a nursing home administrator, a private practitioner who provides clinical services to seniors and their families, and a social work researcher who studied kinship caregivers. A member of the Hood College psychology faculty spoke on funeral and grief rituals in the African American community. The experiences and feedback suggest that these efforts are worthwhile. However, faculty must ensure that the address specific social work skills, knowledge, and attitudes needed by the generalist practitioner. The point is not just to add aging, but to link each presentation to other curricular needs as well.

For example, a doctoral student described the results of her qualitative research study of low income, inner city grandmothers and other older caregivers who are raising their grandchildren or other young relatives. The presentation occurred in the first class in the HBSE sequence, which focuses on early to middle childhood, families, and cultural issues. It provided the students with an example of integrating research and practice, and the benefits of qualitative research in providing a rich picture of people's struggles and daily concerns were quite evident. One student noted that the presentation helped her realize the "stereotypes placed on African American grandmothers" while another noted that the she learned something about the complexity of research and that she benefited from the personal descriptions of grandmothers, their children, and the environments in which they live.

In the "macro" unit of Methods II, a course that focuses on social work with families, groups, and communities, a panel of administrative social workers discussed various administrative issues related to management style and how social workers can make change on a macro level. A BSW who has been a director of social work in several nursing homes participated on the panel. Generally, the students had a favorable reaction to this panel.

CONCLUSIONS

As one of 67 social work education programs involved in the GeroRich project, Hood College has committed to both pervasiveness of aging content and sustainability of these changes. Hood College's geriatric enrichment project has provided social work students and faculty with the opportunity and impetus to change the approaches and the mindset about what constitutes "good" preparation for beginning generalist practice.

There are three important lessons learned from the pilot testing of new activities and learning strategies that were introduced as a result of "bringing the community in." First and foremost, there is no substitute for actual exposure to a new or stigmatized population, as research has shown (Quinn, 1999; Kropf, Schneider, & Stahlman, 1993; Scharlach, Damron-Rodriguez, Robinson, & Feldman, 2000). The community providers' recommendations about wide-ranging and varied exposure to older adults dovetail with research that shows that students' attitudes towards and desire to work with older adults after graduation is influenced by positive interactions with older adults (Angiullo, Whitbourne, & Powers, 2001; Cummings & Galambos, 2002; Gorelik, Damron-Rodriguez, Funderburk, & Solomon, 2000).

A second lesson relates to program size and program mission, which is to create competent generalist social work practitioners. In the efforts to create aging savvy social workers, we cannot ignore other curricular knowledge and skill areas. Thus, it is important to look for learning strategies that teach more than one dimension of social work knowledge and skill. Finally, networking must be continuous and vibrant with respect to the gerontology community, for all programs new to infusing aging content, but most especially for small programs where the faculty cannot be expert in everything and cannot offer the students a variety of viewpoints and social work experience. The ability to go beyond their own academic department and to seek experts in other departments is a critical channel to the community.

External focus groups, interviews and surveys led to new assignments, which were incorporated in a more fluid manner with social work curriculum, as well as new connections in the community. Specialists from the community now comprise a growing list of experts available for: speaking to students or field instructors, field trip opportunities, panels or advisory committees, and field placements.

Comments from students and focus group data reveals that actual experience with the aging population was the most potent, effective intervention to changing student attitudes and knowledge base. Increased education of the faculty and the development of outcome expectations, with input and support from the gerontology community, are critical to provide clear goals and expectations to social work students. Ongoing feedback from student assignments, field evaluations, and aging activity evaluation forms from field instructors and students is crucial to a shift from a fragmented addition of an aging assignment here and there, to a more cohesive curriculum that includes aging content as well as specific social work topics such as the ethics related to end-of-life issues, communication with diverse populations, social justice and policy concerns, and interviewing skills. For a small faculty, at least two areas must always be addressed at once. For example, one scenario might be a role-play in class with a Latino family with an aging grandparent living in the home, where the student can practice her interviewing and assessment skills.

Creativity, collaboration, the faculty's willingness to learn, and engaging the students, other faculty and practice community have all contributed to an essential, and hopefully permanent change to the social work curriculum at Hood College. It is possible to infuse gerontology into the social work curriculum of a small two-faculty social work program with the help of community partners, and the program will continue to use their support, knowledge, and feedback to produce aging-savvy generalist social workers.

REFERENCES

Angiullo, L., Whitbourne, S. K., & Powers, C. (2001). The effect of instruction and experience on college students' attitudes towards the elderly. *Educational Gerontology*, 483-495.

Council on Social Work Education. (2000, June). Some findings from SAGE-SW. Council on Social Work Education. Available: www.cswe.org/sage-sw/resrep/somefindings.htm#TOP [2002, October 15].

Council on Social Work Education. (2002). Educational Policy and Accreditation Standards. *Council on Social Work Education* [2002, October 18].

Cummings, S. M., & Galambos, C. (2002). Predictors of graduate students' interest in aging-related work. *Journal of Gerontological Social Work*, *39*(3), 77-94.

Drumm, R. D., & Suppes, M. A. (2000). Small social work programs: Strengths and challenges in student development and delivery of curriculum. *Journal of Baccalaureate Social Work*, *6*(1), 1-17.

Durfee, M. (1999). The small, remote, or odd college: Making the most out of your new teaching position. *Political Science & Politics*, *32*(1), 109-112.

Forte, J. A., & Mathews, C. (1995). Potential employers' views of the ideal undergraduate social work curriculum. *Journal of Social Work Education*, *30*(2), 228-240.

Gorelik, Y., Damron-Rodriguez, J., Funderburk, B., & Solomon, D. (2000). Undergraduate interest in aging: Is it affected by contact with older adults? *Educational Gerontology*, *26*, 623-638.

Hartford Geriatric Enrichment in Social Work Education. (2003). Preparing Aging-Savvy Social Workers. *University of Washington School of Social Work*. Available: http://depts.washington.edu/gerorich [2003, September 28].

Johnson, H. W., & Hull Jr., G. H. (1992). Autonomy and visibility in undergraduate social work education. *Journal of Social Work Education, 28*(3), 312-321.

Kropf, N. P., Schneider, R. L., & Stahlman, S. D. (1993). The status of gerontology in baccalaureate social work education. *Educational Gerontology, 19*, 623-634.

Maryland Department of Aging. (2003). Demographics: Maryland's 60 + Population Projections by Jurisdiction, 2000-2030. *Maryland Department of Aging.* Available: http://www.mdoa.state.md.us/demogtable1.html [2003, September 28].

Morrow, D. F. (2000). Gatekeeping for small baccalaureate social work programs. *Journal of Baccalaureate Social Work, 5*(2), 67-80.

Scharlach, A., Damron-Rodriguez, J., Robinson, B., & Feldman, R. (2000). Educating social workers for an aging society: A vision for the 21st century. *Journal of Social Work Education, 36*(3).

doi:10.1300/J083v48n03_07

Preparing Social Work Students to Work with Grandparents in Kinship Care: An Approach to Infusion of Content Materials into Selected Core Social Work Courses

Patricia Johnson-Dalzine, PhD, LSW

SUMMARY. Grandparents in kinship care represent an expanding population of older adults assuming primary parenting responsibilities for their grandchildren at a time when many grandparents may also be experiencing developmental changes accompanying their own aging process. Research documents a lack of social workers prepared to respond to the needs of an aging population in general, and grandparents in kinship care in particular, as curricular content on this population has been limited in undergraduate and graduate social work programs. This article describes an infusion model proposed for an undergraduate social work program's GeroRich Project designed to introduce content on an aging population in four foundation courses to expand students' knowledge of older adults and grandparents as kinship care providers. doi:10.1300/J083v48n03_08 *[Article copies available for a fee from The Haworth Document Delivery Service:*

The model was developed for the Department of Social Work's CSWE-Hartford GeroRich Project, Wright State University, Dayton, Ohio.

[Haworth co-indexing entry note]: "Preparing Social Work Students to Work with Grandparents in Kinship Care: An Approach to Infusion of Content Materials into Selected Core Social Work Courses." Johnson-Dalzine, Patricia. Co-published simultaneously in *Journal of Gerontological Social Work* (The Haworth Press, Inc.) Vol. 48, No. 3/4, 2007, pp. 405-420; and: *Fostering Social Work Gerontology Competence: A Collection of Papers from the First National Gerontological Social Work Conference* (ed: Catherine J. Tompkins, and Anita L. Rosen) The Haworth Press, Inc., 2007, pp. 405-420. Single or multiple copies of this article are available for a fee from The Haworth Document Delivery Service [1-800-HAWORTH, 9:00 a.m. - 5:00 p.m. (EST). E-mail address: docdelivery@haworthpress.com].

1-800-HAWORTH. E-mail address: <docdelivery@haworthpress.com> Website: <http://www.HaworthPress.com> © 2007 by The Haworth Press, Inc. All rights reserved.]

KEYWORDS. Kinship care, grandparents, older adults, grandchildren, aging, infusion model, social work students

INTRODUCTION

Grandparents in kinship care today are receiving increased public attention from service providers, advocacy groups, politicians, and others because their numbers have expanded as they have assumed long-term roles as primary parents for their grandchildren. These roles present new challenges for them and their grandchildren (U.S. Census Bureau, 2000; Roe & Minkler, 1999; Bryson, 2001; Minkler, Fuller-Thompson, Miller, & Driver, 1997) and service systems, which do not have social workers in sufficient numbers with training in gerontological social work to respond to the needs of an aging caregiver population (Scharlach, Damon-Rodriguez, Robinson, & Feldman, 2000). Grandparents are providing care for over four million children under the age of 18, and some 2.4 million of them have primary parenting responsibilities for their grandchildren and many grandparents are over age 65 (U.S. Census Bureau, 2000; Generations United-Online).

Kinship care is defined as "the full-time nurturing and protection of children who must be separated from their parents by relatives, members of their tribes or clans, godparents, stepparents or other adults who have a kinship bond with a child" (Child Welfare League of America, 1994, p. 2). As part of extended kin network, grandparents often help their adult children with the care of their grandchildren either living in their household or providing day care, or by providing full time custodial care (Ruiz & Carlton-LaNey, 1999; Taylor, Chatters, & Jayakody, 1997; Emick & Hayslip, 1996; Jendrek, 1994). Informal kinship placements, arranged by family members, have had a long history among some ethnic groups, especially African Americans, Hispanics, and Native Americans. These placements are intended to maintain their children's connection to the kin networks, limit contact with formal agencies, and reduce the impact of discriminatory practices within formal service systems (Hegar, 1999; Garcia-Preto, 1996; Sutton & Broken Nose, 1996; Cross, 1986).

Custodial care grandparents in kinship care are the focus of attention as they have assumed long-term care responsibilities through the formal placement process usually involving a public child welfare agency. This long-term caregiving for grandparents has been attributed to numerous problems with their adult children including AIDS, divorce, substance abuse, child abuse and/or neglect, death, incarceration, domestic violence, abandonment, teenage pregnancy, unemployment, financial, and physical and mental health problems that rendered the grandparents' own children incapable of performing their parenting duties (Sands & Goldberg-Glen, 2000; Pruchno, 1999; Barnhill, 1996; Pinson-Milburn, Fabian, Schlossberg, & Pyle, 1996; Minkler & Roe, 1996; Dowdell, 1995; Kelley & Danato, 1995; Dressel & Barnhill, 1994; Jendrek, 1994). Researchers examining the impact of caregiving on grandparents have identified a number of problems which they experience that can be categorized in terms of health (Cox, 2002; Fuller-Thomson & Minkler, 2000; Minkler et al., 1997; Burnette, 1999), social isolation (Burnette, 1999; Burnette, 1997; Roe & Minkler, 1999), financial hardship (Kelly, Whitley, Sipe, & Crofts-Yorker, 2000; Christian, 2000; Burnette, 1997; Minkler & Roe, 1996), and legal problems (Cox, 2002; Bobroff, 2000; Flint & Perez-Porter, 1997; Hartfield, 1996; Karp, 1996; de Toledo & Brown, 1995; Turner, 1995). In response to the difficulties grandparents are experiencing in caring for their grandchildren, a wide range of services are now available to grandparents to assist them in maintaining their own well-being while providing care for their grandchildren.

However, obtaining these services requires them to be able to negotiate and master interactions with many service systems such as financial, health care, legal/courts, schools, and social services (Cox, 2002; Bobroff, 2000; Rothenberg, 1996; Takas, 1995; Turner, 1995).

Grandparents in kinship care constitute a special population of vulnerable older adults assuming primary parenting roles at a time when many may also be experiencing developmental changes accompanying their own aging process. Social workers responding to this population's needs must be sensitive and competent in utilizing broad knowledge and skills in identifying grandparents' needs and linking these individuals with services, coordinating these services, acting as advocates for services, and assisting grandparents in being empowered to secure services (Cox, 2002; Thompson & Thompson, 2001; Jones & Kennedy, 1998; Cox & Parsons, 1994).

NEED FOR SOCIAL WORKERS

Kinship care places social workers in a unique position of responding to the needs of an older population having assumed the role of primary caregiver for their grandchildren. However, research documents an insufficient number of social workers who are adequately prepared to work with an expanding older population in general (Council on Social Work Education [CSWE]

SAGE/SW, 2001; Rosen & Zlotnik, 2000; Scharlach et al., 2000), and especially grandparents in kinship care (U.S. Census Bureau, 2000; Bryson, 2001; Jackson, 1996; Berrick, Needell, & Minkler, 1999; Berrick, Barth, & Needell, 1994). Students preparing for a career in social work in undergraduate and graduate programs have been reported as having limited exposure to content on gerontology in the curriculum (Damron-Rodriguez & Lubben, 1997).

The Council on Social Work Education, with funding from the John Hartford Foundation, initiated a major project *Strengthening Aging and Gerontology Education for Social Work (CSWE/SAGE-SW)* to fill the void in gerontological social work content in both undergraduate and graduate programs (CSWE/SAGE-SW, 2001).

CSWE/SAGE-SW in partnership with the Hartford Geriatric Social Work Program Initiative awarded grants to BSW and MSW programs grants to develop learning experiences to equip students with knowledge to work with older adults and sponsored training for social work educators through its Faculty Development Programs (CSWE/SAGE-SW, 2001). These projects are expected to influence curriculum development, expand the pool of faculty with gerontological expertise, expand students' knowledge to work with an aging population, and increase the number of students who will be prepared to respond to the service needs of this population (CSWE/SAGE-SW, 2001; Scharlach et al., 2000; Singer, 2000).

INFUSION MODEL

This article discusses a method that could be used by faculty in undergraduate programs to infuse gerontological content into existing courses. It is based on a proposal the author submitted to a CSWE funded undergraduate GeroRich Project. The purposes of the project were (a) to enrich the social work curriculum with gerontology content, addressing the health and well-being of older adults and (b) to increase the gerontology competencies of baccalaureate social work graduates thereby improving the quality of services to older adults.

The infusion model, consistent with the goals of the Social Work Geriatric Enrichment Initiative, introduces content materials on aging into social work foundation courses (CSWE, 2001). This approach offers a viable method through which social work programs may begin to prepare social workers to work with populations of older adults and the multi-dimensional challenges that are encountered in providing services to a vulnerable population of older adults (Cummings & Kropf, 2000). Consistent with the goals of the GeroRich Project, grandparents in kinship care was the targeted aging population for infusion of content materials into foundation courses. The purpose in using this population was to describe a method for contributing to social work students' preparation to respond to the diverse service needs of this group of older adults. Specific content addressing various service needs of grandparents and how social workers and service systems should respond to these needs are suggested for selected courses consistent with established course descriptions, learning outcomes, and assignments. Singer (2000), in observing how aging content may be addressed, notes that "it is possible to open the door to aging content inclusion without specific mention in either goals or objectives" (p. 4). Singer cites an example of a program objective which states that "Students will demonstrate an understanding of human development in the social environment and be able to apply that knowledge to practice" (p. 4). An implication of Singer's view is that aging content may be expected as part of the life span content materials. For faculty who are concerned with the freedom to develop their course goals and objectives, using the infusion approach to include content on aging is not threatening. It gives the faculty member broad options for content materials from which to select those most beneficial for the students' learning experiences and meeting the goals and objectives for their courses.

When the content focuses on particular issues for a designated population of older adults, such as grandparents in kinship care, faculty who lack requisite expertise will need access to specific materials and methods for the utilization of this material. Materials clearly developed and easily accessible for utilization by faculty help them in selecting specific information that may be useful for infusing into their courses (CSWE/SAGE-SW, 2002).

The model used four courses from three content areas for infusion of content on grandparents in kinship care. The courses were Generalist Practice with Individuals, Generalist Practice with Families, Human Behavior and Social Environment, and Social Welfare Policy. In proposing content materials, existing course syllabi were reviewed and supportive elements for infusion of content materials were identified in the course descriptions, learning outcomes, and course assignments.

Content materials on grandparents in kinship care can contain general information, which is useful for lectures across the four courses in addition to content specific to certain issues that may be addressed in the courses. General content is an option for exposing students to background information on grandparents in kinship care. This type of content could include demographics, types of grandparent caregiving, impact of caregiving, factors contributing to grandparents' caregiving, and information on the health, financial, legal, and emotional needs of grandparents in kinship care. Specific content information for inclusion in a course, such as social welfare policy, could include a review of legislation or court decisions that have had an impact on kinship care focusing on issues that made them necessary. One example of a key court decision is *Miller v. Youakim, 1979*, which requires states to provide the same financial assistance to relative foster parents as non-relative foster parents (Gleeson, 1999). The Indian Child Welfare Act, 1978 which mandated relatives as first consideration for children being removed from their biological parents' is an example of an important piece of legislation that could be infused into a policy course (Hegar, 1999; Matheson, 1996; Cross, 1986).

Course descriptions, learning outcomes, and course assignments were broad enough that general and specific content materials offer many opportunities and choices for faculty to select materials for learning experiences they deem suitable based on the structure of their courses.

SELECTED COURSES

The courses, Generalist Practice with Individuals, Generalist Practice with Families, Human Behavior and Social Environment, and Social Welfare Policy, as noted earlier, are from an undergraduate social work curriculum. Course descriptions, learning outcomes, and course assignments offer opportunities for faculty to select content on grandparents in kinship care as a way of satisfying some of the course requirements. Each course is discussed in the paragraphs that follow.

Generalist Practice with Individuals

Course Description

The description for this course as stated in the syllabus provides support for infusion of content materials on grandparents in kinship care. The course was described as designed to promote skills for generalist social work practice with individuals based on a strengths perspective. Content materials that address empowerment work and help students develop knowledge and awareness of the need for social workers to assist grandparents in their role as kinship caregivers, are ideal for infusion into a generalist practice with individuals course. Such a course should prepare social workers to assist grandparents to be empowered to use their strengths, abilities, and competencies to secure resources necessary for them to manage the multiple difficulties they experience in kinship care (Cox, 2002; Thompson & Thompson, 2001; Cox, 2000; Cox & Parsons, 1994).

Learning Outcomes

Four learning outcomes from the course syllabus are points of consideration for infusion of content on grandparents in kinship care (a) understand and apply the concepts of strength-based social work practice with individuals, (b) understand and apply the relationship-building, interviewing, and planned change skills necessary to work with individual clients, (c) demonstrate knowledge of particular issues for social work practice with clients representing populations at risk, and (d) demonstrate awareness of the importance of advocacy in social work with individuals. These outcomes support infusion of specific content materials for two areas, individual work with grandparents and system focused work that have an impact on services delivered to this population. On the individual level, work is directed at helping grandparents develop empowerment approaches to negotiating key service systems (Cox, 2002; Christian, 2000; Cox, 2000; Cox & Parsons, 1994). For the system level, content materials are focused on empowerment actions directed at changes to be made by practitioners, agencies, and administrators as they seek to respond to the needs of this population. This content provides opportunities for learning experiences that expose students to knowledge about advocacy work for micro-level, mezzo-level, and macro-level changes needed for working with this older population. Students develop awareness of the need and responsibility of organizational cultures to be supportive at different levels within service systems participating in the empowerment process for kinship care providers (Cox, 2002; Thompson & Thompson, 2001; Eastman, 1995; Cox, 1994; Staples, 1990).

Course Assignment

The course assignment provides another avenue for infusion of content on grandparents in kinship care. The course had an assignment that involved students doing a personal interview with a client and developing a comprehensive plan for action based on this interview. For one component of the assignment, *The Client-Driven Service Plan,* the syllabus stated the following objectives (a) students are expected to design a service and support plan for clients identifying needs with the highest priority, (b) the plan is to include impact goal, service objectives, tasks, activities, or interventions required for accomplishing the goal and objectives at micro, mezzo, or macro levels, and (c) identify actors or persons responsible for carrying out the tasks, activities, or interventions. One option for the students' target population for the assignment could be a grandparent in kinship care. This population experiences multiple difficulties with their own physical and mental well-being, finances, and legal problems, and need multiple services cross systems such as social service, health care, financial, educational, and legal service systems. This component of the assignment directly engages students in developing knowledge about this group of older adults and provides an in-depth learning experience in developing a service plan with a grandparent.

Generalist Practice with Families

Course Description

Three points in the description of this course were avenues for consideration of infusion of content materials as stated in the syllabus (a) the course is designed to provide students with opportunities to understand the family as a system and as a unit of attention in generalist practice, (b) attention will be given to family functioning, family dysfunctioning, and the concept of change as it relates to families encountered in social work practice, and (c) the course will explore the importance of identifying the strengths and limitations of the family as the bases for intervention. Infusing content on grandparents in kinship care that examines the origin and contributing factors of that care, complexities and problems experienced and the resilience of grandparents, provides students with opportunities to learn about the multiple elements that affect families' ability to function and the need for social work intervention (Cox, 2002; Kelley, Yorker, Whitely, & Sipe, 2001; O'Brien et al., 2001; Christian, 2000; Fuller-Thomson & Minkler, 2000; Kelley et al., 2000; Minkler & Roe, 1999; McLean & Thomas, 1996).

Course Learning Outcomes

Two learning outcomes are noted as supportive of infusion of content on grandparents in kinship care (a) identify and assess situations where the relationship between client systems and social institutions need to be initiated, enhanced, restored, protected, or terminated and (b) link clients with systems that provide them with resources, services, and opportunities.

Infusing content on the multiple and diverse service systems such as social service, education, court/legal, financial, and health care, which grandparents in kinship care must negotiate, exposes students to knowledge of problems and difficulties that this population of older adults experiences and provides information to help them understand the kind of assistance that these types of family units need to function and maintain themselves (Cox, 2002; Cox, 2000; Strom & Strom, 2000; Burnette, 1999; Smith, Dannison, & Vacha-Hasse, 1998; McLean & Thompson, 1996; Pinson-Milburn et al., 1996; Jones & Kennedy, 1996; Turner, 1995; Jendrek, 1994; Wilson, 1994).

Course Assignment

The course assignment offers another structured opportunity that supports infusion of this content. The assignment from the actual syllabus includes a family analysis paper for senior social work majors who are in their advanced practicum experience. One of the goals for the assignment, as stated in the syllabus, was to help students understand how important family functioning is for its members and their subsequent behavior. The guidelines for completion of the assignment have students addressing key elements with the target family such as demographics, family history, family group relationships, community involvement, family strengths, and considering how the students' own families have influenced them today.

Infusion of content on grandparents in kinship care provides students with an abundance of knowledge about the functioning of such families. It allows students to demonstrate their assessment skills, provides an opportunity for faculty to evaluate the level of assessment skill being demonstrated in analyzing this family, and provides insight into how students view their own family's influence on them.

Human Behavior and Social Environment

Course Description

This course description, as stated in the syllabus, offers support for infusion of content on kinship care.

The course is designed to assist students in their integration of knowledge about the life span development of individuals and the impacts resulting from membership in families, groups, organizations, and communities; the relationship of biological, psychological, cultural, social, and spiritual influences (systems) as they impact upon and are impacted by human behavior; and, the celebration of diversity in ethnic background, race, class, sexual orientation, gender, and culture in a pluralistic society.

Infusing content on grandparents in kinship care is a conduit for broad and specific knowledge across racial and ethnic groups about the significance of family relationships with their cultural, ethnic, and spiritual connections (Hegar, 1999; Garcia-Preto, 1996; Sutton & Broken Nose, 1996; Cross, 1986). The literature documents problems with services to kinship care relatives and especially relatives of color (Ehrle & Green, 2002; DHHS, 2000; Burnette, 1999; Danza & Jackson, 1997; Scannapieco & Jackson, 1996; Matheson, 1996; Zambrana, R., 1995).

Focusing on grandparents in kinship care exposes students to a group of older adults who are likely to be culturally, ethnically, and racially different and require social workers who are competent to work with these populations (Lum, 2003; McPhatter & Ganaway, 2003; NASW, 2001; McPhatter, 1997; Scannapieco & Jackson, 1996).

Course Learning Outcomes

Three learning outcomes from the syllabus support infusing content on kinship care (a) identify and assess situations where the relationship between client systems and social institutions needs to be initiated, enhanced, restored, protected, or terminated, (b) demonstrate understanding of the relationship between bio-psycho-social-cultural-spiritual systems as they impact upon and influence human behavior over the life span, and (c) demonstrate an understanding of the impact of diversity on human functioning. Content materials on grandparents in kinship care addressing unmet needs, elements that influence their use of formal services, and how formal service systems respond to their needs, provide broad learning experiences for students. Such content could include information on interactions with service systems in several ways including the influence of diversity, factors influencing service utilization by grandparents, and the formal systems' response to the needs of grandparents (Cox, 2002; DHHS, 2000; Berrick et al., 1999).

Course Assignment

One course assignment selected from the syllabus, *Personal is Political Projects,* provides another conduit for infusion of content on grandparents in kinship care. This assignment required students to choose a specific life course stage, then select someone, a person or group of persons currently living that specific life course stage to observe and/or interview for one hour. The life course stage for this assignment could be the older adult as a grandparent in kinship care attending a grandparents' support group. This assignment involves students directly with this population and exposes them to a group of older adults who assumed a new role and who will share their role experiences, their problems and problem-solving skills, and the needed nurturance and support they have gained from other grandparents (Cohen & Pyle, 2000; Strom & Strom, 2000; Cohen, 1997; Pinson-Milburn et al., 1996; Strom & Strom, 1993).

Social Welfare Policy

Course Description

Support for infusion of content on grandparents in kinship care is demonstrated in the course's description:

- The course is designed to develop beginning knowledge and skill in the development and/or analysis of social welfare policy. Social work values, knowledge, and skills will be applied to current social welfare policies and programs that provide for social needs beyond the capacity of individuals and families to provide for them.

- Many of the required content elements as described for the course can be gleaned from exposure to the issues, court decisions, and legislation leading to the development and implementing of federal and state policies that influenced and shaped kinship care services. Legal decisions such as the Supreme Court Decision, *Miller v. Youakim* (1979) and federal legislation such as the Adoption Assistance and Child Welfare Act of 1980, Title IV of the Social Security Act, the Indian Child Welfare Act, the Adoption and Safe Families Act of 1997, *Troxel v. Granville* (2000) clearly document how kinship care has been influenced by the courts and legislation with significant impact on children and relatives (Leos-Urbel, Bess, & Green, 2002; Bobroff, 2000; CWLA-Online). Students gain insight into the legal debates and advocacy efforts among supporters of kinship care from these litigants' challenges against the public child welfare agencies that have resulted in laws and legislation which have significantly influenced services to grandparents and other relatives in kinship care.

Course Learning Outcomes

Three outcomes from the course syllabus support infusion of content on grandparents in kinship care (a) to understand the roles and obligations of generalist practitioners in developing or changing social welfare policies and (b) to develop and utilize a beginning framework for social welfare policy development or analysis, and (c) to utilize research and other empirical knowledge in evaluating a policy's effectiveness for social work practice. These outcomes are achieved by focusing on policies that affect kinship care on both the federal and state levels, which provide students with diverse knowledge and facilitates their understanding of the need for social welfare policies and programs for this population. Content materials on federal and state legislation and court decisions that affect kinship care policy could be infused in the course. Two examples of federal court decisions that can be useful are *Miller v. Youakim, 1979*, which required states to provide the same financial assistance to relative foster parents as non-relative foster parents, and *Troxel v. Granville, 2000*, which addressed grandparents' visitation (Bobroff, 2000; Gleeson, 1999). An example of a court decision at the state level could be the Illinois case, *Reid v. Suter, 1992*, which required priority consideration of relatives for placement of children and a stronger appeal process for relatives challenging a denial of approval or placement of a child in their home (Gleeson, 1999). Several examples of legislation on the federal level have significance for kinship care, the Indian Child Welfare Act, 1978, which mandated relatives as first consideration for children being removed from their biological parents (CWLA, 2000; Hegar, 1999; Bending, 1997; Matheson, 1996), the National Family Caregiver Support Program as part of the Older Americans Act Amendments of 2000, which makes a myriad of social services available to grandparents and other older relatives caring for children under the age of 18 (Generations United, 2001; Beltran, 2001), and The Adoption Assistance and Child Welfare Act 1980, Title IV of the Social Security Act, and the Adoption and Safe Families Act of 1997 (CWLA-Online).

Course Assignment

The course assignment, a policy analysis paper, offers another opportunity of infusing this content as students are to select and analyze a particular social welfare policy for its impact on clients and programs of services. Federal and state policies affecting grandparents in kinship care can be used to meet this assignment. A general classroom examination of these policies with an accompanying in-depth, student-assigned examination of a particular policy's impact on grandparents in kinship care can provide the students with awareness and understanding of why this population requires such policies and programs and may need additional ones in the future.

CONCLUSIONS

The intent of this article is to offer a model for infusing content on an aging population, grandparents in kinship care, using existing course descriptions, learning outcomes, and assignments as conduits of support for infusion of content materials. The article makes suggestions for infusing content into selected core social work foundation courses to assist faculty with exposing students to this population of older adults and to help students acquire knowledge and develop the skills necessary to provide services to grandparents in kinship care and their grandchildren. The content materials are relevant for the courses based on the course descriptions, learning outcomes, course assignments, and CSWE standards for these core courses (CSWE, 2001). This model complies with the purposes of the social work program's GeroRich Project.

REFERENCES

Administration for Children and Families, Administration on Children, Youth & Families, Children's Bureau. (2000). *Report to the congress on kinship foster care. Part I: Research review, Part II: Secretary's report to the congress.* Washington, D.C.: United States Department of Health and Human Services. Retrieved February 15, 2001, from http://aspe.hhs.gov/hsp/kinr2c00/full.pdf.

Barnhill, S. (1996). Three generations at risk: The imprisoned women, their children, and the grandmother caregiver. *Generations, 20,* 39-40.

Beltran, A. (2001). *A guide to the National Family Caregiver Support Program and its inclusion of grandparents and other relatives raising children.* Washington, D.C.: Generations United.

Bending, R.L. (1997). Training child welfare workers to meet the requirements of the Indian Child Welfare Act. *Journal of Muticultural Social Work, 5*(3-4) 151-164.

Berrick, J.D., Needell, B., & Minkler, M. (1999). The policy implications of Welfare Reform for older caregivers, kinship care and family configuration. *Children and Youth Services Review, 21,* 9-10.

Berrick, J.D., Barth, R.P., & Needell, B. (1994). A comparison of kinship foster homes and foster family homes: Implications for kinship care as family preservation. *Children and Youth Services Review, 16,* 33-63.

Bobroff, R. (2000). The survival of grandparent visitation statues. *Journal of Poverty Law and Policy, 34*(5), 284-296.

Burnette, D. (1997). Grandparents raising grandchildren in the inner city. *Journal of Contemporary Human Services,* Sept/Oct., 489-99.

Burnette, D. (1999). Custodial grandparents in Latino families: Patterns of service use and predictors of unmet needs. *Social Work, 44,* 22-34.

Bryson, K. (2001). *New census data on grandparents raising grandchildren.* Paper presented at a Generations United congressional staff briefing. Washington, D.C.: Generations United.

Child Welfare League of America (1994). *Kinship care: A natural bridge.* Washington, D.C.: CWLA North American Kinship Care Policy and Practice Committee.

Child Welfare League of America. Frequently asked questions. Retrieved March 22, 2005 from http://www.cwla.org/programs/kinship/faq.htm.

Christian, S. (2000). Helping kin care for kids. *State Legislatures, 26*(10), 20-23.

Cohen, C.S., & Pyle, R. (2002). Support groups in the lives of grandmothers raising grandchildren. In C.B. Cox (Ed.), *To grandmother's house we go and stay: Perspectives on custodial grandparents.* New York: Springer Publishing.

Cox, C.B. (2002). Empowering African American custodial grandparents. *Social Work, 47*(1), 45-54.

Cox, C.B. (2000). Empowering grandparents raising grandchildren. In C.B. Cox (Ed.) *To grandmother's house we go and stay: Perspectives on custodial grandparents.* New York: Springer Publishing.

Cox, E.O., & Parsons, R.J. (1994) *Empowerment-oriented social work practice with the elderly.* Pacific Grove, CA: Brooks/Cole Publishing Company.

Cross, T. (1986). Drawing cultural traditions in Indian child welfare practice. *Social Casework, 67,* 283-289.

CSWE/SAGE-SW (2001). Strengthening the Impact of Social Work to Improve the Quality of Life for Older Adults and their Families: *A Blueprint for the New Millennium.* Alexandria, VA: Council on Social Work Education.

CSWE/SAGE-SW (2002). *Strengthening the capacity to teach aging content: Teaching resource kit.* Alexandria, VA: Council on Social Work Education.

CSWE (2001). *Educational Policy and Accreditation Standards.* Alexandria, VA: Council on Social Work Education.

Cummings, S.M., & Knopf, N.P. (2000). An infusion model for including content on elders with chronic illness in the curriculum. *Advances in Social Work, 1*(1), 93-105.

Damron-Rodriguez, J., & Lubben, J.E. (1997). The 1995 White House Conference on Aging: An agenda for social work education and training. *Journal of Gerontological Social Work, 27*(3), 65-67.

Danzy, J., & Jackson, S. (1997). Family preservation and support services: A missed opportunity for kinship care. *Child Welfare, 76*(1), 31-44.

De Toledo, S., & Brown, D.E. (1995). *Grandparents as parents: A survival guide for raising a second family.* New York: The Guilford Press.

Dowdell, E.B. (1995). Caregiver burden: Grandparents raising their high risk children. *Journal of Psychosocial Nursing, 33*(3), 27-30.

Dressel, P.L., & Barnhill, S.K. (1994). Reframing gerontological thought and practice: The case of grandmothers with daughters in prison. *The Gerontologist, 34*, 685-691.

Eastman, M. (1995). User first: Implications for management. In R. Jack (ed.) *Empowerment in Community Care.* London: Chapman and Hall.

Ehrle, J., & Green, R. (2002). Children cared for by relatives: What services do they need? In *New Federalism: National Survey of American's families.* Washington, DC: The Urban Institute.

Emick, M., & Hayslip, B. (1996). Custodial grandparenting: New roles for middle aged and older adults. *International Journal of Aging and Human Development, 43*(2), 135-154.

Flint, M.M., & Perez-Porter, M. (1997). Grandparent caregivers: Legal and economic issues. *Journal of Gerontological Social Work, 28*(1), 63-76.

Fuller-Thomson, E., & Minkler, M. (2000). African American grandparents raising grandchildren: A national profile of demographics and health characteristics. *Health & Social Work, 25*(2), 109-118.

Garcia-Preto, N. (1996). Latino families: An overview. In M. McGoldrick, J. Giordano, & J.·Pierce (Eds.), *Ethnicity and family therapy* (2nd ed.) (pp. 141-154). New York: Guilford Press.

Glesson, J.P. (1999). Kinship care as a child welfare service: Emerging policy issues and trends. In R. L. Hegar & M. Scannapieco (eds.) *Kinship Foster Care.* New York, NY: Oxford Press.

Hartfield, B.W. (1996). Legal recognition of the value of intergenerational nurturance: Grandparent visitation in the nineties. *Generations*, 53-56.

Hegar, R.L. (1999). The cultural roots of kinship care. In R.L. Hegar & M. Scannapieco (Eds.) *Kinship Foster Care: Policy, Practice, and Research.* New York: Oxford University Press.

Jackson, S. (1996). The kinship triad: A service delivery model. *Child Welfare, 75*(5), 583-599.

Jendrek, M.P. (1994). Grandparents who parent their grandchildren: Circumstances and decisions. *Gerontologist, 34*, 206-216.

Jones, L., & Kennedy, J. (1996) Grandparents united: Intergenerational developmental education. *Child Welfare, 75*(5), 636-650.

Karp, N. (1996). Legal problems of grandparents and other kinship caregivers. *Generations*, Spring, 57-60.

Kelley, S.J., Crofts Yorker, B., Whitley, D.M., & Sipe, T.A. (2001). A multimodal intervention for grandparents raising grandchildren: Results of an exploratory study. *Child Welfare, 80*(1), 27-49.

Kelley, S.J., & Danato, E.G. (1995). Grandparents as primary caregivers. *Maternal and Child Nursing, 20,* 326-332.

Kelley, S.J., Whitley, D.M., Sipe, T.A., & Crofts-Yorker, B. (2000). Psychological distress in grandmother kinship care providers: The role of resources, social support, and physical health. *Child Abuse and Neglect, 24*(3), 311-321.

Leos-Urbel, L., Bess, R., & Green, R. (2002). The evolution of federal and state policies for assessing and supporting kinship caregivers. *Children and Youth Services Review, 24*(1-2), 37-52.

Lum, D. (2004). *Social Work Practice and People of Color: A process-stage approach.* (5th ed.) Belmont, CA: Thomson Brooks/Cole.

Matheson, L. (1996). The Politics of the Indian Child welfare Act. *Social Work, 41*(2), 232-235.

McLean, B., & Thomas, R. (1996). Informal and formal kinship care populations: A study in contrasts. *Child Welfare, 75*(5), 489-505.

McPhatter, A.R. (1997). Cultural competence in child welfare: What is it? How do we achieve it? What happens without it? *Child Welfare, 76*(1) 255-278.

McPhatter, A.R., & Ganaway, T.L. (2003). Beyond the rhetoric: Strategies for implementing culturally effective practice with children, families, and communities. *Child Welfare, 82*(2), March/April., 103-124.

Miller v. Youakim, 440, U.S.125 (1979).

Minkler, M., Fuller-Thomson, E., Miller, D., & Driver, D. (1997). Depression in grandparents raising grandchildren. *Archives of Family Medicine, 6,* 445-542.

Minkler, M., & Roe, K.M. (1996). Grandparents as surrogate parents. *Generations, 20,* 34-38.

O'Brien, P., Massat, C.R., & Gleeson, J.P. (2001). Upping the ante: Relative caregivers' perceptions of changes in child welfare policies. *Child Welfare, 80*(6), 719-748.

Pinson-Milburn, N. Fabian, E.S., Schlossberg, N.K., & Pyle, M. (1996). Grandparents raising grandchildren. *Journal of Counseling & Development*, July/August, *74,* 548-554.

Pruchno, R. (1999). Raising grandchildren: The experiences of black and white grandmothers. *The Gerontologist, 39*(2), 209-211.

Roe, K.M., & Minkler, M. (1999). Grandparents raising grandchildren: Challenges and responses. *Generations,* Winter 1998-1999, 25-32

Rosen, A.L., & Zlotnik, J.L. (2000). *Social work education and practice for a growing aging population* (Paper presented at the IFSW/IASSW Conference).

Rothenberg, R. (1996). Grandparents as parents: A primer for schools. *Eric Digest.* Retrieved August 3, 2000 from www.npinil.crc.uiuc.edu/digests/dr-gra96.html.

Ruiz, D.S., & Carlton-LaNey, I. (1999). The increase in intergenerational African American families headed by grandmothers. *Journal of Sociology and Social Welfare, 26*(4), 71-86.

Sands, R.G., & Goldberg-Glen, R.S. (2000). Factors associated with stress among grandparents raising their grandchildren. *Family Relations, 49*(1), 97-105.

Scannapieco, M., & Jackson, S. (1996). Kinship care: The African American response to family preservation. *Social Work, 41*(2), 190-196.

Scharlach, A., Damron-Rodriguez, J., Robinson, B., & Feldman, R. (2000). *Journal of Social Work Education, 36*(3) Retrieved September 24, 2002 from www.cswe.org/sage-sw/resrep/educsws.htm.

Singer, T.L. (2000). *Structuring education to promote understanding of issues of aging.* CSWE/SAGE-SW. Retrieved July 8, 2003 from www.cswe.org/sage-sw/resrep/understandaging.htm.

Smith, A., Dannison, L., & Vacha-Hasse, T. (1998). When grandma is mom: What today's teachers need to know. *Childhood Education, 75*(1), 12-16.

Strom, R., & Strom, S. (2000). Meeting the challenge of raising grandchildren. *International Journal of Aging and Human Development, 51*(3), 183-198.

Takas, M. (1995). *Grandparents raising grandchildren: A guide to finding help and hope.* Crystal Lake, IL: National Foster Parent Association.

Taylor, R.J., Tucker, M.B., Chatters, L.M., & Jayakody, R. (1997). *Recent demographic trends in African American family structure.* In R.J. Taylor, J.S. Jackson, & L.M. Chatters (Eds.) Family Life in Black America. Newbury Park, CA: Sage.

Thompson, N., & Thompson, S. (2001). Empowering older people. *Journal of Social Work, 1*(1), 61-76. Thousand Oaks, CA: Sage Publications. Retrieved from http://jsw.sagepub.com/content/vol1/issue1.

Troxel v. Granville, 530 U.S.57 (2000).

Turner, L. (1995). Grandparent-caregivers: Why parenting is different the second time around. *Family Resource Coalition Report, 14*(Spring-Summer), 6-7.

U.S. Census Bureau. (2000, March). *America's families and living arrangements.* (Current Population Reports). U.S. Department of Commerce. Washington, D.C.: U.S. Government Printing Office.

Zambrana, R. (1995). *Understanding Latino families.* Thousand Oaks, CA: Sage Publications.

doi:10.1300/J083v48n03_08

Joy of Living:
A Community-Based
Mental Health Promotion Program
for African American Elders

Sandra Edmonds Crewe, PhD, MSW

SUMMARY. African American elders are often acknowledged for their resilience in overcoming discrimination. Because of their unique historical experience, many have relied upon family support and spirituality to address mental health problems and have shunned professional mental health services. Despite the strengths of African American elders, there are mental health needs that require professional intervention. This article specifically discusses a mental health promotion program sponsored by the Mental Health Association of the District of Columbia. It provides a description of the program and an evaluation of its outcomes. An analysis of pre and post intervention evaluations (n = 228) shows success of the intervention in raising participant awareness of normal and abnormal mental health as well as resources available to them. doi:10.1300/J083v48n03_09 *[Article copies available for a fee from The Haworth Document Delivery Service: 1-800-HAWORTH. E-mail address: <docdelivery@haworthpress.com> Website: <http://www.HaworthPress.com> © 2007 by The Haworth Press, Inc. All rights reserved.]*

The author would like to thank Shelita M. Snyder, MSW, PhD, who served as research assistant on this project. Dr. Snyder is currently Adjunct Assistant Professor for the Howard University School of Social Work.

[Haworth co-indexing entry note]: "Joy of Living: A Community-Based Mental Health Promotion Program for African American Elders." Crewe, Sandra Edmonds. Co-published simultaneously in *Journal of Gerontological Social Work* (The Haworth Press, Inc.) Vol. 48, No. 3/4, 2007, pp. 421-438; and: *Fostering Social Work Gerontology Competence: A Collection of Papers from the First National Gerontological Social Work Conference* (ed: Catherine J. Tompkins, and Anita L. Rosen) The Haworth Press, Inc., 2007, pp. 421-438. Single or multiple copies of this article are available for a fee from The Haworth Document Delivery Service [1-800-HAWORTH, 9:00 a.m. - 5:00 p.m. (EST). E-mail address: docdelivery@haworthpress.com].

KEYWORDS. African American elders, spirituality, mental health

INTRODUCTION

Resilience is a strength often associated with African American families, especially elderly members. Martin and Martin (1995) describe a resilient culture among African American enslaved people that was highly adaptable to practically any situation regardless of how extreme it was. "Black people had a strong faith and belief in powers to endure and overcome ..." (Martin & Martin, p. 212). There is a relationship between resilience and the sense of need and acceptance of formal mental health care. Surviving in a hostile environment nurtured the sense of self-reliance and skills at masking pain. Paul Laurence Dunbar, an African American poet, uses his poem "We Wear the Mask" to explain resilience (http://www.poets.org).

> *We wear the mask that grins and lies,*
> *It hides our cheeks and shades our eyes,*
> *This debt we pay to human guile;*
> *With torn and bleeding hearts we smile,*
> *And mouth with myriad subtleties.*
> *Why should the world be over wise,*
> *In counting all our tears and sighs?*
> *Nay, let them only see us, while*
> *We wear the mask.*
> *We smile, but, O great Christ, our cries*
> *To thee from tortured souls arise.*
> *We sing but oh the clay is vile*
> *Beneath our feet, and long the mile;*
> *But let the world dream otherwise,*
> *We wear the mask!*

The poem depicts a social reality for Blacks that allowed little or no room for self-attention. While laws ended many discriminatory practices, changing longstanding customs of self care has proven to be more difficult. As we focus on eliminating health disparities, more innovative ways are needed to convince African Americans of the value of mental health care.

"African Americans occupy a unique niche in the history of America ..." according to the U.S. Surgeon General's Report on *Mental Health: Culture, Race and Ethnicity* (USHHS, 2001, p. 53). The report acknowledges the resilience within the African American community but underscores the role of discrimination in their current social and economic standing. This is especially true for African American elders who reached adulthood during the era of legalized racial segregation. Many have carried its harmful effects into their later life. Black men and women who were middle aged during the Civil Rights movement and reached retirement during the late 1970s and 1980s have emerged with social, economic, and health deficits relative to their White elderly cohorts (Siegel, 1999). In their lifetime they have seen the injustices of Jim Crow. Consequently, current generations of African American elders are often characterized as resilient or able to "make a way out of no way" because many have endured hardships and remained focused.

To survive and meet new challenges, many African Americans relied upon their internal strength, their family, and their faith which are sometimes referred to in literature as the nurturing community. Dilworth-Anderson and Burton (1999) also document that the mental well-being of African Americans was primarily tied to these three resources. Gray-Little and Hafdahl (2000) believe that this practice explains why many African Americans do not suffer from low self-esteem despite the racial assaults and mundane extreme environmental stress they experience. Literature is rich with description of the collective identity and mutual support networks within the African American community (Crewe, 2003; Dilworth-Anderson & Burton, 1999; Martin & Martin, 1995). It is this resilience that presents a challenge in working with this population. The historical pattern of African Americans using informal versus formal networks for mental health care makes outreach and promotion more complex. There is stigma and shame associated with mental illness therefore many African Americans are not looking to self-impose another barrier to their often fragile well-being. Also, access to culturally competent mental health providers has been a barrier along with shame, stigma, discrimination, and mistrust (USHHS, 2002).

This article discusses the barriers to mental health care for older persons with particular focus on African Americans. It also presents findings from a mental health promotion program for African American elders.

OLDER ADULTS AND MENTAL HEALTH

"Millions of older Americans–indeed the majority–cope constructively with the physical limitations, cognitive changes, and various losses such as bereavement, that frequently are associated with late life" (U.S. H.H.S. Surgeon General, 2000, p. 335). Despite the resilience of older Americans to successfully respond to end of life losses, the Surgeon General's report states almost 20% of the 55 and older age group experience specific mental disorders that are not a normal part of aging. The report also noted that unrecognized or untreated mental disorders such as depression, Alzheimer's disease, alcohol and drug abuse and misuse, anxiety, late life schizophrenia and other conditions can be severely impairing and fatal in some instances. Suicide is reported higher among older adults and it is well documented that suicide is a consequence of depression. The question that must be asked and answered is why given these data there is inadequate attention to the mental health needs of older persons. According to Atchley (1985) and Rosen and Perksy (1997) ageism and stigma help to define mental health services for older persons. The belief that older persons are too old to benefit from mental health services results in them being denied services (NASW, p. 322). This is evidenced by the fact that while 13% of the population is over 65, they only account for 6 percent of people treated in community mental health centers (Colenda & van Dooren, 1993). Comorbidity of health and mental health exacerbate the inadequate care of many elderly persons (NASW, 2003; Kramer et al., 1992). Changes in general health conditions and cognitive capacities often mask mental disorders. Too often, the older person's difficulties are diagnosed as age related and providers fail to explore alternative explanations. In fact, mental disorders are the number one reason for institutionalization of our elders. Other reasons that older persons are not readily treated for mental health disorders include affordability and accessibility.

The failure of society to address the mental health needs of older persons creates other burdens. Families find themselves caring for individuals who have mental disorders that have been overlooked. Untreated mental disorders make caregiving particularly burdensome. This is especially important for African American families who carry more of the caregiving responsibilities for elders. Thus, it is very important to understand how African American elders react to the mental health care network.

RACE, AGEISM, AND MENTAL HEALTH

Forty years ago the National Urban League (1964) issued a report titled *Double Jeopardy* that addressed the confluence of ageism and racism for Blacks in America. The report stated that "age merely compounded those hardships accrued ... as a result of being Negro." It posed the question, "Can we not, while lifting their level of living, also lift their spirits?" (p. 19). The report stated that there was an obligation to make sure that older Blacks did not continue to face life burdened by the accumulated hardships of lifetimes that placed them in double jeopardy. The historic 1964 *Double Jeopardy* report explained that today's aged Negro is different from today's aged White because he is Negro ... and this alone should be enough basis for differential treatment. For he has, indeed, been placed in double jeopardy: first by being Negro and second by being aged. Age merely compounded the hardships accrued to him as a result of being a Negro (1964, p. I).

Forty years later, we continue to see evidence of cumulative disadvantage in the form of health disparities among African Americans. Nowhere is this more evident than for many African American elders who have experienced the indignity of aging in a hostile social system (Lindsay, I & Hawkins, B.D., nd). This lifetime of marginalization not only affected their physical health, but for some it has also resulted in poor mental health. Although the NUL report "Double Jeopardy" addressed race and poverty as co-conspirators, one can also view double jeopardy from the perspective of the historical difficulty Blacks have had with *accessibility* and *affordability* of health and mental health care.

There is a dearth of literature on the mental health disorders of older African Americans. According to the Surgeon General's (2001) report on *Mental Health: Culture, Race and Ethnicity*, what is known is that there are higher rates of cognitive impairments; many residing in nursing homes need psychiatric care (Class et al., 1996); 27% of older African Americans living in public housing need mental health treatment (Black et al., 1997); and older Blacks in long term care are less likely to use available community services and have elevated symptoms of depression (Mui & Burnette, 1994). Because of these and other barriers, new approaches are necessary to address the mental health needs of African American elders.

Because of the unforgiving nature of the institution of slavery, many African American elders enter old age with both inadequate knowledge and access to mental health resources. Having already been stigmatized by race, many older Blacks endure mental discomfort rather than to risk adding yet another label to an already overburdened psyche. Thus, many African American elders undoubtedly suffer in silence rather than divulge anything that might be perceived as a weakness of character. Private suffering is indeed part of their spirituality. Spirituals such as "What a Friend We Have in Jesus" often are used to describe their coping process. The following verses from this often referenced spiritual help to describe the heavy reliance on faith:

> *Are we weak and heavy ladened, cumbered with a load of care?*
> *Precious savior still our refuge, Take it to the Lord in prayer*
> *Do thy friends despise, forsake thee, Take it to the Lord in prayer*
> *In his arms, he'll take and shield thee, thou will find solace there.*

Often, African American elders rely upon their spirituality and do not feel the need to seek professional help. To counter this, effective ways of health promotion, outreach and service delivery that incorporate spirituality are needed. Martin and Martin (2002) emphasize the importance of spirituality in working with African Americans. Although public policy cannot completely erase the historical cumulative disadvantage of double jeopardy, it can double its efforts to put in place more programs that build upon their collective strengths. A recent report by the National Center and Caucus of the Black Aged (2003) emphasized that "one important area that needs immediate improvement for tackling the health disparities issue is to close the current information gap" (p. 39). It is important to use the knowledge about the strengths and inherited disadvantages of the group and design culturally sensitive information dissemination programs that make Blacks more receptive to mental health care.

ADDRESSING THE MENTAL HEALTH NEEDS OF ELDERS

The National Association of Social Workers (NASW) is a leader in documenting the mental health needs of older persons. Through policy recommendations, they have called attention to the importance of mental health care and the barriers that many individuals face in receiving care. Lin (1995) in an article in the *Encyclopedia of Social Work* noted that the mental health service delivery system must do a better job in responding to the twin problems of affordability and quality of services. She challenged the mental health system to integrate mental health services with existing networks to ensure maximum use of the services. The NASW (1994) policy statement reaffirmed the need for "a continuum of care that includes community-based services, prevention, short and long-term hospitalization, outpatient services, outreach and emergency services, and supportive services to families with mental disorders" (p. 1,709). The article further called for the profession of social work to move beyond the traditional therapeutic models and embrace new ways of assessment and treatment. The most recent NASW mental health policy statement (2003-2006) also documents that some subgroups of the population, including women, members of racial and ethnic groups, and those of the lowest socioeconomic status have been poorly or underserved. Racism, ageism, and classism, according to *Social Work Speaks,* have resulted in biased diagnoses and treatment. This was documented by the Institute of Medicine's (2002) report titled *Unequal Treatment: Confronting Racial and Ethnic Disparities in Health Care.* Ironically, the findings that African Americans are treated differently often with negative outcomes will place more of a burden on the health and mental health system to *regain* the trust of a group that was already somewhat suspect of their care.

Recognizing the importance of mending and bridging the health and mental health service disparity gap, the NASW mental health and senior health, safety, and vitality policy statements (2002-2006) include a number of position statements that specifically address the need to provide better mental health care for older persons of color. NASW states that:

- social workers should recognize outreach services as an important part of mental health;
- the preventive functions of social work practice, including education, consultation and early intervention, should be recognized and fully funded, with the goal of maximizing individual and family wellness and fostering resilience;
- culturally responsive treatment in the most therapeutic and last restrictive environment, including use of the consumer's native language, should guide the practice of social work;
- social workers should take the lead role in advocating for viable, comprehensive, community-based mental health services; and
- social workers play a key role in educating the public about mental illness as a means of fostering prevention, encouraging early identification and intervention, promoting treatment, and reducing the stigma associated with mental illness. This responsibility includes efforts to influence public policy in ways that will foster improved prevention and diagnosis and promote comprehensive, continuous treatment of mental illness for all individuals who need these services and not only those who might be considered a threat to society.
- promotion of wellness, prevention, early intervention and outreach services instead of sickness care in health and social services programs for seniors and their families;
- promotion of and advocacy for improved access to mental health services for older adults;
- promotion of policies and funding programs that reduce the incidence of suicides in our senior population; and
- encouragement of social work research, professional publications, and community of best practices in services to older persons and their families.

Putting these policy statements into action will produce a new model of service delivery for African American elders and their unique needs. Programs that are proactive will supplant the disease model. The U.S. Surgeon General agrees with the need to change our approach to meeting the mental health needs of older persons. The 2000 report identifies a new model that postulates that successful aging is contingent on three elements: (1) avoiding disease and disability, (2) sustaining high cognitive and physical function; and (3) engaging with life (Rowe & Kahn, 1997). According to the report, these three elements act in concert to produce successful aging. Attention must be given to all three simultaneously to ensure quality of life. To do this, it is important to broaden delivery mechanisms to include more health promotion. This is especially important for African American elders who are doubly at risk because of cumulative racial disparities.

JOY OF LIVING PROGRAM

The Mental Health Association (MHA) of the District of Columbia created *Joy of Living: Keeping Healthy Mentally* as an educational program for African American older adults through the faith-based community and the District of Columbia's aging network. They formed an advisory group to provide consultation on program curriculum, design, and evaluation. The group represented members of the faith-based community, MHA DC Board members, local government personnel and mental health professionals with expertise in gerontology. The Mental Health Association contacted faith-based senior center/programs as well as senior center operated by the District of Columbia's Office on Aging. Using this process, six facilities agreed to sponsor the program.

CURRICULUM

The *Joy of Living* program considered four key elements for working with the African American community. It acknowledges the importance of using existing community programs to disseminate information. It avoided mistrust by linkage with known programs. Secondly, the program used culturally competent presenters. Using African American experts helped to ensure that the message was couched in strengths versus pathology framework. The third element stressed the inclusion of faith and spirituality in reaching cohorts of African Americans. The fourth element of the program was the use of self-help principles through the integration of sharing circles (Figure 1).

This pilot program helps to develop a model of the fundamental aspects of an integrated mental health and senior center program (Depla et al., 2003). The *Joy of Living* program consisted of a series of three workshops focusing on health and its relationship to mental health, memory loss, and depression. The three workshops were:

- Workshop I. Keeping Mentally Health (Phase I) The Relationship Between Mental & Physical Health (Phase II)
- Workshop II. Memory Loss and Alzheimer's (Phases I & II)
- Workshop III. The Blues: Depression (Phases I & II)

FIGURE 1

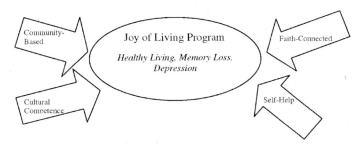

The series of three workshops were held at six sites serving senior citizens. During Phase I, the pilot program, two faith-based senior centers were used. In Phase II, four additional sites were located. Three of the senior centers were operated by the District of Columbia's aging program. There was also an additional faith-based senior center. The format of the presentation was relatively consistent across the six sites and the 18 sessions. The one exception was that Workshop I for Phase I focused on keeping healthy mentally and in Phase II the workshop focused on the relationship between mental and physical health. They shared some content but they were different enough to report separately on them. The sessions lasted about two hours and used the following general format:

- Introduction of topic
- Distribution of five question pretest
- Speaker on Topic
- Sharing Circles
- Wrap Up (including Posttest and Evaluation)

Expert guest speakers presented the three topics. Speakers included a psychiatrist, a professor from Howard University, a retired social worker, and a mental health professional for the Capitol Alzheimer's Association. Sharing circles composed of 7-10 participants followed each group presentation. Each group had a facilitator and a recorder/reporter (different from speakers); these groups were planned to help participants learn to share their feeling and stories. The groups' recorders reported back to the reassembled larger groups. The guest presenter made closing remarks to reemphasize learning focus. Also handouts were given to participants at each session. The handouts included materials on the topic such as brochures on depression, memory loss, etc.

Program Goals and Objectives

The primary goal of the program was to improve the mental health of older African Americans. Key Objectives:

- To differentiate between normal and abnormal mental health
- To increase comfort in talking to doctor about problems
- To increase knowledge of causes, symptoms and treatment of poor mental health
- To increase knowledge of resources available to get help
- To learn new strategies to address specific problems (i.e., memory loss, depression)

PARTICIPANTS

The program participants were predominantly African American. No descriptive data were collected, however, based upon knowledge and observation of the program participants, a substantial majority were African American (99%) and about 80% female. All were over 65 years of age and capable of managing with little or no assistance. The centers had cognitively impaired elderly persons who attended the presentations but did not complete forms or participate in sharing circles or focus groups.

RESEARCH DESIGN

Each session was evaluated using the pre and posttest questions related to the topic. The pretest included five questions related to the specific topics. The true-false pretest was given before the presenter addressed the topic. Their surveys were collected. The posttest queried individuals about the same content in the pretest; however, the questions were presented in different formats. Using different questions made it more difficult to analyze change because some questions could have been interpreted differently, thus not measuring the exact same thing. An example of a pre and posttest question follows:

Pretest Question
Older persons get irritable and crabby with old age.   True   False

Posttest Question
Which of the following is not a part of the aging process?

a. irritability   b. mild forgetfulness
c. body slows down   d. gray hair

In addition to pre and posttests, all participants were asked to evaluate each workshop using the following seven questions: They were asked for yes or no responses (questions 1-6).

Session Evaluation questions
1. Did you find the workshop useful?
2. Did you find the workshop interesting?
3. Did you learn anything new about the signs of (topical area)?
4. Did you learn anything new about the causes of (topical area)?
5 Did you learn anything new about the treatment of (topical area)?
6. Would you talk to your doctor about your concerns?
7. Comments
Items 1-6 were yes or no responses

In addition to the quantitative pre and posttest measures, qualitative evaluation measures were used. Participant observation was used to capture evaluative information from the sharing circles. The evaluator participated in six of these circles to understand their value. Additionally focus groups were conducted by the same evaluator at three locations–one faith-based senior center and two city senior centers. Both the sharing circles and the focus groups provide more information about the effectiveness of the program. The qualitative measures were probably most effective because the quantitative instruments had some design limitations and their unique quality of gaining perceptions of the target group.

RESULTS

Workshops	Phase I (2 sites)	Phase II (4 sites)	Total
Workshop I. Keeping Healthy Mentally	34	51	85
Workshop II. Memory Loss and Alzheimer's	15	55	70
Workshop III. The Blues: Depression	36	37*	73
Total	85	143*	228

* There were an additional 40 surveys that were lost.

Phase I (2001)

Collectively, there were 85 completed evaluation forms. All (100%) workshop participants found their workshop very useful and interesting. Almost all respondents recognized the importance of speaking with their doctor about mental health concerns. Among the 70 persons responding to the question, 99% (98.6%) said they would talk to their doctor about any concerns. Only one (1.4%) individual reported that she/he would not talk with her/his doctor (about memory loss).

Eighty-three percent of the participants in the Keeping Healthy Mentally workshop learned how to detect signs of poor mental health; 80% developed awareness about where to seek help if needed; and 82% (81.5%) were educated about how to talk to their doctor about keeping mentally healthy. Pretest questions verified that there was some lack of knowledge about mental health and older persons. For example, during the pretest almost half (47%) of the respondents believed that older people get irritable and crabby with advancing years. The posttest measure showed that almost 70% felt that irritability was not a normal part of aging. During the pretest 55% felt that serious mental illness was most common in older persons. The posttest findings showed that only 28% still believed this. Thus, there was some change noted in their knowledge.

The participants in the Not a Normal Part of Aging: Memory Loss workshop learned new things about detecting the signs of memory loss (96.2%), identifying the causes of memory loss (95.7%), and effective ways to improve their own memory (100%). Pretest scores showed that over 50% of participants felt that memory loss was a normal part of aging. Also, over 80% felt that there was nothing that could be done about memory loss. Interestingly 5% understood that mild memory loss might be due to physical conditions. Also, 90.7% knew that Alzheimer's disease was not the only reason for memory loss. This could be attributed to strategies to stay mentally healthy being addressed in the first session. Just over 60% of the group was unaware that African Americans were at higher risk for memory loss than Whites. It was most notable that 80% in the pretest did not feel that memory loss was a normal part of aging. Also, the higher prevalence of memory loss among African Americans was not known. For the most part all posttest answers were correct. During the posttest 100% of participants recognized that African Americans were at a higher risk of developing memory loss.

The Blues: Depression and Older Adults workshop yielded similar findings. Participants discovered new insight pertaining to: recognizing the signs of depression (100%), identifying the causes of depression (88.5%); and effective ways to treat depression (100%). The pretest indicated that there was considerable lack of knowledge about depression. For example, almost 16% believed that depression was a personal weakness, 65.9% believed that it was normal to be depressed a long period after the loss of a loved one, 58.1% believed that it was normal for older persons to be depressed and 36% did not understand that medications could be responsible for causing depressive symptoms. The posttest documented a positive change in their knowledge. Whereas 58.1% during the pretest believed that depression was a normal part of aging, only 13.8% felt this way after the workshop. Equally important, the posttest measure showed that nearly 60% recognized the common signs of depression.

Phase II (2002)

Overall, 143 evaluations were received from the three workshops. All participants found the workshops useful and interesting, with the majority (97.5%) indicating a strong positive response. More than 90% said they would talk to their doctor about any concerns. Just over 8% were uncertain and two persons indicated they would *not* talk with their doctor about any concerns.

In The Relationship Between Mental & Physical Health workshop (n = 51), 94% learned something new about treating poor mental health; 98% had a better understanding of the relationship between mental and physical health; and 96% learned something new about the brain's involvement with mental health. The pretest showed that there was a good understanding of the relationship between mental and physical health. In four out of the five questions, over 90% answered correctly. During the pretest, almost one third of the participants felt that poor mental health was mostly caused by poor judgment. The posttest measures showed that there was generally new knowledge learned in that the participants were able to clearly identify factors other than poor judgment that contribute to mental illness.

The Memory Loss and Alzheimer's workshop participants learned new things about Alzheimer's disease (98.1%), detecting signs of memory loss (98%), and the necessary steps to take in dealing with memory loss (98.2%). Prior to the workshop, most (96%) were aware that there were effective ways to deal with Alzheimer's disease and that there was no cure (90%). However, just over 30% felt that memory loss and Alzheimer's disease were virtually the same. Posttest results showed that 90% were comfortable with discussing memory loss with their physician and knew the steps to take to address memory loss.

In The Blues: Depression workshop, participants discovered new insight pertaining to recognizing the signs of depression (96.6%), identifying the causes of depression (96.3%); and effective ways to treat depression (96%). Prior to the workshop nearly 20% did not believe that depression was a medical condition. Almost half felt that feeling sad or depressed over the loss of a loved one is a sign of severe or clinical depression. Also, almost one third felt that clinical depression affects almost every adult. Although posttest results showed some changes in knowledge, there was still considerable misunderstanding of depression, thus indicating the need for additional sessions or activities.

The following selected direct statements from participants in Phase I & II add to the understanding of the value and outcomes of the program.

> I think meetings (seminars) are important and helpful. You reaffirm yourself that you are not there by yourself.

The workshop was very timely in as much as we are getting older. The discussion will help us identify memory loss sooner.

I'm looking forward to improved health as a result of this. It was very interesting and made me feel more comfortable.

Although the program is geared toward seniors, it may be good to include younger persons who are facing so many challenges.

I really enjoyed all three sessions. It would be nice if we could have some more. It was really very interesting.

SHARING CIRCLES

The sharing circles were rich with exchange. The facilitator queried participants about their experiences related to the topical area and asked them to share some of their coping strategies. Most of the participants actively participated. They not only shared their experiences but also were very open to listening to others and trying to help them. There was a great deal of empathy demonstrated. For example, in the sharing circle for one of the depression workshops, one member patiently explained to someone that she had gone through the same things and felt the same way at one time. The other participant burst out in tears because she was so relieved that she was not the only one having the problem. When it was time to go back to the larger group, individuals lingered and continued to talk with each other and share experiences. This sharing continued in the larger group and it was somewhat difficult to get the group centered again. It was clear that the sharing circles were meeting an important need for peer support.

FOCUS GROUPS

In the focus groups individuals also shared the value of the workshops. The group indicated that the sessions made them more mentally aware and helped to keep them calmer. It also had the benefit, according to the group, of helping them see things in the right perspective.

Based upon their comments, they had retained much of the information presented and were able to use it. For example, one participant specifically noted that she tries to keep her mind more active. Another indicated that in order to keep her mind stimulated she writes things down. Interestingly, another participant indicated that she had stopped allowing a friend to stress her out–she now referred them to the Mental Health Association. Most indicated that they enjoyed the session on depression the most. This seems to relate, in part, to their experiences with this area. One individual indicated that he never understood depression and the workshop helped him. Others focused on their new knowledge about the relationship between depression and physical health. They generally agreed that the most valuable aspect of the workshop was the strategies that they learned and seem to be putting to use. The groups also liked the structure of the sessions. They discussed the value of the sharing circles, especially as it related to their greater awareness of fellow senior center members' personal "stories."

The groups identified several topics for future discussions. They suggested more sessions on mental health, sexuality, and how to live in a stressful world (session took place approximately one month after terrorists attacks on the U.S.). The participants also seemed to be interested in the topic of death and dying. Surprisingly they also expressed and interest in knowing more about mental health topics for children.

The workshops were effective in helping the participants differentiate between normal and abnormal health. Their pre and posttests proved evidence of this. For example, almost all of the participants stated in their evaluation that they would be comfortable in talking to their doctor about their problems. The posttest was probably most effective in capturing the participants' knowledge of symptoms and treatment of poor mental health. Although it is not clear how much of it was new knowledge, the evaluations overwhelmingly indicated that there is some awareness of causes and symptoms. The participants reported that they learned new resources. In fact, one focus group participant stated that she gives out the Mental Health Association number to individuals who call her and seem to need help. This also addressed the value of the sessions in providing new strategies to participants.

CONCLUSIONS AND FUTURE DIRECTIONS

There is a growing demand for evidence to support the effectiveness of program innovations. It is often difficult to measure success in service oriented environments. This program is such an example. The evaluation instruments while imperfect begin to support this program model. The participants were open to learning new things and the tests confirmed that there was a change in their knowledge in all of the sessions. It builds upon the well established correlation between education and health outcomes and adds to the accumulating evidence that makes the case for learning as health promotion (Cusack, Thompson & Rogers, 2002). Cusack, Thompson and Rogers also endorse the need for mental fitness research for older person because of their status as life long learners and the significant improvements in depression that have been documented.

As previously stated the model focuses on using a community-based facility (a natural setting) to educate consumers about mental health concerns. It confirms the special value of programs based on the unique needs of the community and the importance of mobilizing existing resources (Cooley, Ostendorf & Bickerton, 1979). Partnerships emerged that will continue to yield benefits. The *Joy of Living* model also used experts who were culturally competent to address the topics. Using African American presenters helped to address the concern of racial bias and insensitivity. Also, the model included self-help opportunities through sharing circles. Allowing individuals to share their stories made the sessions more responsive to individual needs and it also promoted self-help and mutual support that are core to the African American community. Finally there was the recognition of the importance of faith-based linkages. The presenters used spirituality in their discussions and some facilities were themselves faith based. The presenters noted no difference in the spirituality at the faith-based versus city-run facilities. It was clear that regardless of the setting, the message had to recognize the community's faith connectedness. The Surgeon General's report on *Mental Health: Culture, Race and Ethnicity* emphasize that efforts to promote mental should build on "intrinsic community supports such as spirituality, positive ethnic identity, traditional values, educational attainment, and local leadership" (p. 168).

There were other important lessons learned from this program. In addition to reaffirming the general merit of the model, the evaluation documented some particular strengths. The model used a three-workshop model. Rather than the one time presentation, it scheduled a series of sessions that built upon each other. There was overlap that proved to be useful. Participants talked about knowledge gained from one session to the other.

Also the sharing circles were particularly noteworthy because they engaged the participants in meaningful dialogue. Using the self-help process empowered the participants to use their recently attained knowledge. It freed them to talk about their unique experiences free of shame or embarrassment. This sentiment was echoed several times by members of the focus group. One member stated that they spend a lot of time with each other in the center, but most of it is so programmed they never get to really know and help one another. The centers learned that group discussions work. Not only do seniors need to hear from experts, they are experts themselves because of their life experiences. They are willing to use this knowledge to help others. The sharing circles spurred me to create an assignment in social gerontology called learning partners. All students are asked to identify an older person (65 and older) and dialogue with them weekly on various topics covered in class. They maintain a journal and use the learning partner dialogues to enrich the learning experiences. The assignment has also been shared with HBSE classes as part of John A. Hartford Foundation and Council of Social Work Education Geriatric Enrichment in Social Work Education program.

The final important observation was that older persons are interested in issues that affect their families. Often programming at senior centers focuses on the needs of older persons. Yet, the focus groups indicated that they needed more information on the mental well-being of younger groups. During all three focus groups, participants sought to better understand issues like ADHD in children; the effect of violence on children; and children's responses to death and dying. It should be noted that one focus group was held shortly after September 11th, 2001 and another in October 2002 around the time of the sniper scares in the District of Columbia. Older persons were looking for strategies to help their younger family members. This is consistent with literature that notes the intergenerational characteristics of African American families. African American grandparents show high rates of stress and depression that can possibly be attributed to their caregiver roles (Crewe, 2003; Crewe & Stowell-Ritter, 2003). Therefore, it is sound programming that considers their concerns about their grandchildren and children.

The *Joy of Living* program made an important contribution to educating African American elders about key mental health issues. It responds to the Surgeon General's call to expand and improve services to deliver culturally and geographically accessible programs. How well did it do? The participants endorsed the program and gave it the highest compliment–they asked the program to continue. I have taken the liberty of allowing a participant to offer the closing evaluative statement about the *Joy of Living* program:

> We were provided with a lot of information. The presentations were excellent. It was a learning experience. I truly enjoyed the workshop. Thanks for making us more aware.

REFERENCES

Atchley, R. (1985). *Societal forces an aging* (4th ed.). Belmont, CA: Wadsworth.

Black, B.S., Rabins, P.V., German, P., McGuire, M., & Roca, R. (1997). Need and unmet need for mental health care among elderly public housing residents. *The Gerontologist, 37*, 717-728.

Class, C.A., Unverzagt, F.W., Gao, S., Hall, K.S., Baiyewu, O., & Hendrie, H.E. (1996). Psychiatric disorders in African American nursing home residents. *American Journal of Psychiatry, 153*, 677-681.

Colenda, C., & van Dooren, H. (1993). Opportunities for improving community mental health services for elderly persons. *Hospitals and Community Psychiatry, 44*, 531-533.

Cooley, R.C., Ostendorf, D., & Bickerton, D. (1979). Outreach services for elderly Native Americans. *Social Work*, 151-153.

Crewe, S.E., & Stowell-Ritter, A. (2003). *Grandparents raising grandchildren in the District of Columbia: AARP focus group report*. Washington, DC: AARP.

Crewe, S.E. (2003). African-American grandparent caregivers: Eliminating double jeopardy in social policy. In T. Bent-Goodley, Ed., *African American Social Welfare Policy.* The Haworth Press, Inc.

Crocker, J., & Major, B. (1989). Social stigma and self-esteem: The self protective properties of stigma. *Psychological Bulletin, 96,* 608-630.

Cusack, S.A., Thompson, W. J., & Rogers, M.E. (2003). Mental fitness for life: Assessing the impact of an 8 week mental fitness program on healthy aging. *Educational Gerontology, 29,* 393-403.

Depla, M.F. (2003). Integrating mental health care into residential homes for the elderly: An analysis of six Dutch programs for older people with severe and persistent mental illness. JAGS, 51: 1275-1279. American Geriatrics Society.

Dilworth-Anderson, P., & Burton, L. (1999). Critical issue in understanding family supports in older minorities. In *Full Color Aging* (Toni Miles, Ed.). pp. 93-107. A publication of the Gerontological Society of America.

Gray-Little, B., & Hafdahl, A.R. (2000) Factors influencing racial comparisons of self-esteem: A quantitative review. *Psychological Bulletin, 126,* 26-54.

Kramer, M., Simonsick, E., & Lima B., & Levav, I. (1992). *The epidemiological basis for mental health care in primary health care: A case for action.* New York: Tavistock/Routledge.

Lin, A.M. (1995). Mental health overview. In *Encyclopedia of Social Work,* 19th ed. pp. 1705-1711. Washington, DC. Author.

Lindsay, I., & Hawkins, B.D. (n.d.). Research issues related to the Black aged. Available from author.

Martin, E., & Martin, J. (1995). *Social work and the Black experience.* Washington, DC: National Association of Social Workers.

Mui, A.C., & Burnette, D. (1994). Long term care use by the frail elders: Is ethnicity a factor? *The Gerontologist, 34,* 190-198.

National Association of Social Workers (2003). *Social work speaks: National Association of Social Workers policy statements 2003-2006,* 6th edition. Washington, DC: Author.

National Caucus and Center for the Black Aged (2003). *The health status of older African Americans.* Washington: Author.

National Urban League (1964). *Double jeopardy: The older Negro in America today.* New York: Author.

Rosen, A., & Persky, T. (1997). Meeting mental health needs of older people: Policy practice issue for social work. *Journal of Gerontological Social Work, 27,* 45-54.

Rowe, J.W., & Kahn, R.L. (1997). Successful aging. *Gerontologist, 37,* 433-440.

Siegel, J.S. (1999). Demographic introduction to racial/Hispanic elderly populations. In Toni Miles (ed.) *Full Color Aging,* pp. 1-17.

U.S. Department of Health and Human Services (2001). *Mental health: Culture, race and ethnicity*–A Supplement to Mental Health: A Report of the Surgeon General. Rockville, Md.

U.S. Department of Health and Human Services (2000). *Mental health: A Report of the Surgeon General.* Rockville, MD.

doi:10.1300/J083v48n03_09

Filipinas as Residential Long-Term Care Providers: Influence of Cultural Values, Structural Inequity, and Immigrant Status on Choosing This Work

Colette V. Browne, DrPH
Kathryn L. Braun, DrPH
Pam Arnsberger, PhD

SUMMARY. This exploratory study investigated reasons why Filipinas in Hawai'i have become the primary caregivers of elders in residential care homes and if they thought their children would follow them in this profession. A random sample of 173 Filipina care home operators (CHO), of which 95% were first-generation immigrants, was interviewed using telephone survey methods. Data were collected: to profile caregivers; to identify motivations for becoming a care home operator; and to gauge if

The authors gratefully acknowledge the assistance of Dr. Eldon Wegner and the Honorable Dennis Arakaki for their encouragement, Daisy Ascuncion for data entry, Heidi Wong, Lyn Mulrooney, Alissa Rogers, Michael Tamashiro, and Debra Vandergriend for data collection.

This research was funded through a grant from the College of Social Sciences, University of Hawai'i.

[Haworth co-indexing entry note]: "Filipinas as Residential Long-Term Care Providers: Influence of Cultural Values, Structural Inequity, and Immigrant Status on Choosing This Work." Browne, Colette V., Kathryn L. Braun, and Pam Arnsberger. Co-published simultaneously in *Journal of Gerontological Social Work* (The Haworth Press, Inc.) Vol. 48, No. 3/4, 2007, pp. 439-455; and: *Fostering Social Work Gerontology Competence: A Collection of Papers from the First National Gerontological Social Work Conference* (ed: Catherine J. Tompkins, and Anita L. Rosen) The Haworth Press, Inc., 2007, pp. 439-455. Single or multiple copies of this article are available for a fee from The Haworth Document Delivery Service [1-800-HAWORTH, 9:00 a.m. - 5:00 p.m. (EST). E-mail address: docdelivery@haworthpress.com].

439

they or their children would continue in this line of work. The sample was composed of middle-aged Filipina CHO with training and experience in elder care who concurred that the job fit their cultural values. About a third also felt that this job was open to immigrants and helped them buy a house. Twenty percent or less felt discriminated against because of this work. Although half the sample felt that women were better caregivers than men, only 38% felt that caregiving was primarily the responsibility of women. Almost 90% planned to continue with this work, but only 12% said it was likely that their children or grandchildren would become CHO, supporting the notion that choosing this profession had less to do with cultural values and gender expectations than with economic opportunities available to the current cohort of CHO. Given these findings, Hawai'i's capacity to meet future residential long-term care needs is discussed. doi:10.1300/J083v48n03_10 *[Article copies available for a fee from The Haworth Document Delivery Service: 1-800-HAWORTH. E-mail address: <docdelivery@haworthpress.com> Website: <http://www.HaworthPress.com>*

KEYWORDS. Filipino Americans, geriatric foster care, elderly, long-term care, workforce development

INTRODUCTION

It is well documented that families meet the bulk of care and assistance needs of the nation's frail elderly population (Noelker & Bass, 1995; Pearlin et al., 1990). Nonetheless, when elders and their families need assistance, they turn to a wide range of paraprofessionals that provide home and personal care (Dorfman et al., 1998; Penning, 1995). Given the rapidly growing aging population and the increased need for personal and assistant services, paid caregiving for the aged is one of the fastest growing service occupations in the U.S. In fact, the demand for these types of jobs will increase by 63.5 percent by the year 2010 (U.S. Department of Labor, 2003).

In Hawai'i, families that can no longer provide in-home care to vulnerable older adults often turn to small (four-to-five bed) care homes, which are family homes that provide 24-hour residential care to dependent adults with custodial and personal care needs. Payment depends on the client's level of care and payer, and operators can earn more for clients with higher-care needs and private-paying clients. In other locales, these homes are called hostels, foster homes, and board-and-care homes (e.g., Kane, 1991). According to the Hawai'i Department of Health (2000), 97% of the 563 licensed small care homes in the

City and County of Honolulu are operated by Filipinas. An under-researched minority, Filipino Americans comprise one of the nation's most rapidly growing Asian American populations, now numbering more than 2 million (U.S. Census, 2000).

The predominance of Filipinos in low-paying service jobs is an international phenomenon (Chang & Ling, 2003; Lim, 1998) and has led to a number of explanatory theories, e.g., the influence of gender and cultural values, discrimination to other employment sites, and immigration status and patterns (Glenn, 1999; Marchand & Sisson Runyan, 2003; Stoller & Gibson, 2000). Globally, Filipino women have emerged as a major group of paid caregivers of the aged in developed countries in Europe, Canada, Asia, and the Middle East (Chang & Ling, 2003; Youngs, 2003). In the U.S., the clearly bifurcated long-term care labor force relies heavily on ethnic minority women, immigrant women, and lower social class women to fill generally low-paid paraprofessional positions (Department of Labor, 2003; Glenn, 1999; Tung, 2000).

In this study, we examined the specific case of Filipinas in Hawai'i who work as care home operators (CHO) to describe this population of long-term care providers and to understand their motivations for choosing this work, their expectation for continuing to operate a care home, and their thoughts about their own children becoming CHO in the future. Clearly, understanding the needs of women who provide this care "an important area of study in its own right" has implications for how frail elders will be cared for in the future, especially in light of the growing number of older adults in the U.S.

CONCEPTUAL FRAMEWORK

A possible motivation for operating a care home is Filipino culture. Culturally-linked values and norms of caring for the aged may be related to the value an ethnic group places on elder care (Braun & Browne, 1998; McBride, 1998; Young & Kahana, 1995). Similar to any population, there exists great heterogeneity among Filipinos based on age, gender, socioeconomic status, level of acculturation, immigration history, and other factors (McBride, Morioka-Douglas & Yeo, 1996). Nonetheless, universal Filipino values elevate eldercare to an honorable profession, including *utang no loob* (debt of gratitude to those who have helped you), the importance of family and intergenerational interdependence, and *pakikisama* (harmony in personal relationships) (Agbayani-Siewert, 1994; McBride, 1999). Dissimilarly to Confucian cultures, Filipino culture is more egalitarian than patriarchal and, as such, women and women's roles are not considered less important than men and men's roles in Filipino culture (Agbayani-Siewert, 1994), and there is a relatively low level of ethnocentrism.

Another possible motivator for becoming a CHO relates to structural barriers to other employment. The low-paid long-term care service network is sexualized (i.e., there is a predominance of females) and racialized (i.e., there is a predominance of ethnic minority and immigrant women) (Tung, 2000). Structural barriers to better-paying jobs include lack of English-language skills, low educational attainment, lack of opportunity, and perceived and real employment discrimination (Glenn, 1999). A more focused examination of the evidence provides support for Asian Americans' experience of discrimination (Min, 1995), and research on Filipinos supports this hypothesis (Pratt, 2002; Tung, 2000). Rather than choosing to become a CHO, perhaps this occupation was the best available job considering language-, race-, gender-, and opportunity-based barriers.

A related reason that Filipinas may predominate in the long-term care industry (and perhaps the care home industry as well) speaks to the relationships among the continuing high levels of poverty in the Philippines, this country's reliance on foreign currency sent home by Filipinos living abroad, and the globalization of the economy (Marchand & Sisson, 2002; Pratt, 1999). The population of the Philippines continues to grow at a rapid rate, despite significant reductions in population growth in neighboring Asian countries. Supporting a family member to work outside the country so that he/she can send home foreign currency is a common way to supplement a family's income and afford education and property. In fact, 7.3 million overseas Filipinos remitted $7.2 billion back to the Philippines in 2000, representing 9% of the country's gross national product (Go, 2002). Some Filipinos have immigrated permanently to the U.S., and Hawai'i CHO fall in this category. However, many other Filipinos reside in the U.S. as temporary and/or illegal workers. They have left family members behind, including young children, to whom they send as much as 75% of their income to raise the family's standard of living, with plans to return to the Philippines after a number of years, e.g., after all children have completed their schooling (Tung, 2000).

In summary, 97% of Hawai'i care homes are operated by Filipina, yet very little is known about these women. The general lack of information about these caregivers is compelling for at least two reasons. First, we need to learn more about this group to see why they predominate in this profession, if they plan to continue in it, and if they expect their progeny to continue in this field? If Filipinas have chosen this profession because it is one of the few avenues open to first-generation immigrant women, it would be reasonable to assume that their children, born and educated in the U.S., would have a broader range of career opportunities. This leads to a second question: Who will provide this care in the future, as the numbers of the aged dramatically grow, and need for long-term care services increases? To address these questions, we investigated the role of gender, cultural values, structural inequalities (i.e., workplace discrimination), and immigration status on occupational motivation among Filipina care home operators. With such data, states may be better equipped to understand who is attracted to elder care as a paraprofessional occupation and how to develop a responsive labor force for the future cohort of older adults.

METHODS

Sample

From the state's 2000 listing of 563 licensed four-to-five-bed care homes, we deleted operators without Filipino surnames, leaving 548 potential respondents. We hoped to interview a third of this group, thus we chose every third name on the list and then over-sampled by approximately 5% using the same procedure with names not originally chosen. Of the 203 individuals selected for the sample, 23 refused to participate, five could not be contacted after five attempts, and two did not finish the interview. Completed interviews were obtained for 173 (85%) of the 203 Filipinas in the sample, representing 32% of Hawai'i's licensed CHO.

Measures

We asked for age, marital status, birthplace, level of education, and degrees earned, length of time in the job, and type of work done previously. Operators were asked about their net monthly income and if they felt that CHO were paid adequately. We recorded data on the number of residents and their care level and payer (state or private) and on others (family and non-family) that helped to provide care and/or run the care home.

The project's theoretical orientation and findings from focus groups with Filipina CHO guided the development of 22 items tapping motivation for operating a care home, and these related to personal skills, cultural values, gender expectations, immigration, and discrimination (see Table 4). Items were scored on a five-point Likert-type scale and coded so that the higher score reflected a higher level of endorsement of the construct. We also asked open-ended questions about the best and worst things about the job. We asked whether they would be continuing as a CHO, whether they would like to see their children do this same work, and their estimate of the likelihood that a child or grandchild might enter the field.

Procedures

Prior to the study, meetings were held with a state legislator known for his support of care homes and the leaders of the two major CHO associations to introduce the study. These associations also provided recommendations that were adapted into the survey instrument. On their direction, a letter explaining the study and encouraging participation was mailed to each of the 203 CHO, and this letter was signed by the study investigators, the key legislator, and the associations' presidents. Graduate students were trained in the telephone interview protocol and met weekly with the investigators to resolve emerging data collection issues. Each member of the sample was telephoned up to five times to arrange an interview. A summary of findings was mailed to each participant, along with a thank-you letter and a $10 gift certificate.

Analysis

Data were managed and analyzed in SPSS version 11. First, we calculated frequencies and means to profile the sample. Next, we examined relationships between hypothetically potential predictor or explanatory variables and the three outcome variables: (a) Do you plan to continue as a care home operator? (yes/no), (b) Would you like to see your children and grandchildren do the same work? (on a scale from 1-5), and (c) How likely would it be that your children or grandchildren will go into this same work? (on a scale from 1-10). For ease of analysis, responses to these outcome variables were post-coded into dummy variables, with yes or very likely coded as "1" and all other responses coded as "0." Open-ended responses to questions about the best and worst things about the job were post-coded by investigators.

The 22 Likert-scored motivational items were subjected to principal component analysis, which is the most computationally simple approach to factor analysis with small item pools (Kim & Mueller, 1978). The Promax rotation with the Kaiser (eigenvalue greater than one) criterion was chosen, as the output then includes the results from both the orthogonal and the Promax rotations. Factors were analyzed for internal reliability. Factors retained were then treated as continuous variables and analyzed to examine the relationship between these factors and the three outcome variables of interest.

RESULTS

The characteristics of the sample are presented in Table 1. The mean age of respondents was 55, 86% were born in the Philippine, 82% were married, 90% were home owners, and 84% reported at least one other family member living in the house. For those born in the Philippines, the mean number of years since immigration was 30. All had completed high school, and 74% had post-high-school training. Of these 121 women, 107 (88%) had studied something related to

TABLE 1. Care Home Operator Demographics (N = 173)

Variable	Mean (range)	N (%)
Mean age of respondent	54.9 (31-82)	
Years as care home operator	15.6 (1-40)	
Married		141 (81.6)
Born in the Philippines		166 (96.0)
Years living in US, since immigration	30.5 (9-60)	
Home ownership		155 (89.6)
Hawai'i		152 (87.9)
Outside of Hawai'i		27 (15.6)
Highest educational attainment (n = 171)		
High school diploma		45 (26.3)
Some college or technical school		67 (39.2)
College degree		59 (34.5)
Area of study post-high school (n = 121)		
Nursing		55 (45.5)
Certified Nurse Aide course		17 (14.0)
Care home operator course		12 (9.9)
Other health-related field (midwifery, nutrition, lab tech)		23 (19.0)
Other (non-health related)		14 (11.6)
Place of post-high school study (n = 121)		
Philippines only		46 (38.0)
Hawai'i and/or US mainland only		46 (38.0)
Philippines and Hawai'i/US mainland		29 (24.0)
Previously did similar work in another setting		121 (69.9)

healthcare or care home operation, including 55 (46%) who had studied nursing and 17 (14%) who were certified nurse aides. Fully 62% of women who reported taking post-high-school courses had studied in Hawai'i and/or the U.S. mainland. On average, these women had been operating their care homes for 16 years; almost 70% previously had done similar work (caring for dependent adults) in a different setting, e.g., in a hospital or nursing home or with a home or community-based project.

On average, respondents were caring for 4 residents (not shown in table) with a mean age of 70; 57% of clients were male and 43% were female. For 72% of clients, CHO were paid from government sources, through the mechanisms of Social Security and Supplemental Security Income. Among homes with other family members in residence, 85% of caregivers said that these family members assisted with operations, specifically by watching the residents when the operator had to be away, assisting with meals, and cleaning the house. Almost half (45.8%) of the operators also were paying non-family members to assist. The most-often named task for this paid group (unlike the presumably unpaid family members) was to provide personal care. Only 52 respondents answered the question on monthly income after expenses and responses varied, with some operators claiming virtually no profit and others claiming profits of up to $9,500 month. Due to low response and high variability, this variable was dropped from further analysis.

The distributions of responses to the three outcomes variables are shown in Table 2. Almost 90% of respondents planned to continue operating their care homes. Although 37% would like to see their children and grandchildren do this same work, only 13% felt it was very likely that they would do so.

Caregivers were asked to name the three best and three worst things about the job (Table 3). Things they liked best were working with older people (55.4%), spending time with family (49.1%), helping others (45.7%), and working at home (44.0). The things they liked least were the confining 24-hour-a-day nature of the job (79.4%), client health and behavior crises (45.5%), and conflict with clients' family and the health professionals helping them (34.0%). Additionally 19.8% were frustrated by the government requirements for paperwork and inspection visits, and 19.6% were unhappy with the job's low pay and poor benefits.

Shown in Table 4 are the items means and the number and percent of respondents that either agreed or strongly agreed with each of the 22 motivation-related statements. Among the items in the "culture and caring" category, 4 items were agreed to by 94% or more of the sample, including "in my culture, showing

TABLE 2. Chance that Operators and Their Progeny Will Continue in This Work

Outcome variables	n (%)
I plan to continue as care home operator. (n = 172)	
Yes	154 (89.5)
No	18 (10.5)
I would like to see my children and grandchildren do this same work. (n = 171)	
Agree or strongly agree	64 (37.0)
Neutral	33 (19.1)
Disagree or strongly disagree	74 (42.7)
Likelihood that my children and grandchildren will work as care home operators (n = 165)	
Very unlikely (scores 1-3)	91 (55.2)
Not sure, maybe (scores 4-6)	53 (32.1)
Likely or very likely (scores 7-10)	21 (12.7)

TABLE 3. Best and Worst Things About Being a Care Home Operator

Best things about the job		Worst things about the job	
Working with older people	55.4%	Confining 24-hour nature of job	79.4%
Spending time with children/family	49.1%	Client health and behavior problems	45.4%
Helping others	45.7%	Conflict with family, MD, SW	34.0%
Working at home	44.0%	Government demands and inspections	19.8%
Good pay and benefits	16.8%	Poor pay and benefits	19.6%
Being your own boss	14.5%	Too much responsibility	10.4%
It fits my experience and training	12.1%	No time for self and family	5.2%
Flexibility and low stress	12.2%		
Steady work, hard to find new job	11.0%		

respect to elders is very important" and "this job allows me to show respect to my elders"; and 83% said they chose this job because they liked working with older people. Related to gender and caring, half the sample felt that women were better caregivers than men, but only 38% felt that caregiving was primarily the responsibility of women. More than 94% agreed that they had the skills and training for this work, although only 24% felt it was easy to establish their business. About a third also felt that this job was open to immigrants and helped them buy a house. Among items related to discrimination, 34% felt they had been treated poorly due to English-language difficulties, but only 21% felt they had been treated poorly because of the work they did and only 17% would rather be working in another field. Contrary to our expectations, 92% agreed that people who provide care to older adults get a lot of respect in the U.S.

In factor analysis of the 22 motivational items, 6 factors emerged when extraction was based on eigenvalues, however 9 items either loaded on more than one factor or not at all. These tended to be items that were global (e.g., "I think new immigrants experience discrimination.") and/or related to gender (e.g., "Caring for others is primarily the responsibility of women."), and were eliminated. The subsequent free analysis yielded four factors; however, the number of items per factor was small, and the fourth factor was not conceptually meaningful. We forced a three-factor solution that was conceptually and statistically sound. As shown in Table 5, the three factors were: (a) the job fits my qualifications, training, and culture ($\alpha = .7403$); (b) the job has helped me as an immigrant to work and buy a house in the U.S. ($\alpha = .6933$); and (c) I have

TABLE 4. Motivations for Choosing This Work

Items	Item mean	n (%) agreed
Items related to culture and caring		
I think caring for older adults is an important job.*	4.3	166 (95.9)
This job allows me to show respect to my elders.	4.3	169 (97.2)
The people I care for become like family members to me.	4.3	163 (94.2)
I chose this job because I like to work with older people.	3.9	149 (83.2)
In my culture, showing respect to elders is very important.	4.3	168 (97.1)
It is the duty of young people to care for those who need help, especially older family members.*	3.7	127 (73.5)
God does not give you a job that you cannot do.*	3.6	124 (71.6)
Items related to gender and caring		
Caregivers can be women or men.*	3.3	63 (36.4)
Caring for others is primarily the responsibility of women.*	2.8	66 (38.2)
When it comes to caring for older people, I think women do a better job at it than men.*	3.4	84 (48.5)
Items related to job skills and fit		
It was easy to open this business.	2.3	41 (23.7)
I have enough training to do this job.	4.1	162 (93.6)
I am qualified for this job.	4.2	167 (96.5)
Items related to immigrant status		
This is a good job for people who have recently arrived in the U.S.	2.8	54 (31.2)
This is a good job for people who didn't have the chance to go to college in the US.	2.7	54 (31.2)
This job has helped me buy a house.	2.6	51 (29.5)
Items related to discrimination and structural inequity		
I chose this job because it was hard for me to find something else.	2.2	22 (15.6)
I think new immigrants experience discrimination in the workforce.*	3.3	48 (27.8)
I have been treated poorly in the US because I don't speak English well or because I speak w/an accent.	2.7	58 (33.5)
I think people treat me poorly because I do this kind of work.	2.5	36 (20.9)
I think people who provide care to older adults get a lot of respect in this country.*	2.0	159 (91.9)
(Because of discrimination) I'd rather be working in another field.	2.4	30 (17.4)

* Items eliminated due to ambiguous or non-loading.

TABLE 5. Factor Loadings and Reliability Coefficients for Three Motivational Factors

	Factor loadings		
	1	2	3
The job fits my qualifications, training, and culture. (α = .7399)			
I am qualified for this job.	.882	2.079	.088
I have enough training to do this job.	.805	2.094	.169
The people I care for become like family members to me.	.707	2.114	2.068
This job allows me to show respect to my elders.	.649	2.060	2.294
In my culture, showing respect to elders is very important.	.548	2.076	2.206
I chose this job because I like to work with older people.	.391	2.022	2.227
Mean for sum of 6 items = 25.1			
The job has helped me as an immigrant to work and buy a house in the U.S. (α = .6933)			
This is a good job for people who didn't have the chance to go to college in the US.	2.014	.775	.159
This is a good job for people who have recently arrived in the US.	2.006	.717	.028
I chose this job because it was hard for me to find something else.	.067	.632	.018
This job has helped me buy a house.	2.377	.629	.310
It was easy to open this business.	2.261	.601	.173
Mean for sum of 5 items = 12.5			
I have had negative experiences as an immigrant and in this job. (α = .5287)			
I have been treated poorly in the US because I don't speak English well or because I speak w/an accent.	2.118	.071	.734
I think people treat me poorly because I do this kind of work.	2.031	.116	.718
I would rather be working in another field.	2.082	.168	.603
Mean for sum of 3 items = 7.5			

Extraction Method: Principal Component Analysis.
Rotation Method: Promax with Kaiser Normalization.

had negative experiences as an immigrant and in this job (α = .5287). The three factors were not intercorrelated (r between 2.10 and .15), and together the factors explained 49.7% of the variance.

Although three motivation factors were confirmed, they were minimally associated with the three outcome variables (not shown in table). Respondents who planned to continue as care home operators, who would like to see their children in the same work, and who felt it was likely that their children would enter the field had similar scores on the three factors: about 25 (out of 30) for the "fit" factor; about 12.5 (out of 25) for the "good job for an immigrant" factor; and about 7.5 (out of 15) for the "negative experience" factor. Only one association was significant: respondents who would like to see their children become CHO scored higher on "good job for an immigrant" scale than respondents who would not like to see their children in this job (F = 4.92, p = .028). The minimal differences were due in part to the lack of variance in the outcome variables, e.g., 90% of respondents planned to continue as CHO and only 13% felt is was likely that their children would enter the field.

Despite the lack of variance, we attempted to search for other variables that would distinguish between CHO who planned to continue in this type of work from those who would not. There were no significant associations, but several approached significance (not shown in table). Respondents who said they would continue in this work were more likely to report enjoying the work and report having a spouse who provided substantial assistance. Respondents who were not planning to continue were more likely to own a home outside Hawai'i and were more likely to feel that the job was not providing an adequate income.

DISCUSSION

Our exploratory study examined the phenomena of first-generation immigrant women from the Philippines and their predominance as operators of small residential care homes in Hawai'i. We attempted to profile this group and to explore motivations for becoming CHO, looking at the role of culture, structural inequity, and immigrant status. Our analysis suggests that Filipina CHO in Hawai'i are primarily middle-aged women who chose this work because it fit their skills and their cultural values. About 30% also agreed that this work was a good avenue for first-generation immigrants and that this job had helped them buy a home in Hawai'i. Being able to help elders while spending more time with one's own family were among the best-liked things about the job. The vast majority (90%) planned to continue in this work.

Since we did not compare various ethnic groups with one another, we can not say that this sample enjoys working with older adults more so than other ethnic groups. We were impressed, however, that more than 95% of the sample agreed that caring for older adults was an important job and that their residents "became like family members." However, it was clear that the job also "fit" this group's skill set and needs. Many respondents had experience and/or training directly applicable to their jobs as CHO, e.g., 70% had done similar work in another setting and 69% had studied nursing and/or was a certified nurse aide. The job allowed them to fulfill other family obligations while making a living and to establish themselves in the U.S. Although only 30% said the job helped them buy a home, in fact, 90% of the CHO were homeowners, an amazingly high rate for first-generation immigrants, especially in Hawai'i where the cost of living is quite high.

The ability of the job to allow these women to care for their own families while caring for older adults and making an income is also interesting and speaks to a greater theoretical understanding of the complex ways in which home and family are situated differently by groups of women, often discussed by feminist thinkers (P. H. Collins, 1991). A transnational view may well allow us to see that this type of work can be both exploitive as well as empowering to women. Gender remains an important variable in this study; i.e., it is worth noting again that it is not Filipino men but women who work as CHO.

The findings from this study may have applicability to other locales. Although other states may not have a population of CHO with similar ethnic and immigrant status, we do know that growing numbers of Filipinas are employed in long-term care in other U.S. communities albeit in somewhat different capacities. Some are professionals (primarily as RNs), but a growing number are migrant laborers. A study in California, where 52% of U.S. Filipinos reside, revealed an extensive network of Filipina migrant workers as providers of in-home eldercare, estimating that Filipina migrants comprised 75% of all such providers in Los Angeles (Tung, 2000). These women, even if legally residing in the U.S., were not licensed or registered to provide eldercare and were paid "under the table," thus adding to the challenges of studying them. Few had health insurance, none owned homes in the U.S., and all planned to return to the Philippines. On average, these women remitted 75% of their income back to their families in the Philippines. Similarly to our study, Tung (2000) found that migrant Filipina eldercare workers felt that the job "fit" them. For example, they reported great confidence in their skills to provide care, they maintained that the people they cared for became like family members, and the job allowed them to send home enough money to increase their own family's standard of living and give their own children a broader range of opportunities. Canada appears to be depending on a similar source of help, having recently passed the controversial Live-in Caregiver Program, whereby immigrants, primarily Filipina, live with a Canadian family as a care provider to its frail members. Not considered immigrants, they retain their residency in their country and have few rights (Pratt, 1999).

Returning to our study, 87% of these first-generation immigrant CHO doubted that their children and grandchildren would choose the same work. They likely hoped that their immigration to the U.S. and the sacrifices that they are making as the first generation will give their children more opportunities so that they can obtain an even higher standard of living. Suggested reasons why caregivers would not recommend the job to their progeny include the 24-hour nature of work, dealing with residents' difficult health and behavior issues, conflicts with other family members and others involved in the residents' care, demands of the government offices that inspect and license care homes, and inadequate pay.

If second-generation Filipinos will not enter this field, what group will emerge to operate residential care homes in Hawai'i? Should Hawai'i investigate expanding immigration opportunities for Filipino families? Currently, federal policies in the Philippines support the continued exportation of Filipino labor, but as migrant labor, i.e., Filipinos can relocate temporarily for purposes of earning income, but must leave their families behind (Chang & Ling, 2003; Marchand & Runyan Sisson, 2003). The 1994 Technical Skills Development and Education Act passed by the Philippine government, which aimed to increase the education of its citizens and to decrease the numbers of the poor, has helped fuel the outflow of migrant laborers (Liban, 1999). Through its Technical Education and Skills Development Authority, more than 150 training centers operate to train Filipinas as caregivers of children and the elderly. Graduates leave their country (and their own families) to provide care and earn money to send home.

In contrast to these more recent immigrants (who have no chance of citizenship rights in the country in which they work), earlier waves of immigrant women (our sample) came to the U.S. to establish themselves, to earn a living, to buy a home, and to build a good life for their families. Providing residential long-term care services helped them meet these goals. Migrant workers may do well at meeting in-home eldercare needs, as long as states continue to allow the provision of such care by undocumented and/or unlicensed workers, but will not be able to establish residential care homes. Policy makers in Hawai'i need to consider what will happen when the current CHO cohort retires. Does the state look to new immigrant groups to fill this role? Which other ethnic/cultural groups have the same combination of skills, values, and ambitions?

Our attempt confirmed that Filipina CHO hold positive feelings toward eldercare, and that these are linked to culture. Second, the gender items did not load in the model or loaded on more than one factor. This may suggest that caregiving is not the exclusive domain of women in the Philippines. However, given that Filipino laborers in long-term care are predominantly female, we suspect that the problem could lie in inadequate construction of items to tap this domain. The discrimination scale was weak, in part because some of the theorized items loaded in the second factor ("good job for an immigrant") and took a positive spin. Thus, our measures need to be improved upon. However, we believe that we have established a foundation for continued examination of the competing influences of culture, gender, immigration, and discrimination on job choice in long-term care.

Although beyond the scope of this paper, these questions beg for an in-depth discussion of long-term care policy in the U.S. Should eldercare continue to be relegated as a job that is so unimportant and invisible that it is left in the hands of unpaid family members, low-paid migrant workers, or new immigrants (Glazer, 1990; Glenn, 1992; Tung, 2000)? Or, as is our hope, can the government, private insurers, and industry begin to pay a decent wage for caregiving so that the work is economically feasible for all who have the skills and the desire to do it?

This is an area ripe for further study. Few researchers have tried to quantify the intersection of gender, ethnicity and social class in the paraprofessional long-term care industry. Even fewer are asking questions about quality care for elders and how not to exploit those who provide it. While positive regard for older adults may well be a culturally-linked values (McBride & Parreno, 1996), we question this oversimplification for why Filipinas provide this type of work for two reasons. First, and as others have noted, there is great heterogeneity among Filipinas due to SES, nativity, acculturation levels, and other variables (McBride, Morioka-Douglas, & Yeo, 1996). Second, the idea that Filipinas are "natural nurturers" is a comparable argument posed by conservative theorists to describe women's similar "natural" role as unpaid caregivers in this country. In the end, this essentialist framework may legitimize the low pay of personal and home care workers by arguing that it is the nature of women and of certain cultural populations to provide this type of work. In contrast, we strongly suspect that it s a combination of economics (both the global economy and the national economy), immigrant patterns, cultural values, and traditional gender roles that result in this phenomenon.

As the size of American's older adult population grows, so will the demand for home-based long-term care and for low-paid personal care and home health workers (Department of Labor, 2003). Who will accept these jobs? Long term settings and home care requires all kinds of workers, especially those who provide the important personal care so needed by those who can no longer manage alone. This study suggests that our present strategy of relying on immigrant women, even those who value working with older adults, may be problematic. As a nation, we are faced with a complex balancing act between the need to have a labor force trained to assist the frail aged and the rights of those who provide the care. In the end, if we truly care about the well-being of older adults and the women who provide this care, there is a need to develop mechanisms to make the work attractive and economically rewarding for those who seek it.

REFERENCES

Agbayani-Siewert, P. (1994). Filipino Americans culture and family: Guidelines for practitioners. *Families in Society, 75,* 429-433.

Braun, K.L., & Browne, C.V. (1998). Perceptions of dementia, caregiving, and help seeking among Asian and Pacific Islander Americans. *Health and Social Work, 23,* 262-274.

Chang, K.A., & Ling, L.H.M. (2003). Globalization and its intimate other: Filipina domestic workers in Hong Kong. In M. Marchand and A. Sisson Runyan (Eds.), *Gender and global restructuring* (pp. 27-43). London: Routledge.

Collins, P.H. (1991). *Black feminist thought: Knowledge, consciousness, and the politics of empowerment.* New York: Routledge.

Dorfman, L.T., Holmes, C.A., & Berlin, K.L. (1998). Attitudes toward service use among wife caregivers of frail older veterans. *Social Work in Health Care, 27,* 4, 39-64.

Glazer, N. (1993). *Women's paid and unpaid labor: The work transfer in health care and retailing.* Philadelphia, PA: Temple University Press.

Glenn, E.N. (1999). The social construction and institutionalization of gender and race: An integrative framework. In M. M. Ferree, J. Lorber, & B. B. Hess (Eds.), *Revisioning gender* (pp. 3-41). Thousand Oaks: Sage.

Glenn, E.N. (1992). From servitude to service work: Historical continuities in the racial division of paid reproductive labor. *Journal of Women in Culture in Society, 18,* 1-43.

Go, S. (May 2002). Remittances and international labor migration: Impact on the Philippines. Paper presented at Metropolis Seminar on Immigrants and Homeland, Dubrovnik, Croatia. *www.international.metropolis.net/events/croatia/Dubrovnik_paper.doc* (accessed 10/5/03).

Kane, R.A., Kane, R.L., Illston, L.H., Nyman, J.A., & Finch, M.D. (1991). Adult foster care for the elderly in Oregon: A mainstream alternative to nursing homes? *American Journal of Public Health, 81,* 1113-1120.

Kim, J., & Mueller, C.W. (1978). Factor analysis: Statistical methods and practical issues. Newbury Park: Sage.

Liban, D.V. (1999). Bridging technical education to higher education for the Men in Blue (MIB). *http://www.tesda.gov.ph/events/speeh3.asp* (accessed 9/20/03).

Marchand, M.H., & Sisson Runyan, A. (2003). *Gender and global restructuring: Sightings, sites and resistances.* London: Routledge.

McBride, M., Morioka-Douglas, N., & Yeo, G. (1996). *Asian/Pacific Islander American elders* (2nd ed.). SGEC Working Paper #3, Stanford, CA: Stanford Geriatric Education Center.

McBride, M. (1999). *Health and health care of Filipino American elders. Http://www.stanford.edu/group/ethnoger/filipino.html* (accessed 9/20/03).

McBride, M., & Parreno, H. (1996). Filipino American families and caregiving. In G. Yeo and D. Gallagher-Thompson (Eds.), *Ethnicity and the dementias*. Washington, DC: Taylor and Francis.

Min, P.G. (Ed.) (1995). *Asian Americans: Contemporary trends and issues*. Thousand Oaks, CA: Sage.

Noelker, L.S., & Bass, D.M. (1995). Service use by caregivers receiving case management. *Journal of Case Management, 4,* 4, 1442-149.

Pearlin, L.I., Mullan, J.T., Semple, S.J., & Skaff, M.M. (1990). Caregiving and the stress process: An overview of concepts and measures. *The Gerontologist, 30,* 5, 583-594.

Penning, M.J. (1995). Cognitive impairment, caregiver burden, and the utilization of home health services. *Journal of Aging and Health, 7,* 2, 233-253.

Pratt, G. (2002). Collaborating across our differences. *Gender, Place, and Culture, 9,* 2, 195-200.

Pratt, G. (1999). Is this really Canada? Domestic workers' experiences in Vancouver, BC. In J. Momsen (Ed.), *Gender, migration, and domestic service* (pp. 23-42). London: Routledge.

State of Hawai'i, Department of Health, Care Home Data, 2000.

Stoller, E., & Gibson, R. (2000). *Worlds of difference: Inequality in the aging experience*. Thousand Oaks: Sage.

Tung, C. (2000). Cost of caring: The social reproductive labor of Filipina live-in home health caregivers. *New Frontiers,* 60-67.

U.S. Department of Labor, Bureau of Labor Statistics, 2003. *Occupational Outlook Quarterly, http://bls.gov* (accessed 9/25/03).

Youngs, G. (2003). Breaking patriarchal bonds: Demythologizing the public/private. In M. Marchand & A. Sisson Runyan (Eds.), *Gender and global restructuring* (pp. 44-58). London: Routledge.

doi:10.1300/J083v48n03_10

Listening to Seniors:
Successful Approaches to Data Collection
and Program Development

Waldo C. Klein, PhD, MSW
Cheryl A. Parks, PhD, MSW

SUMMARY. This paper provides guidelines for high quality data collection with community-residing older adults with illustrations drawn from the authors' practice. A mixed-method approach is described as a means to obtain the highest quality information from the sample. This approach combines focus groups and interviews along with mailed, closed-ended surveys to access both the "depth" of the seniors' responses as well as the "breadth" of responses; that is, the qualitative aspects provide the opportunity to identify and define relevant issues in the voices of respondents, while mailed surveys provide the kind of coverage necessary to make accurate predictions to the larger population of community-residing seniors. doi:10.1300/J083v48n03_11 *[Article copies available for a fee from The Haworth Document Delivery Service: 1-800-HAWORTH. E-mail address: <docdelivery@haworthpress.com> Website: <http://www.HaworthPress.com> © 2007 by The Haworth Press, Inc. All rights reserved.]*

KEYWORDS. Data collection, mixed-method, needs-assessment, older adults, survey

---

[Haworth co-indexing entry note]: "Listening to Seniors: Successful Approaches to Data Collection and Program Development." Klein, Waldo C., and Cheryl A. Parks. Co-published simultaneously in *Journal of Gerontological Social Work* (The Haworth Press, Inc.) Vol. 48, No. 3/4, 2007, pp. 457-473; and: *Fostering Social Work Gerontology Competence: A Collection of Papers from the First National Gerontological Social Work Conference* (ed: Catherine J. Tompkins, and Anita L. Rosen) The Haworth Press, Inc., 2007, pp. 457-473. Single or multiple copies of this article are available for a fee from The Haworth Document Delivery Service [1-800-HAWORTH, 9:00 a.m. - 5:00 p.m. (EST). E-mail address: docdelivery@haworthpress.com].

INTRODUCTION

The voices of consumers are an essential element in planning and evaluating senior service programming activities. Yet, it is often difficult for social workers to secure the kind of information on which sound programmatic decisions should be made. Questions about selecting from the range of research methods, drawing representative samples, and conducting meaningful analysis all cause hesitation for many program managers. Too often, program planners settle for using scattered anecdotal information often resulting in a few "squeaky wheels" getting a disproportionate share of a program's "oil."

Yet, for most senior program planning and needs assessment purposes, neither the data collection methodologies nor the analytic procedures are so complex that most motivated and conscientious social work program managers would be unable to undertake such research in a credible manner. This paper demystifies the fundamental considerations involved in data collection with community-residing older adults and provides the reader with illustrative examples from the authors' own practice. In particular, a multi-method approach involving both qualitative and quantitative methods is described (Morgan, 1998). We believe that the highest quality information can be gained from community-residing older adults through a combination of qualitative and quantitative research approaches. More specifically, we find great value in using focus groups and interviews along with mailed, closed-ended surveys in order to access both the "depth" of the seniors' responses as well as the "breadth" of responses; that is, through focus groups and interviews respondents are provided with the opportunity to identify and define issues relevant to the study that are meaningful to them. Equally important, respondents are able to express these ideas in their own voice and vernacular. In turn, mailed surveys provide the kind of coverage that is necessary to make accurate predictions about the degree to which varying perspectives are held among community seniors.

Total response rates in these mailed surveys among senior center participants have ranged to over 90% with usable response rates nearly as high. As will be discussed below, each of these methodological approaches plays an important role in providing an accurate and comprehensive picture of the senior community. Using reliable and valid information gathered from seniors through this multi-method approach will enhance the quality of modifications to current programs or design of programs for future delivery. Such programs will "connect" more fully with the needs or interests of senior participants because they were grounded in the voice and experience of the senior consumers.

The literature has for too long reflected the debate over the relative merits of qualitative and quantitative approaches to conducting research. "Science" is really a cyclical process that involves two fundamental components. First, it moves from observations through generalizations and on to the suggestion of explanations (theories) for these observations–the inductive and largely qualitative side of science. From these theories, good science is able to draw hypotheses that are put to the test by making more real-world observations– the deductive and largely quantitative side of science. To argue that one of these essential sides is more important than the other is foolishness. If we are interested in providing quality services to older adults, we have no time for foolishness.

PURPOSE OF FOCUS GROUPS AND INTERVIEWS

Focus groups or interviews may be undertaken either as free-standing tools for data collection and research, or as a mechanism in which they are used to develop and refine closed-ended items for other survey use. Use in this latter capacity should in no way be taken to suggest that these qualitative tools are in any way inferior or secondary to the use of quantitative survey methods. As suggested above, we do not subscribe to this artificial debate. Instead, we see focus groups and interviews as opportunities to work in concert with quantitative methods so that the results of the investigation might have both the rich meaning associated with traditional qualitative methods along with the capacity to generalize across larger populations that depends more fully on quantitative methods.

The world of social research and community needs assessment would be so much simpler if researchers and program planners always knew the correct questions to ask as well as the right people to ask. If that were the reality, it would be an uncomplicated matter to find those people and ask the questions. However, while it is very often true that gerontological professionals may know many questions (and for that matter, answers), they can never presuppose to have all of the accurate insights without testing their "reality" against that of the older adults who they are seeking to serve. Focus groups and interviews provide the opportunity for this reality check.

In the process of conducting community-based senior needs assessments, focus groups and interviews serve two general purposes. First, consumers are provided with the opportunity to identify those issues that are important to them as individuals, including the subtle nuances that are often unrecognized when a planner's focus is on the "big picture." To this end, focus groups and interviews offer slightly different avenues. In short, interviews will provide higher quality data if the topic area being considered is one in which individual responses may be guarded or suppressed through public expression. If the exposure of one's views might in any way be threatening to the respondent, a personal interview will yield better data. On the other hand, if the topic of interest is one in which opinions and attitudes might be expressed more fully through the synergy of a group process, clearly, this is the route to take. Whichever of these choices is made, the goal is to understand and appreciate the topic area more fully through the voices of the older adult respondents.

A second purpose that is served by the use of focus groups or interviews is to identify the specific–and especially unique–language that is used by respondents. It has been our experience while working with older adults in different communities that local language has developed to describe specific places or activities. By hearing and seeking a clear understanding of this *local language* researchers and planners are able to incorporate it into subsequent data collection efforts. This in turn offers two further benefits. First, the use of this familiar language enhances the clarity of communication and hence, the validity of the data. When questions are more fully understood, answers are more valid. Second, the use of *local language* enhances the credibility of the questioner, again enhancing the validity of answers and, perhaps, encouraging a higher response rate. With these thoughts in mind, we turn to the use of focus groups in survey item development.

GOALS OF FOCUS GROUPS IN SURVEY DEVELOPMENT

Consistent with the more general goals of focus groups, the specific goals for the use of focus groups in this application are to generate new areas of inquiry that are relevant to the population, to refine existing questions in terms of language or focus for a better "fit" with the population of interest, and to informally "pre-test" new or revised items that might be used in a subsequent survey. Nassar-McMillan and Borders (2002) provide an excellent overview of the use of focus groups in the development of items to be used in a subsequent survey instrument. Krause (2002), too, recommends the use of focus groups as a part of a process to develop closed-ended survey items. A clear advantage to the use of focus groups in this way is that they provide direct access to the feelings and thoughts that people have about the topic at hand; feelings and thoughts that are unencumbered by the researcher's expectations. Beyond this, focus groups allow the researcher to capture the actual words and phrases people use to describe their experiences for use in the newly designed survey.

Along with these advantages, focus groups carry certain likely limitations. First, if many focus groups are to be used, they can be quite time intensive. The necessary preparations, actual facilitation of the groups, and the management and analysis of data can involve very significant amounts of time. Too often, those who are unfamiliar with this methodology mistakenly assume that little more than the time to conduct the group is involved. A second major limitation to focus groups and qualitative methods in general is a severe constraint on the ability to generalize to some larger population. Again, novices to this methodology often neglect this basic requirement of logic and critical thinking. When working with older adults, individuals' circumstances around mobility and accessibility often further reduce the degree to which generalizations might be made.

Preliminary Planning: Identifying and Preparing for Participants

Of course, the first step of any research process is to be clear about the purpose for which the study is being undertaken. From this well-defined purpose, determine who your relevant stakeholders are. Stakeholders are all of those people who have any kind of significant investment in the topic area to be explored. In the case of most community-based senior needs assessments, stakeholders might include senior center personnel, other aging network members, health service providers, community decision makers and certainly, seniors themselves. In a given locality, there are likely to be other relevant stakeholders. While it is not necessary to *include* all of the stakeholders in one of the focus groups, it is necessary to *consider* all stakeholders. Which of them has the most direct contribution? Which of them offers a unique perspective that is not likely to be offered by anyone else? To intentionally or unintentionally exclude relevant stakeholders is to eliminate this "voice" from consideration.

Coupled with the decision about which stakeholders to invite to participate (and how many representatives from any one stakeholder group might be appropriate) is the practical decision about how many focus groups to hold and the desired size of each. While making hard decisions about who to involve becomes easier as the number of available seats increases, the task of critical analysis of focus group data increases geometrically with increases in the number of participants/groups. Pragmatic considerations about the time available to conduct focus groups and subsequent analysis, the accommodations that might be available for group meetings, and other resource issues will also influence these decisions.

Concomitant with these decisions, it must be decided if the study purposes will be better served with groups that are relatively homogeneous, as contrasted to those that are more heterogeneous, in terms of characteristics (e.g., gender, age, stakeholder role, etc.) critical to the study focus. Homogeneous groups may allow for greater comfort and spontaneity among respondents, based upon their similarities in experience and perspective and the absence of perceived "outsiders" from whom judgment or dissension may be anticipated. Thus, a more open and wide-ranging discussion of the particular stakeholder perspective may be obtained. Homogeneity may, however, also act to suppress expression of the more unique or critical perspectives held among otherwise like-minded peers. In contrast, while heterogeneous groups may afford greater access to a broader range of stakeholder perspectives, the role or implicit "power" of some participants (e.g., providers, community leaders) might easily overwhelm the voices of those having less formalized authority (e.g., community seniors).

Once the number of participants and the general stakeholder types has been determined, a specific recruitment strategy for recruiting potential group participants must be identified. At the most simple, this may involve nothing more than picking up the phone and calling individuals who emerge as "obvious" choices to request their participation. This may be especially true if one is seeking "key informant" type participants. However, careful attention should be paid to avoid relying on the selection of "obvious" choices for all participants. Just as the researcher's own views and predispositions can shape the development of questions asked and the interpretation of answers given (issues of major importance to be avoided), the construction of a group that mirrors one's own views will create a parallel "group think" approach that reflects the group's biased composition. Indeed, the goal here is to seek out and include the other voices that are too often neglected when developing new programs. Personal contact and sincere solicitation of those who are able to represent these often neglected groups may require careful consideration of community dynamics. As before, if these voices are not included in the discussion, they will not be represented in the findings.

Planning for all focus groups must also include the specification of the general questions to be addressed by the groups. The ideal set of questions will provide parameters within which the group's discussion will take place, but not be so limiting as to exclude the identification of issues that had not occurred to those planning the focus group. Certainly, a primary purpose of conducting focus groups is to identify such emergent topics. As with other qualitative interviewing procedures, questions should be ordered from those that are more general and move to those that are more specific.

The identification of a facilitator or small number of facilitators (depending on the number of groups you have decided to hold) is extremely important. Group facilitators must obviously be familiar with the purpose of the study and with the composition of the groups. Facilitators must also be able to guide group discussion without directing or controlling it. There is an advantage to the uniformity of facilitation style that accompanies using only one facilitator; however, reasonable training can provide assurance that multiple facilitators can manage different groups with adequate comparability. Facilitators must also be comfortable with the means of recording group sessions that has been decided upon. Tape recordings provide the easiest means of securing a verbatim record of the discussion and are strongly suggested here. An alternative that can provide reasonable results is a co-facilitator who is responsible for writing detailed notes. If the staff power is available, simultaneous audio recording and note-taking by a co-facilitator provides the opportunity for the co-facilitator to note and record observations of group dynamics, while the audio recording can capture the specific words and phrases used.

All of the standard requirements of informed consent apply to the use of focus groups. Respondents must be told of the nature of the study and the specifics of their involvement. In addition to making the commitment to hold all information obtained from the group in confidence, the use of the group method requires that participants also be asked to commit to holding information acquired from other groups members in confidence; it is appropriate to point out that the facilitator has no control over individual group participants and cannot assure that every member will respect the confidence of the group. Finally, individual participants must understand that participation in the group is voluntary and that there will be no negative sanctions should they choose not to participate or to withdraw. A written informed consent statement should be provided to each participant and reviewed with the group prior to starting focus group discussions.

Conducting the Groups

While involvement as a participant may seem like a fairly straightforward experience, some members are likely to feel some apprehension or anxiety. It is important that the facilitator arrive early in order to welcome all participants, make individual introductions, and respond to any initial anxiety that may be present. The availability of very modest refreshments (e.g., coffee, cookies) enhances a more relaxed and welcoming atmosphere as participants arrive. When all participants are present, use the informed consent process to put people at ease with their participation. Review the purpose and structure of the group by way of introducing the informed consent statement and requesting each participant's signature. If audio taping is the desired means of recording group discussions, it is important to ask for and receive consent from each participant before proceeding with the group interview. As indicated above, the facilitator should start the work of the group by posing a very general open-ended question about the topic. "What have been your experiences with ... ?" or "What are your thoughts about ... ?" provide comfortable openings in most cases. As the group's conversation evolves, the facilitator should progressively funnel to more narrow topics as indicated by the planned focus group interview schedule. Probes should be used to elicit details as needed. It is very important to monitor participants so that all members are getting an opportunity to respond and that no one is monopolizing the discussion. Care should also be taken to ensure that the group process stays within the agreed upon time. Several minutes before the scheduled ending, participants should be offered the opportunity to ask questions or to express ideas "that we may not have explored but would be important for us to consider" in the effort to understand the topic at hand.

Analyzing and Making Use of the Qualitative Data

The "raw data" generated out of each focus group may include an audio taped verbatim record of the discussion, a facilitator generated post-session record of group dynamics, a detailed within-session written record of the group discussion and dynamics, or some combination of all three. Audiotapes should be transcribed, and all data compiled and identified by group, for review following completion of each focus group session. This timely and systematic organization of qualitative data will facilitate its use and integration within subsequent phases of the overall study.

Initially, data from each focus group should be reviewed for its utility in conducting each subsequent focus group session. Practical issues, such as any problems in quality of the audio recording and assuring accuracy in the record of group dynamics, are most productively addressed earlier rather than later in the data gathering process. In addition, material generated out of the first or subsequent focus groups may suggest areas of inquiry to explore further with groups to follow. Because the purpose of the focus group is to obtain depth of understanding about the topic, this type of addition to the interview format is not problematic to the integrity of the study.

As subsequent focus groups are conducted, data are continuously reviewed for two purposes: identification of *the major themes/issues* raised within and across groups and extraction of the *local language* used by stakeholders. Both are incorporated into the construction of questions and response sets of a survey instrument. The use and value of *local language* was discussed previously and needs no further elaboration. Identification of *major themes* helps to define important content areas for question development; commonalities and contrasts in the perspectives of different stakeholder groups around these themes helps to define the response set appropriate to each question. If new or preexisting survey items were discussed or "pre-tested" within the focus groups, review of feedback regarding these questions may also be extracted for use in refining a survey instrument.

Finally, analysis of the body of qualitative data generated as a whole provides a contextual backdrop to the interpretation and discussion of the survey results. The generalized, issue-focused analytic approach described by Weiss (1994) provides a helpful structure to this process. The *major themes/issues* identified during the ongoing data review provide a good starting point. Data excerpts from all of the data records are coded and sorted into files according to the topic, theme or issue being addressed. Excerpts within each file are sorted again into narrower topic areas (e.g., contrasting perspectives, divergent views of different stakeholder groups). This process of coding and sorting allows identification of trends that link the experiences or perspectives of different participants. As the subsequent survey data are analyzed, the identified trends and connections between data categories, as well as the quoted voices of individual respondents, provide an added depth and meaning to the survey numbers.

PURPOSE OF CLOSED-ENDED SURVEYS

While focus groups are an excellent tool for developing a rich understanding of the context in which senior services take place and eliciting information about the nuances of consumer interest, they cannot, under normal circumstances, provide the information that allows one to make accurate inferences about the population from which the sample of respondents was drawn. On the other hand, while closed-ended mail surveys tend to provide high levels of reliability and the ability to generalize back to a larger population, this may come at the cost of failure of the data to capture the contextual tapestry in which respondents are wrapped. The procedure recommended here of starting the needs assessment process with focus groups provides the opportunity to better understand respondents' context and to incorporate that contextual understanding into the closed-item survey items. Use of familiar language, clear wording and appropriate survey design are always essential elements, however, this is especially true when surveying older adults. While the focus of this paper is on data collection from community-residing seniors in general, Gruman and associates (2000) have cautioned that survey methodology may not be appropriate for use with frail home-bound seniors in need of home care services. To that end, special care should be taken to ensure clarity of meaning when surveying older adults.

Such well-constructed closed-ended mail surveys provide an effective way to gather information from groups that are too large to directly observe. When accurate predictions or generalizations to a population of older adults are desired–as is the case with much program planning–mail surveys are a cost-efficient means for collecting the perspectives of a large sample. In contrast to face-to-face interviews or a large series of focus groups, mail surveys may be conducted relatively cheaply. Excellent sources providing the technical details for conducting mail surveys are readily available (Dillman, 2000; Erdos, 1983) and the reader is encouraged to consult them for detailed guidance. Among these are consideration of appropriate colors and font size to accommodate potential vision impairment. As with virtually all community surveys, care must also be taken to ensure that the reading level reflected in surveys of older adults is appropriate. Generally, clarity–and thus, reliability and validity–is enhanced when the reading level is held quite low.

Identifying the Questions

As indicated in the previous sections, we start the process of identifying questions for inclusion in the mailed survey by interviews with key stakeholders and through the use of focus groups. These mechanisms ensure that the appropriate domains are being investigated and also support the use of the most locally meaningful and relevant language. When writing survey items, it is important to keep them tightly focused on the topic and to use language that will be clear to the respondent. Unlike interviewing or focus groups, mailed surveys offer no opportunity to provide clarification to the respondent. In general, shorter items that avoid the use of jargon or negative phrasing are most clear. Biased terms or phrasing, and skip patterns or contingency questions should also be avoided. A somewhat lengthy but very thorough discussion of item development is provided by Sudman and Bradburn (1982).

Designing the Instrument

Instrument design involves the determination of the actual survey instrument layout as well as the ordering of items, the development of response sets, and the wording and placement of instructions. Perhaps the most important consideration in deciding upon item ordering is to begin with the item or set of items that is most likely to be interesting to the respondent. Remember that the survey is competing with everything else in the respondent's life for time and attention. By starting with a question that is stimulating and engaging, it is more likely that the respondent will complete and return the survey. One of the most common mistakes of inexperienced survey designers is to begin the instrument with demographic questions. While these are easy and non-threatening (also good qualities for initial items), they do not engage the respondent in an interesting task. Demographic items are probably best placed at the end of the instrument. If respondents find themselves getting tired as they approach the end, these easy-to-complete items are more likely to be completed than those that might require more significant cognitive processing. Also, if the respondent simply chooses to skip the demographic items, they may still return responses to the more substantive items already completed.

The manner in which respondents record their answers should also be easy to use. *Recognition* responses that involve selecting an answer from choices that are given are generally much easier for respondents than *recall* responses that require the respondent to survey his/her memory for an answer. All recognition response sets should be mutually exclusive and exhaustive. This means that every respondent should have one ("exhaustive") but only one ("mutually exclusive") response that they should be comfortable using. *Ratings* that don't involve too many choices (e.g., more than three or four) are fine; however, rankings are much more difficult for respondents. *Rankings* involving more than three ranks should never be used. Similarly, if *Likert-type* response sets are used, the number of choices should be kept low. Of course, Likert response sets must always be balanced with an equal number of positive and negative options so that respondents are not provided with a greater number of response choices in either the positive or negative direction.

Instructions for completion of the instrument are also important. Instructions, like the items themselves, should be clearly worded and reflect the use of local language as appropriate. If the instrument is comprised of multiple parts, each section should include instructions specific to that portion of the instrument. When a set of items and instructions has been fully developed, a thorough pretest is worthwhile. Submitting the instrument to a group of older adults similar to those who will be participating in the actual survey will help to identify areas that may be confusing or lack clarity. A pre-test will also provide the opportunity to determine the average amount of time required to complete the survey instrument. Surveys that require more than ten to 15 minutes are probably too long for general purposes. Unless a lengthy survey is investigating an area that is of particularly high salience to the respondent, the response rate is likely to be unacceptably low. Again, once a mail survey is distributed, there is no opportunity to address the issues that should have been identified in a pre-test.

In designing the layout of a mail survey instrument, we have had very positive results with a format that uses an 8.5 × 14 inch page in a landscape format. This page is folded such that it yields four 7 × 8.5 inch "pages." In general, the first page is used as a cover; however, if additional space is necessary, the actual items can be started on this page. We have found that with careful attention to the use of response sets, an instrument formatted in this way provides ample space for an aesthetically pleasing instrument. One of the additional benefits of using this survey format is that the survey booklet may be inserted into a #10 business envelop by folding it vertically only once.

Finding and Engaging the Respondents

Because the purpose of a mailed survey is to generalize to a larger population it is imperative that the sample used be representative of the population of interest. Because the degree to which any sample is actually representative of a population can never be known, the method by which a sample is secured is generally taken as indicative of the degree to which it might be representative. To this end, random samples are generally accepted as representative of the population, or more particularly, the sampling frame from which they were drawn. In the case of senior needs assessments, we have utilized random samples drawn from registered voters over a particular age, and random samples drawn from senior center memberships. Note that these two sampling procedures *do not* yield equivalent samples. Rather, each sample is representative of a larger population (registered senior voters community-wide or members of a given senior center) that may be of interest.

When a sampling procedure is being planned, the target sample size must be considered. The binomial sampling distribution provides a simple approach to determining a basic target sample size. This approach estimates sample size through calculations incorporating the desired confidence level (conventionally .05 in social science research), the tolerable margin of error (expressed in percentage terms), and the anticipated proportion of one outcome (e.g., 50% in a random binomial probability). A more complete discussion of this procedure can be found in Cournoyer and Klein (2000). Note that if predictions are made for subgroups within the sample, these same calculations can provide estimates of the confidence level and margin of error that will be present with the reduced number of cases included in the subgroup.

When moving from the sample size suggested by the binomial sampling distribution to the number of surveys that will actually be mailed, it is important to remember that the number of survey packets sent out and the number returned will not be the same! Table 1 provides the results of six separate survey procedures. While all of these usable response rates are well within the range of acceptability and some are exceptionally high, in one case (the voter registration sample in site 2), nearly 40% of those initially contacted failed to provide a usable response. Unfortunately, this same sample included a very high number of "undeliverable" instruments. Thus, the difference between the initial mailing sample size and the number of responses actually received was especially large. This decreases the certainty with which generalizations to the population might be made in unknown ways and to unknown magnitudes. (We will return to this point in the following paragraph.) Because these things can never be known in advance, it is important to target a higher number than is

TABLE 1. Response Rates from Six Samples (Three Sites)

	Site 1 Senior Center	Site 1 Voter Reg.	Site 2 Senior Center	Site 2 Voter Reg.	Site 3 Senior Center	Site 3 Voter Reg.
Total Surveys Sent	78	122	130	170	200	300
Less "undeliverable"	–2	–2	–10	–40	–4	–4
Viable Survey Contacts	76	120	120	130	196	296
Total Surveys Returned	70	108	104	84	180	226
Total Response Rate	92%	90%	87%	65%	92%	76%
Less "unusable"	–6	–11	–7	–3	–6	–8
Total Usable Returns	64	97	97	81	174	218
Usable Response Rate	84%	81%	81%	62%	89%	74%

actually desired. We take a fairly conservative position here and generally seek responses from twice as many respondents as we will ultimately need.

While securing a large sample size is important, a small proportion of responses from a large mailing *cannot* be assumed to be as representative as a larger proportion of responses from a smaller mailing. The 64 responses (an 84% response rate) in the Site 1 Senior Center sample above may well be more fully representative of the population from which they were drawn than are the 81 responses (a 62% response rate) in the Site 2 Voter Registration sample. Thus, engaging potential respondents so that they will complete and return the instrument is of primary importance. We now turn our attention to the dynamics that enhance a high response rate.

While some people are intrinsically more motivated to respond to mailed surveys than others, we view the decision of whether or not to respond to a given survey as the culmination of a whole series of component decisions. The first of these is made when one becomes the recipient of a mailed survey. The envelope in which the survey arrives should carry the return address of an organization that is recognized and respected by the potential respondent. For older adults, we have used business return addressed envelopes for the local senior center, town government, or other recognized survey sponsors. We always use real first class stamps rather than metered postage. We prefer envelopes that are addressed directly rather than using gummed labels. All three of these contribute to a recognition of our survey materials as something *other than* junk mail. The goal at this point is to get the potential recipient to open the survey packet.

Survey packets include a cover letter, the survey itself, an incentive for participation, and a self-addressed stamped envelop (SASE) for the returned survey. All of these things fit comfortably in a standard #10 business envelope and present a professionally appearing packet to the respondent. A #9 business envelope is used for the SASE. Use of a #9 envelope contributes to the professional appearance of the packet as well as avoids the amateurish folding that is necessary if a #10 envelope is used for the return.

The cover letter is probably the most important part of the survey packet. As with the overall packaging of the survey packet, the most important single quality of the cover letter is to engage and motivate the respondent, and to communicate the importance of the survey. Assuming the survey is being sponsored by a recognized senior-friendly organization, printing the cover letter on the letterhead of the sponsoring organization enhances the credibility of the survey. The cover letter should explain the purpose of the survey and how the respondent was selected for participation as well as provide a general estimate of the time that will be required to complete the instrument. Finally, the cover letter should assure confidentiality to the respondent and communicate appreciation for the respondent's willingness to participate. Personal signatures by a recognized representative of the sponsoring organization as well as the researcher (if different) are appropriate. Respondents should be invited to address any questions to one of these signatories and a direct contact telephone number should be included for this purpose.

Research evidence supports the use of incentives in survey work, and money is an especially effective incentive (Erdos, 1983). In our experience, uncirculated $1 bills are easy to handle and have produced excellent results. In the overall context of the survey preparation, administration, and analysis, the "cost" of dollars is also relatively modest. Dillman (2000) has suggested that the use of token financial incentives creates a sense of trust by the potential respondent. The increased motivation to respond created by providing the response incentive is also consistent with basic exchange theory.

There is also clear evidence supporting the use of follow-up mailings. The results presented in Table 1 were obtained using a follow-up post card approximately one week following the mailing of the initial packet. The timing of this reminder card is intended to be soon enough following the initial mailing that the instrument has not yet found its way to the recycling bin. In monitoring our own returns, the positive impact of this reminder has been repeatedly confirmed. About two weeks following the reminder card, a complete survey packet should be mailed to all sample members from whom a response has not been received. (Coding numbers on the return envelope or directly on the survey provide a convenient means to track returns.) In this final mailing, the cover letter reiterates all of the points made above with the additional acknowledgement of the (hopefully) high early response rate. We do not include an incentive to respond in this final mailing.

GROUP ADMINISTERED SURVEYS

Occasionally, the opportunity presents itself to survey groups of seniors aggregated in place and time. For this to truly be an opportunity, the group at hand must legitimately represent a sample that is representative of some larger group and *not* just a sample of convenience. For example, we have had two occasions to meet with large groups (>100) of nursing home resident council presidents. As representatives elected by their peers, these groups offer a unique view into the experience of nursing home residents more generally. On these occasions, we have employed a group survey procedure that involves an instrument constructed in a manner similar to that which might be used for a mailed survey, but then administered to the group in an open format.

When doing so, respondents have been grouped at tables that will accommodate the completion of the survey instrument. We have projected survey items onto a large screen and then "talked our way through" the instrument. Because the sample has included persons with various levels of physical impairment, we have also arranged to have assistance available to each small group. Obviously, the specific arrangements that might be necessary will be dictated by the needs of the respondents. This procedure has the advantage of being able to offer clarification for questions that might arise. Additionally, it is a very time-efficient approach to collecting a substantial data set.

The foremost need in approaching data collection in this manner is the identification of an appropriate group. *Appropriate* in this sense refers to the requirement that the group legitimately offer a representative view of the population to whom it is hoped to extend the findings. This is a more demanding standard than it might initially seem. Typically, issues such as self-selection impinge on the legitimacy of generalizations that might be made. While it would be unlikely that a random selection process is used to define the membership of any intact group, critical thought should be given to the process by which participants were selected with special attention to the biases that may exist.

Analyzing and Making Use of the Quantitative Data

Data analysis can be as sophisticated or as basic as is needed to support the intended programmatic decisions. A tremendous amount of high quality information can be secured using basic descriptive statistics and frequencies. While it is arguably more fun to be surprised by findings, it is also valuable to have those things that might have been *assumed* confirmed in the data. Knowing the programming interests of different subgroups in the senior population allows planners to develop and target programs with an understanding of the consumer groups who might be most interested. In one assessment in which we were involved, knowledge about the specific subgroups who were interested in a weekend senior center expansion guided program staff to develop the kinds of programs that would appeal to these identified subgroups. Of course, even the identification of these appealing programs was suggested by the needs assessment data.

More elaborate multivariate modeling can also be used with data collection efforts such as have been described here. We do caution the reader that such statistical procedures should not be used as a *fishing expedition* but rather as a guided examination of variables based upon the study's hypotheses or questions. As with all deductive research methods, relationships to be tested should be hypothesized in advance and consistent with the rules of logic that are implicit in the statistical techniques. It has been our experience that the kinds of needs assessment described in this paper are usually undertaken for more basic purposes rather than sophisticated model testing.

CONCLUSION

The important purpose of this paper has been to describe a process by which program planners can *listen to seniors*; first by using qualitative focus groups to identify salient programming issues and the language that communicates most clearly about these issues, and then by using mailed survey procedures to enable generalizations and predictions about those issues to the larger population of older adults. Program and policy decisions are often based on professional judgments or opinions of what older adults want or need. When these judgments and opinions are flawed, the resultant policies and programs are less effective than they might otherwise be. Good data support good decision making, and good data can be secured for a reasonable cost through the procedures outlined in this paper.

REFERENCES

Cournoyer, D., & Klein, W. (2000). Research Methods for Social Workers. Needham Heights, MA: Allyn & Bacon.
Dillman, D. (2000). Mail and internet surveys (2nd ed.). New York: Wiley.
Erdos, P. (1983). Professional mail surveys. Malabar, FL: Krieger.

Gruman, C., Porter, M., Curry, L., & Bowers, B. (2000). Limitations in Understanding of Health Care and Satisfaction Terminology by Frail, Older Adults: Results from a Consumer Survey Among Participants of the Connecticut Home Care for Elders Program. Unpublished manuscript.

Krause, N. (2002). A comprehensive strategy for developing close-ended survey items for use in studies of older adults. *Journal of Gerentology: Social Sciences 57B* (5), S263-S274.

Morgan, D.L. (1998). Practical strategies for combining qualitative and quantitative methods: Applications to health research. *Qualitative Health Research, 8*, 362-376.

Nassar-McMillan, S.C., & Borders, L.D. (2002). Use of focus groups in survey item development. *The Qualitative Report, 7* (1) [online]. Available at: http://www.nova.edu/ssss/QR/QR7-1/nassar.html.

Sudman, S., & Bradburn, N. (1982). Asking questions. San Francisco: Jossey-Bass.

Weiss, R.S. (1994). *Learning from strangers: The art and method of qualitative interview studies.* New York: The Free Press.

doi:10.1300/J083v48n03_11

Mosaic of Difference:
Enhancing Culturally Competent
Aging-Related Knowledge
Among Social Workers

Sandra Owens-Kane, PhD, LCSW

SUMMARY. The professional literature has not adequately addressed the behavioral and social factors that contribute to different coping outcomes for African American elder caregivers as compared to non African Americans. Awareness and understanding of these unique experiences would better prepare professionals to work with such clients. This study examines the predictors of emotional distress among 46 African American women who provide care to dependent elderly parents. Multivariate statistical analyses show that elder caregivers' rating of quality of life, their years of caregiving, as well are their poor heath constitute significant predictors of risk for depression. The results of the study provide support for the inclusion of more culturally appropriate measures of caregiver distress, and provide insights to inform social work practice, policy and research concerning African American female elder caregivers in the 21st century. doi:10.1300/J083v48n03_12 *[Article copies available for a fee from The Haworth Document Delivery Service: 1-800-HAWORTH. E-mail address: <docdelivery@haworthpress.com> Website: <http://www.HaworthPress.com> © 2007 by The Haworth Press, Inc. All rights reserved.]*

[Haworth co-indexing entry note]: "Mosaic of Difference: Enhancing Culturally Competent Aging-Related Knowledge Among Social Workers." Owens-Kane, Sandra. Co-published simultaneously in *Journal of Gerontological Social Work* (The Haworth Press, Inc.) Vol. 48, No. 3/4, 2007, pp. 475-492; and: *Fostering Social Work Gerontology Competence: A Collection of Papers from the First National Gerontological Social Work Conference* (ed: Catherine J. Tompkins, and Anita L. Rosen) The Haworth Press, Inc., 2007, pp. 475-492. Single or multiple copies of this article are available for a fee from The Haworth Document Delivery Service [1-800-HAWORTH, 9:00 a.m. - 5:00 p.m. (EST). E-mail address: docdelivery@haworthpress.com].

Available online at http://jgsw.haworthpress.com
© 2007 by The Haworth Press, Inc. All rights reserved.
doi:10.1300/J083v48n03_12

KEYWORDS. Elder, older adults, caregivers, Blacks, African American, mental health, stress, burden, coping, quality of life, social work practice

INTRODUCTION

The population of elderly African Americans is increasing at a faster rate than the majority culture, and African Americans disproportionately experience and live with a variety of chronic economic and social conditions such as poverty and racial discrimination (Clark & Anderson, 1999; U.S. Bureau of the Census, 2000; U.S. Department of Health and Human Services, 1991). These conditions remain a major quality of life issue and have been linked with several stress-related diseases (i.e., high blood pressure, stroke, cardiovascular disease) life satisfaction, as well as self-esteem (Council of Economic Advisors, 2000; Health United States with Women's Health Chartbook, 1995; Hacker, 1995; Neighbors, 1984). These conditions, in combination, can contribute significantly to stress related health and mental health problems among African Amercan women in general (Gibbs & Fuery, 1994), and caregivers in particular (Lawton, Rajagopal, Brody & Kleba, 1992). Poor morbidity and mortality indicators for these women (Centers for Disease Control and Prevention, 2000; Health United States with Women's Health Chartbook, 1995; Heckler, 1985; Gibbs & Fuery, 1994) point out the need for efforts to improve health awareness, illness prevention, and treatment in this population.

Women more often than men are the primary caregivers for older adults (Briggs, 1998; Golden & Saltz, 1997). Thus, another major yet less visible and less researched health problem among African American women is the potential stress, depression and other negative outcomes associated with years of unpaid, informal elder caregiving. Poor African American women, who typically cannot purchase home health assistance for sick and aging elders, often will become providers of assistance needed by most elderly family members (Chatters, Taylor & Jackson, 1986). As this study will demonstrate, these women become de-facto informal elder caregivers due in part to familial obligation and in great part to the lack of available, accessible, affordable, and culturally appropriate formal eldercare services for poor, African American elderly. The facts that health care costs are rising and that elders are living longer (Health United States with Health and Aging Chartbook, 1999) will undoubtedly add to the duration and extent of burdens experienced by caregiving women.

We can predict, therefore, that African American women as a group will increasingly be faced with informal caregiving duties in the foreseeable future due to a number of societal factors. These factors include: (1) women (i.e., daughters, wives, and other women) represent 72 percent of elder caregivers

(Briggs, 1998), (2) the ethnic minority elderly population needing caregiving, especially those over age 85, is increasing at a faster rate than other elderly Americans (U.S. Bureau of the Census, 1996); and (3) in 1998 in the United States, Blacks had a higher rate of elders living in poverty (26%) than Hispanics (24%) or Whites (11%) (Rank & Hirschl, 1999) thus increasing the financial demands on their African American female informal caregivers.

The present study investigated dimensions of psychological health and illness in a select group of elder Black female caregivers so that health practitioners, social workers and researchers can better target future illness prevention and treatment interventions in this group. Various dimensions of mental health and psychological distress were explored through in-depth, survey interviews with 46 low income, urban African American women who are the primary providers of in-home, informal caregiving to their elderly parents. For the purpose of this study, informal caregiving is defined as that care and assistance that is given to the elder without charges or expenses being formally associated with the care and assistance.

SOCIOECONOMIC STATUS AND HEALTH OF AFRICAN AMERICAN WOMEN

A growing body of knowledge shows that socioeconomic status (SES) is a significant predictor of physical and mental illness and death (Clark & Anderson, 1999; Coriell & Adler, 1996; Monat & Lazarus, 1991; Outlaw, 1993; Pincus, Kallahan & Burkhauser, 1987). The findings from the aforementioned studies consistently suggest that there is a strong inverse relationship between SES and various morbidity and mortality rates, meaning that as one travels up the SES ladder, morbidity and mortality rates generally decrease. Socioeconomic status can be categorized in terms of the relative level of one's income, occupation, education or social class grouping. A 2000 report of national indicators of social and economic well-being by race and Hispanic origin concludes that, in general, Blacks fare worse than any other group, and Native Americans and Hispanics are often disadvantaged in health status relative to Whites (Council of Economic Advisers for the President's Initiative on Race, 2000). Additionally, there is evidence that Blacks who live in very poor urban areas suffer extreme health disadvantages relative not only to non-Hispanic Whites, but also to Blacks who live in poor rural areas or middle class urban neighborhoods (Geronimus, Bound, Waidmann, & Hillermier, 1996). Moreover, research indicates that the SES-health gradient extends to a wide variety of health problems, including heart disease, cancer, stroke, diabetes, hypertension, and mental illness (Coriell & Adler, 1996; Monat & Lazarus, 1991; Outlaw, 1993; Pincus, Kallahan & Burkhauser, 1987).

As a result of social (e.g., access to health care), economic (e.g., poverty) and behavioral (e.g., dietary practices) variables, African American women suffer disproportionately from the aforementioned physical and mental health problems. The health disparity between African American women and other women in the United States is alarmingly wide and growing (Health United States with Women's Health Chartbook, 1995). Yet increasingly African American women are taking on caregiving roles as grandparent and/or elder caregiver; and they are likely to experience adverse physical and mental health outcomes as a consequence of their efforts to cope with the strain of their multiple roles and responsibilities (George, 1990; Golding, 1989).

African American Women as Caregivers

In addition to experiencing the effects of low socioeconomic status, African American women as a group are more likely than their White counterparts to be single parents (U.S. Bureau of the Census, 1999) and grandparent caregivers to grandchildren (Minkler, Roe & Price, 1992). During the past decade there has been increasing research on African American single parents (Jackson, Gyamfi, Brooks-Guin & Blake, 1998; Jackson, 1992; Lindblad-Goldberg, Dukes & Lasley, 1988) and grandparent caregivers (Burnette, 1997; Chalfie, 1994; Burton, 1992; Minkler, Roe & Price, 1992). Similarly, elder caregiver burden has been the subject of multiple research investigations. To date, findings consistently show significant differences between White and ethnic minority caregivers regarding the level of burden or stress associated with providing care to older relatives (Calderon & Tennstedt, 1998; Cox, 1995; Dilworth-Anderson, Williams & Cooper, 1999; Fredman, Daly & Lazur, 1995; White, Townsend & Stephens, 2000) with African American women caregivers reporting lower symptomotology than their White counterparts.

A review of the caregiving literature published from 1986 to 1990 reveals that family caregivers of chronically ill African American elderly, in comparison with other racial/ethnic groups, exhibit less strain in caring for the elderly with dementia (Hines-Martin, 1992). They also institutionalize those elderly to a lesser degree, have a more varied pool of informal caregiver support, and have higher levels of kin contact (Hines-Martin, 1992). Similarly, a narrative review of 59 articles on ethnic caregiving published between 1980 and 2000 determined that caregiving experiences and outcomes varied across racial and ethnic groups, with the majority of research reporting that caregivers to older ethnic minorities use more informal than formal support in their caregiving and that close and distant family members as well as the extended family provide the majority of this support (Dilworth-Anderson, Williams & Gibson, 2002). Several of the reviewed studies found that African American caregivers were less depressed and/or burdened in their role as compared to Whites, whereas others found no differences between the two groups (Dilworth-Anderson, Williams & Gibson, 2002).

The aforementioned findings in comparative studies of caregivers are important because they point to differences by race/ethnicity. However, they fail to explore and explain fully those differences. In-depth, within group comparisons among African American caregivers may be the only means for such an exploration of salient variables associated with positive or negative physical and mental health outcomes.

Despite the several comparative, empirical studies about African American caregivers of dependent adults that have been completed in the last several years, there remain large gaps in the literature about the behavioral and social factors that contribute to different coping outcomes for African American caregivers as compared to non-African Americans. This study is intended to address the gap in the empirical literature concerning possible reasons for differential outcomes in this caregiver population.

Research Questions

The purpose of this research study was to identify and describe the psychosocial factors that explain the psychological outcomes of African American women who are informal caregivers of their dependent parents. A greater understanding of the coping behaviors African American women use to respond to stress (e.g., use of alcohol or informal social supports) will better inform the ongoing efforts to develop theories and approaches that address the physical and mental health needs of African American women elder caregivers. This study was designed to answer the following research questions: (1) how strongly are independent variables such as caregiving burden, perceived quality of life, and physical and mental health characteristics associated with one another and with psychological well-being among African American informal caregivers?; and (2) does caregivers' age, burden, quality of life, alcohol use, years of caregiving, or perceived health have any effect on respondents' level of psychological well-being?

DESIGN AND METHODS

Sample Selection

The site for the study was an urban city in the United States with a population of 23,500. African Americans comprise 42 percent of this urban population,

Latinos 34 percent, and non-Hispanic Whites 12 percent; 9 percent are Asians and Pacific Islanders. These study data collected from African American female elder caregivers living in the city, were obtained via the snowball sampling method. Since it was not economically feasible to obtain a random sample of this population, the study population ultimately consisted of a sample of self-identified Black women currently providing at least ten hours per week of informal caregiving services to a dependent elderly parent or grandparent living in the city. Of the total women determined to have met the criteria for study inclusion (N = 49), only three chose not to participate in the study. Thus, a total of 46 subjects completed the study instrument. The three women who met the criteria for inclusion but did not complete the study reported that they were too busy to meet with the researcher for at least one hour. The response rate for the study sample was 93 percent.

Data Collection Instrument

The survey instrument designed for and utilized in this study included questions about caregivers' socioeconomic status, physical and mental health status, alcohol use, the role of supportive family or friends, and use of informal and formal services to assist in caregiving or emotional support. The survey instrument, which took an average of one hour to administer, included a majority of closed and semi-structured questions and a few open-ended questions. Several items were drawn (with permission) from Minkler and Roe's (1993) seminal study of African American grandmother caregivers in the city of Oakland, California.

A brief alcohol problems screening measure (only four items) was included in the study to test for possible alcohol abuse among the respondents. The Rapid Alcohol Problems Screen (RAPS) (Cherpitel, 1999) includes such questions as "Do you ever take a drink of alcohol when you first get up in the morning?" and "During the last year has a friend or family member ever told you about things you said or did while you were drinking that you could not remember?"

Hudson's (1982) standardized measure of perceived quality of life was adapted to measure caregiver satisfaction with the quality of various aspects of their lives. The original measure had 40 items and a Cronbach's alpha of .92. A six-item adaptation of this measure produced a Cronbach's alpha of .74 for this sample. An original question asking respondents to rate their satisfaction with their caregiving was added to the five-item adaptation and produced a Cronbach's alpha of .72 in the sample population. The mean score for the adapted version of the Hudson (1982) quality of life scale among the sample respondents is 13 (SD = 2.9) out of a possible 28 total points.

The outcome variable, psychological well-being, was created using two well-known, standardized mental health instruments that are appropriate for use with outpatient populations. One of the measures, the Center for Epidemiologic Studies Depression Scale (CES-D; Radloff, 1977), has 20 items designed to measure depression in the general population. Internal consistency represents an estimate of the consistency or homogeneity of items selected to represent a construct (Grinnell, 1997). The CES-D has a good rating of internal consistency, with Cronbach's alphas of roughly .85 for the general population and .90 for the psychiatric population (Radloff, 1977). The CES-D scale received a .85 Cronbach's alpha for the sample of caregivers in the present study. The samples' mean score for the CES-D is 39 (SD = 9.5) out of a possible total score of 60, with higher scores indicating greater depression. Scores of 16 or higher indicate that further follow-up is necessary to determine whether clinical depression may be present in the respondent (Radloff, 1977). It is noteworthy that 21 (46%) of caregivers, in responding to the CES-D item that asked how often they felt depressed during the last week, reported that they rarely or never had felt depressed. However, analyses of this subgroup of 21 caregivers revealed that their mean CES-D score is 33 (SD = 7.2) out of a possible total score of 60. Therefore, everyone in this subgroup (n = 21) of caregivers who reported not being depressed during the last week had a cumulative CES-D score above the score of 16 that suggests the need for follow up for possible clinical depression. Thus, although these caregivers as a sub-group are all exhibiting indications of high levels of depressed feelings, they are reticent to directly report recent depressed feelings, and yet all of them may need to be evaluated for substantiation of clinical depression.

The other standardized scale used as an outcome variable was the Derogatis Symptom Checklist-90-R (DSCL). The DSCL, formerly known as the Brief Symptom Inventory and then the Hopkins Symptom Checklist, records scaled judgments in nine dimensions: somatization, obsessive-compulsive, interpersonal sensitivity, depression, anxiety, hostility, phobic anxiety, paranoid ideation, and psychoticism (Derogatis, 1994). The DSCL has a good rating of internal consistency for the general population, with alphas ranging from a low of .77 for Psychoticism to a high of .90 for Depression. The DSCL scale, for all nine dimensions combined, received a .96 Cronbach's alpha for the sample of caregivers in the present study. All of the test-retest coefficients in the DSCL are between .80 and .90, which is an appropriate level for measures of symptom constructs (Derogatis, 1994). The mean score for the DSCL was 113 (SD = 53) for the sample. The corresponding DSCL standard (normalized) T score for the sample had a mean of 68 (SD = 7.9), and it was very highly correlated with the overall mean score for the DSCL. The T score was used in subsequent analyses because it is familiar to most psychologists, because it simplifies arithmetic operations, and because there are no decimals to deal with (Derogatis, 1994). It should be noted that a T score of 70 on the DSCL places the respondent in approximately the 98th centile of the normative sample. Almost a third of caregivers (32%) had T scores of 70 or more. Thus, these caregivers are reporting alarmingly high levels of psychological symptomatology.

Interviewer

The study was conducted by the author, an African American social welfare researcher and clinical social worker. The author has considerable experience as a social worker and researcher in the African American caregiving communities in Las Vegas, Nevada and San Francisco, California. She designed the survey instrument, hired, trained and closely supervised one African American female caregiver to assist her with the administration of the interviews.

Data Analysis Strategy

The analysis of the relationship between the independent variables, such as caregiver burden, alcohol problem risk, social support, frequency of family caregiving assistance, and caregiver psychological well-being were systematically explored using (1) a bivariate analysis of the various relationships, and (2) an ordinary least squares regression to identify the significant associations with psychological well-being. Although the sample size was adequate for the type of selected data analyses, the wide confidence intervals for some of the variables suggest that findings should be interpreted with caution.

RESULTS

Sample of Caregivers

The 46 African American elder caregivers in this study had a average age of 38 (SD = 10.30), with a range of ages from 21 to 67 (Table 1). More than half (56%) were not married and/or not living in a marriage-like relationship at the time of the study. This sample population had a slightly higher proportion of female headed households with no spouse present, as compared to the national proportion (45%) of African American female householders with no spouse present (U.S. Bureau of the Census, 1999b). The median number of years caregiving respondents was six (SD = 3.88), with a range in years from six months to 18 total years of caregiving to a dependent parent or grandparent.

TABLE 1. Sociodemographic Characteristics of Sample Caregivers (N = 46)

Characteristics	N	%
Demographics		
Age at last birthday		
Less than 30	11	23
30-39	20	43
40-49	10	22
50-59	3	7
60-69	2	4
Marital status		
Married and living with spouse	9	20
Living in a marriage-like relationship	11	24
Widowed	5	11
Separated or divorced	6	13
Single	15	33
Education		
Some high school	3	7
Completed high school	14	30
Some college or junior college	14	30
Completed college degree	10	22
Some post graduate work	3	7
Completed a graduate degree	2	4
Work status		
Employed full-time (35+ hrs)	23	50
Employed part-time	23	50
Total Family Income for 1998		
Under $10,000	4	8
$10,000 - $19,999	21	46
$20,000 - $29,999	12	26
$30,000 - $39,999	5	11
$40,000 and over	4	8
Income under the 1998 poverty level	26	57
Income was not enough for basic need	11	24

Note: Percentages may not total 100 due to rounding.

Correlation Analyses

In an effort to better understand patterns within these data, frequencies and descriptive statistics were computed for salient variables collected in the study. Of the variables assessed in this study, only six variables (burden, quality of life rating, years of caregiving, age of caregiver, presence of an alcohol problem, and excellent health) showed statistically significant correlations with one another and/or with the DSCL and the CES-D measures. It can be observed in Table 2 that the intercorrelations range from near zero to −.57. The strongest relationship with DSCL and CES-D was an inverse relationship with the variable representing caregivers' perceived rating of health (Excelhlth). This result suggests that the poorer the caregiver's rating of health, the greater her psychiatric symptoms and depression. Negative correlations associated with the number of years as a caregiver (Yrscaring) and the DSCL and CES-D measures indicate that the fewer the years providing caregiving assistance, the greater the psychiatric symptoms and depression.

The tendency towards being positive for an alcohol use disorder (Alcoholprob) was moderately related to the DSCL measure. Thus, as the problem drinking increased, so did the likelihood of experiencing psychiatric symptomatology. Similarly, rating the quality of one's life as poor or unsatisfactory was associated with higher CES-D scores. The correlation of .45 between years as a caregiver (Yrscaring) and age of the caregiver (Agecarer) illustrates that as age increased, so did the number of years of giving care. Although these variables are highly correlated, inclusion of both variables did not significantly decrease the strength of the multiple regression model used to explain the total variance in the outcome variables. As discussed below, the relationships between the salient independent and dependent variables provide a benchmark from which to develop subsequent research investigations regarding psychological well-being of African American caregivers. The results of the multivariate analysis of these selected variables are reported next.

TABLE 2. Intercorrelations for the Independent and Dependent Variables (N = 44)

Measure	Caregiver Burden	Quality of Life	Years of Caregiving	Caregiver Age	Alcohol Problem	Excellent Health	DSCL	CES-D
Caregiver Burden		38**	.11	.22	−.18	.01	.04	.00
Quality of Life			.10	.12	.24	−.22	.14	.31*
Years of Caregiving				.45**	−.04	−.06	−.35**	−.30*
Caregiver Age					−.01	−.24	.03	.11
Alcohol Problem						−.01	.34*	.09
Excellent Health							.31*	−.52**

Regression Analyses. Two separate regression analyses were conducted, one on the DSCL (see part (a) of Table 3) and one for the CES-D (see part (b) of Table 3). The multiple correlation for the DSCL analysis was r = .67; for the CES-D analysis it was r = .69. Whereas the correlation coefficients in Table 3 represent the bivariate relationships for all the combinations of the independent and dependent variables, the multiple correlations represent the collective correlation of the independent variables with the dependent variable (SPSS, 1999). That is, each independent variable in the multiple correlation shares in the measured relationship with the dependent variable. The multiple correlation will always be positive in direction, even if the variables have an inverse relationship, and as great or greater than any single bivariate correlation with the dependent variable. It can be seen in Table 3 that the highest bivariate

TABLE 3. Multiple Regression Analysis for Derogatis Symptom Checklist and the Center for Epidemiologic Studies–Depression Scale (N = 44)

	Independent Variable	Coefficient	SE	t	p (2 Tail)
	Derogatis Symptom Checklist				
	Caregiver Burden	.46	.37	1.23	.23
	Quality of Life	.01	.40	.03	98
(a)	Years Caregiving	−1.03	.30	−3.49	*.01
	Caregiver Age	.14	.11	1.26	.21
	Alcohol Problem	16.69	5.05	3.31	*.01
	Excellent Health	−5.36	2.17	−2.47	*.02
		R = .67	R^2 = .44	Adj. R^2 = .35	
	Center for Epidemiologic Studies–Depressed Mood Scale				
	Caregiver Burden	−.37	.41	−.90	.37
	Quality of Life	.86	.44	1.95	*.05
(b)	Years Caregiving	−.85	.32	−2.67	*.01
	Caregiver Age	.14	.12	1.10	.28
	Alcohol Problem	1.04	4.69	−.22	83
	Excellent Health	−9.25	2.41	−3.85	*.01
		R = .69	R^2 = .47	Adj. R^2 = .39	

* = Statistically significant

correlation with the DSCL was −.35, and for the CES-D it was −.52. However, when all of the variables were considered in combination (collectively), the resulting multiple Rs were .67 and .69, respectively (see Table 3). Both multiple Rs can be considered as moderately high for these kinds of data. The computed Adjusted R^2 for the independent variables (primarily years caregiving, having an alcohol use disorder, and not having excellent health) that were regressed onto the DSCL score is .35, indicating that about 35 percent of the total variation in the DSCL score is explained by the regression. Similarly, the computed Adjusted R^2 for the independent variables (primarily caregiver rating of quality of life, years of caregiving, and not being in excellent health) that were regressed onto the CES-D score is .39, indicating that about 39 percent of the total variation in the CES-D score was explained by the regression. In multiple regression analyses, the regression coefficients reveal which variables contribute most to the multiple correlations.

DISCUSSION

It is emphasized that given the high number of chronic and acute stressors experienced by African American women in general (Centers for Disease Control and Prevention, 2000), knowledge about African American elder caregivers is important for future social work policy and practice. These African American female elder caregivers may have developed both adaptive and maladaptive coping mechanisms as a response to the difficult task of caregiving to their elders–who as a group are the fastest growing segment of the elderly population (U.S. Bureau of the Census, 1996) and have the highest rate of poverty among ethnic groups of elders (Rank & Hirschl, 1999). Adverse and adaptive behaviors of African American caregivers pertinent to physical and mental health can affect not only their own morbidity and mortality, but also the lives of the dependent children and elders in their care. Thus, this study of Black female caregivers of dependent elderly explored the relationship between variables such as caregiver burden, health and alcohol use and two psychological well-being outcomes. The study's findings supplement the meager knowledge of the stressful factors experienced by Black female elder caregivers and the coping strategies they develop to ameliorate these stressors. It is anticipated that these findings will also have implications for developing interventions to promote positive physical and mental health outcomes in this population of caregivers.

A large part of the value of conducting research on a select sample population is that the data and findings are directly relevant and may provide meaningful contributions to the conceptualization and amelioration of problems inherent in the sample. This study of elder caregiving provides some valuable and timely information to guide current and future plans for practice, policy and research related to eldercare in the African American community. Specifically, a close examination of the physical and mental health status and behaviors of this sample of Black elder caregivers has revealed preliminary data to inform practitioners, politicians, and social work researchers at the local, state and national levels.

Practice Implications

This study provides valuable information that helps inform social work in direct practice with elders and their caregiving family members. For example, the finding that as a group these caregivers are at high risk for depression indicates the need to provide services related to caregiver psychological assessments, prevention, early intervention and treatment. Oftentimes social workers working with seniors have little interaction with the senior's caregiving family members, other than to arrange for the elder's support services and transportation needs. However, there should be more contact with these caregivers given that the physical and mental health needs and treatment of elders are often inextricably tied to the health and well-being of the elders' caregivers. Practitioners working in the community with minority elders should consider offering culturally specific caregiver support groups, clinical referral services or counseling services, and stress reduction literature to the informal caregivers of the elders they serve.

Social workers should help devise methods to assist caregivers in continuing and/or enhancing their employment endeavors so that they can meet their financial needs and those of their families. Because of the inevitability of the aging process, some of these caregivers may soon be in need of eldercare themselves; providing them with needed support now will therefore help ease the financial strain of elder caregiving, and help enhance the caregivers' long-term physical health and emotional well-being. In short, supporting and strengthening ethnic minority caregivers now will help ensure their own healthier aging experience and may positively impact morbidity and mortality outcomes in these African American women.

Policy Implications

Some services that caregivers may need will require the development of national, state or local policies and procedures. The findings from this study of elder caregivers suggest that many elders and caregivers are living in impoverished households. Caregivers with primary caregiving responsibilities for dependent elders should be eligible for more generous tax credits. The deductible amounts for caregivers claiming dependent elders should be commensurate with the expense of meeting the documented disabilities and limitations in activities of daily living of the elder. Additionally, poor caregivers with primary caregiving responsibilities should be eligible for vouchers and subsidies such as housing, long term care insurance, public transportation (e.g., bus, senior van or taxi) to and from medical appointments. Poor elders could also benefits from receipt of food donated by local grocers or restaurants, although this service would require legislation that would limit the liability of such donors, as well as policies of distribution that would not be undignified for the elders receiving the food donations. Following the model of the Temporary Aid to Needy Families Act, the study findings give some impetus for the proposal for a Temporary Aid to Needy Elders Program which could be administered by the Regional Offices of Aging Services. The Aging Services Offices could also be given authority to help facilitate approval of Department of Motor Vehicles issued handicapped permits for primary caregivers of frail or disabled elders, as well as supplementing the cost of need-based eldercare supplies such as portable toilets, medic-alert bracelets, shower chairs and hand rails, toilet supports and guard rails. This list of policy recommendations may seem overly ambitious but the demand for and benefits of such accommodations are obvious to those working with and researching low-income elders and their caregivers.

Research Implications

Conducting this research on Black elder caregivers has helped to generate new research questions and suggested methodologies. For example, a subject for subsequent research projects with similar populations is the dynamics and impact of the caregiver-elder relationships and the ages of caregivers. The relative youth of this sample of caregivers has raised several questions regarding the impact or cost of elder caregiving across the lifespan. For example, the Harrow, Tennstedt, and McKinlay (1995) study found that providing informal care to elders in the community "costs" the average primary caregiver 19 hours and $163 per week. The total costs of care for elders living with their primary caregivers were greater than that for elders living alone, likely due to greater amounts of informal care provided (Tennstedt, Crawford & McKinlay, 1993). The actual cost of care is even greater for some caregivers, and infinitely greater in terms of its impact on wealth, health and income for some low-income female caregivers such as those participating in this study of elder caregiving.

Additionally, when considering the relatively young mean age (38) of these daughter caregivers of needy elders, it might be useful to explore other questions that emerge this finding. For example, what are the physical and emotional consequences of years of caregiving for these young women?

Will this relatively early, non-normative engagement in elder caregiving duties by American women in their 30's impact their employability, salary levels, and opportunities for advanced education and training? Do they consistently require cash assistance from extended family and community members in order to maintain the elder in the home? Is there any impact on health and well-being of minor children in their care?

Other questions that could be investigated include the following: Do these young caregivers have a more healthy view of the aging process, as compared to young adults with no caregiving obligations who may fear old age or have a sense of hostility towards death and dying? Are these caregivers benefiting emotionally or financially from providing for the daily living activity needs of their elders? Does receipt of emotional and financial support from the elder buffer or mediate feelings of depression in some caregivers? In summary, caregivers' responses regarding their familial relationship to their helpers raise many questions regarding the effects of early elder caregiving on the mental health and well-being of this and possibly other racial and ethnic populations of caregivers.

Finally, the findings of this study of African American female caregivers provide some support for the inclusion of more culturally consonant measures of caregiver burden, and the use of alternative measures indicating caregiver depression and distress, specifically alcohol abuse, number of years caregiving, poor health and low satisfaction with one's quality of life. The findings further suggest that objective measures of alcohol problem use would be more useful for screening in those caregivers who will not admit to problematic alcohol use. Maybe a triangulation of screening measures could be used such that family members, practitioners, and caregivers could all provide their assessments of the caregivers' possible problematic use of alcohol. Additionally, the national prevalence of problem drinkers who are simultaneously providing eldercare duties needs to be determined. The directional relationship between problem drinking and elder caregiving also needs further research. Assessments of the negative impact of drinking on caregiver provision and supervision of elders' activities of daily living are also very important for the safety and welfare considerations of the elderly who are being cared for by women with problematic alcohol use patterns.

It is necessary to obtain larger, more representative, and ethnically diverse samples of female elder caregivers to fully evaluate the influence of these variables on caregiver psychological well-being. Use of a longitudinal research design, and inclusion of a control or comparison group would enhance the strength of the study's findings and improve generalizability. While these are just two areas of suggested expansion of the research inquiry on elder caregiving, this research reveals many factors, issues and concerns that should be considered and integrated into other research inquiries regarding African American female caregivers in this country. The implications provide a benchmark from which to develop subsequent research investigations regarding psychological well-being of African American elder caregivers.

REFERENCES

Briggs, R. (1998). *Caregiving daughters: Accepting the role of a caregiver for elderly parents.* New York: Garland Publishing, Inc.

Burnette, D. (1997). Grandmother caregivers in inner-city Latino families: A descriptive profile and informal social supports. *Journal of Multicultural Social Work, 5*(3/4), 121-137.

Burton, L. M. (1992). Black grandparents rearing children of drug-addicted parents: Stressors, outcomes, and social services needs. *The Gerontologist, 32*(6), 744-751.

Calderon, V., & Tennstedt, S. (1998). Ethnic differences in the experiences of caregiver burden: Results of a qualitative study. *Journal of Gerontological Social Work, 30*(42), 159-178.

Centers for Disease Control and Prevention. (2000). *Women and heart disease: An atlas of racial and ethnic disparities immortality.* [On-line] Office for Social Environment and Health Research, West Virginia University. National Center for Chronic Disease Prevention and Health Promotion, Centers for Disease Control and Prevention. Available: *http//.ftp.cdc.gov/pub/publications/womens_atlas–atlas.pdf.*

Chalfie, D. (1994). *Going it alone: A closer look at grandparents parenting grandchildren.* Washington, D.C.: American Association of Retired Persons.

Chatters, L. M., Taylor, R. J., & Jackson, J. S. (1986). Aged blacks: Choices for an informal helper network. *Journal of Gerontology, 41*(1), 94-100.

Cherpitel, C. J. (1999, September). Screening for alcohol problems in the U.S. general population: A comparison of the CAGE and TWEAK by gender, ethnicity and services utilization. *Journal of Studies on Alcohol, 60*(5), 705-711.

Clark, R., & Anderson, N. B. (1999). Racism as stressor for African Americans: A biopsychosocial model. *American Psychologist, 54*(10), 805-817.

Corriell, M., & Adler, N. (1996). Socioeconomic status and women's health: How do we measure SES among women? *Women's Health: Research on Gender, Behavior, and Policy, 2*(3), 141-156.

Council of Economic Advisers for the President's Initiative on Race. (2000). *Changing America: Indicators of social and economic well-being by race and Hispanic origin.* [On-line] Available: URL: *http/w3.access.gpo.gov/eop/ca/index.html.*

Cox, C. (1995). Comparing the experiences of black and white caregivers of dementia patients. *Social Work, 40*, 343-345.

Dilworth-Anderson, P., Williams, S. W., & Cooper, T. (1999). The contexts of experiencing emotional distress among family caregivers to elderly African Americans. *Family Relations, 48*, 391-397.

Dilworth-Anderson, P., Williams, I. C., & Gibson, B. E. (2002). Issues of race, ethnicity, and culture in caregiving research: A 20-year review (1980-2000). *The Gerontologist, 42*(2), 237-271.

Fredman, L., Daly, M. P., & Lazur, A. M. (1995). Burden among White and Black caregivers to elderly adults. *Journals of Gerontology: Series B: Psychological Sciences & Social Sciences, 50B*(2), S110-S118.

George, L. K. (1990). Caregiver stress studies: There really is more to learn. *The Gerontologist, 30,* 580-581.

Geronimus, A. T., Bound, J., Waidmann, T. A., & Hillemier, M. M. (1996). Excess mortality among blacks and whites in the United States. *New England Journal of Medicine, 333*(21), 1552-1558.

Gibbs, J. T., & Fuery, D. (1994). Mental health and well-being of black women: Toward strategies of empowerment. *American Journal of Community Psychology, 22*(4), 559-582.

Golden, R., & Saltz, C. C. (1997). The aging family. *Journal of Gerontological Social Work, 27*(3), 55-64.

Golding, J. M. (1989). Role occupancy and role-specific stress and social support as predictors of depression. *Basic and Applied Social Psychology, 10,* 173-195.

Hacker, A. (1995). *Two nations: Black and white, separate, hostile, unequal.* New York: Ballantine Books.

Harrow, B. S., Tennestedt, S. L., & McKinlay, J. B. (1995). How costly is it to care for disabled elders in a community setting? *The Gerontologist, 35*(6), 803-816.

Health United States with Socioeconomic Status and Health Chartbook. (1999). Hyattsville, MD: National Center for Health Statistics 1999. [On-line] Available: *www.cdc.gov/nchs/data/huscht98.pdf.*

Health United States with Women's Health Chartbook. (1995). Hyattsville, MD: National Center for Health Statistics. [On-line] Available: www.cdc.gov/nchs/data/ hus_94.pdf.

Heckler, M. M. (1985). *Report of the secretary's task force on black and minority health.* Washington, DC: Department of Health and Human Services.

Hines-Martin, V. P. (1992). A research review: Family caregivers of chronically ill African-American elderly. *Journal of Gerontological Nursing, 18*(2), 25-29.

Hudson, W. W. (1982). *The clinical measurement package: A field manual.* Homewood, IL: Dorsey Press.

Jackson, A. P., Gyamfi, P., Brooks-Gunn, J., & Blake, M. (1998). Employment status, psychological well-being, social support, and physical practices of single Black mothers. *Journal of Marriage and the Family, 60*(4), 894-993.

Lawton, M. P., Rajagopal, D., Brody, E., & Kleba, M. H. (1992). The dynamics of caregiving for a demented elder among Black and White families. *Journal of Gerontology: Social Science, 47,* 156-164.

Lindblad-Goldberg, M., Dukes, J. L., & Lasley, J. H. (1988). Stress in Black, low-income, single-parent families: Normative and dysfunctional patterns. *American Journal of Orthopsychiatry, 58*(1), 104-120.

Minkler, M. M., Roe, K., & Price, M. (1992). The physical and emotional health of grandmothers raising grandchildren in the crack cocaine epidemic. *The Gerontologist, 32*(6), 752-761.

Monat, A., & Lazarus, R. S. (Eds.). (1991). *Stress and coping: An anthology* (3rd ed.). New York: Columbia University Press.

Neighbors, H. W. (1984). The distribution of psychiatric morbidity in Black Americans: A review and suggestions for research. *Community Mental Health Journal, 20,* 169-181.

Neighbors, H. W. (1984). The use of informed help: Four patterns of illness behavior in the black community. *American Journal of Community Psychology, 12*(6), 629-644.

Outlaw, F. H. (1993). Stress and coping: The influence of racism on the cognitive appraisal processing of African Americans. *Issues in Mental Health Nursing, 14* (4), 399-409.

Picus, T., Kallahan, L., & Burkhauser, R. (1987). Most chronic diseases are reported more frequently by individuals with fewer than 12 years of formal education in the ages 18-64 in the United States population. *Journal of Chronic Diseases, 40,* 865-874.

Radloff, L. S. (1977). The CES-D scale: A self report depression scale for researching the general population. *Applied Psychological Measurement, 1,* 385-401.

Rank, M. R., & Hirschl, T. A. (1999). Estimating the proportion of Americans experiencing poverty during their elderly years. *Journal of Gerontology, Series B, 54*(4), 51-84.

Statistical Package for the Social Science. (1999). *SPSS base 10.0 applications guide.* Chicago, IL: SPSS, Inc.

Tennstedt, S., Crawford, S., & McKinlay, J. (1993). Is family care on the decline? A longitudinal investigation of the substitution of formal long-term care services for informal care. *Milbank Quarterly, 71,* 601-624.

U.S. Bureau of the Census. (2000). *Projections of the total resident populations by 5-year age groups, race, and Hispanic origin with special age categories: Middle series 1999-2000; middle series 2050 – 2070.* [Online]. Available: http://www.census.gov/population/projections/nation/summary/np-t4-a.txt.

U.S. Bureau of the Census. (1999a). *Current population survey, March 1999, racial statistics.* [On-line] Available: http://www.CENSUS.gov/population/socdemo/race/black/tabs99/Education/tabs99/tab05.txt/tab12.txt.

U.S. Bureau of the Census. (1999b). *Householders in family households by family, type and race and Hispanic origin.* [On-line] Available: *http//ww.census.gov:80/population/socdemo/race/black/tabs99/tab03.txt.*

U.S. Bureau of the Census. (1996). *Statistical abstract of the United States* (116th Ed.) Washington, D.C.: U.S. Dept. of Commerce, Bureau of the Census.

U.S. Department of Health and Human Services. (1991). *Health status of minorities and low-income groups* (3rd ed.) DHHS Pub. No. 271-848/40085. Washington, D.C.: U.S. Government Printing Office.

White, T. M., Townsend, A. L., & Stephens, M. A. P. (2000). Comparisons of African American and White women in the parent care role. *The Gerontologist, 40*(6), 718-728.

doi:10.1300/J083v48n03_12

Index

BOOK ORDER FORM!

Order a copy of this book with this form or online at:
http://www.HaworthPress.com/store/product.asp?sku= 5932

Fostering Social Work Gerontology Competence
A Collection of Papers from the First National
Gerontological Social Work Conference

—— in softbound at $52.00 ISBN-13: 978-0-7890-3414-4 / ISBN-10: 0-7890-3414-X.
—— in hardbound at $80.00 ISBN-13: 978-0-7890-3413-7 / ISBN-10: 0-7890-3413-1.

COST OF BOOKS _____

POSTAGE & HANDLING _____
US: $4.00 for first book & $1.50
    for each additional book
Outside US: $5.00 for first book
& $2.00 for each additional book.

SUBTOTAL _____

In Canada: add 6% GST. _____

STATE TAX _____
CA, IL, IN, MN, NJ, NY, OH, PA & SD residents
please add appropriate local sales tax

FINAL TOTAL _____
If paying in Canadian funds, convert
using the current exchange rate,
UNESCO coupons welcome.

❏ **BILL ME LATER:**
Bill-me option is good on US/Canada/
Mexico orders only; not good to jobbers,
wholesalers, or subscription agencies.

❏ **Signature** _____

❏ **Payment Enclosed: $**_____

❏ **PLEASE CHARGE TO MY CREDIT CARD:**

❏ Visa ❏ MasterCard ❏ AmEx ❏ Discover
❏ Diner's Club ❏ Eurocard ❏ JCB

Account #_____

Exp Date_____

Signature_____
(Prices in US dollars and subject to change without notice.)

PLEASE PRINT ALL INFORMATION OR ATTACH YOUR BUSINESS CARD

Name _____

Address _____

City _____ State/Province _____ Zip/Postal Code _____

Country _____

Tel _____ Fax _____

E-Mail _____

May we use your e-mail address for confirmations and other types of information? ❏ Yes ❏ No We appreciate receiving
your e-mail address. Haworth would like to e-mail special discount offers to you, as a preferred customer.
We will never share, rent, or exchange your e-mail address. We regard such actions as an invasion of your privacy.

Order from your **local bookstore** or directly from
The Haworth Press, Inc. 10 Alice Street, Binghamton, New York 13904-1580 • USA
Call our toll-free number (1-800-429-6784) / Outside US/Canada: (607) 722-5857
Fax: 1-800-895-0582 / Outside US/Canada: (607) 771-0012
E-mail your order to us: orders@HaworthPress.com

For orders outside US and Canada, you may wish to order through your local
sales representative, distributor, or bookseller.
For information, see http://HaworthPress.com/distributors

(Discounts are available for individual orders in US and Canada only, not booksellers/distributors.)

Please photocopy this form for your personal use.
www.HaworthPress.com   BOF07